Squid's Little Pink Book

Squid's Little Pink Book

A Pocket Guide for Emergency Doctors

Dr Lydia Lozzi
BSci, BMedBSurg (Hons), FACEM
Course Coordinator - Pathology, Masters of Critical Care
Professional Medical Education
Sydney Medical School
The University of Sydney

Staff Specialist, Emergency Medicine
Central Coast Local Health District
Australia

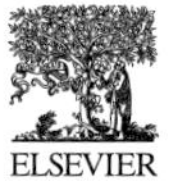

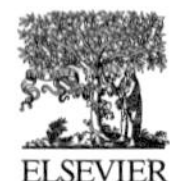

Elsevier Australia. ACN 001 002 357
(a division of Reed International Books Australia Pty Ltd)
Tower 1, 475 Victoria Avenue, Chatswood, NSW 2067

ISBN: 978-0-7295-4376-7

Notice

Knowledge and best practice in this field are constantly changing. As new research and experience broaden our understanding, changes in research methods, professional practices, or medical treatment may become necessary.

Practitioners and researchers must always rely on their own experience and knowledge in evaluating and using any information, methods, compounds, or experiments described herein. In using such information or methods they should be mindful of their own safety and the safety of others, including parties for whom they have a professional responsibility.

With respect to any drug or pharmaceutical products identified, readers are advised to check the most current information provided (i) on procedures featured or (ii) by the manufacturer of each product to be administered, to verify the recommended dose or formula, the method and duration of administration, and contraindications. It is the responsibility of practitioners, relying on their own experience and knowledge of their patients, to make diagnoses, to determine dosages and the best treatment for each individual patient, and to take all appropriate safety precautions.

To the fullest extent of the law, neither the Publisher nor the authors, contributors, or editors, assume any liability for any injury and/or damage to persons or property as a matter of product liability, negligence or otherwise, or from any use or operation of any methods, products, instructions, or ideas contained in the material herein.

National Library of Australia Cataloguing-in-Publication Data

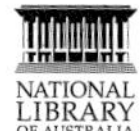

A catalogue record for this book is available from the National Library of Australia

Content Strategist: Larissa Norrie
Content Project Manager: Sukanthi Sukumar
Edited by Leanne Peters
Proofread by Tim Learner
Permissions Processor: Regina Lavanya Remigius
Cover Designer: Natalie Bowra
Index by SPi Global
Typeset by New Best-set Typesetters Ltd
Printed in China by RRD

Last digit is the print number: 9 8 7 6 5 4 3 2 1

About this book

This book is specifically written and designed for the pocket and to be carried everywhere by the busy emergency doctor. It is for quick reference and memory jogging when standing at a patient's bedside postulating a diagnosis. It is for those panicked moments when you feel out of control or when you just need a friend to back you up. It is to be your guide to the questions you need to already have answered before you make the consult and get grilled by the specialty team. And just being in your pocket, it is to make you feel like you are not alone even if there is nobody else around and the computers are down.

How to use this book

This book was designed to be used by any doctor, from student doctor to intern to specialist. Because of this, management plans start with the basics and progress to more advanced care and sometimes will include things that only an emergency specialist would do. Don't follow any management plans (e.g. giving drugs or performing procedures) unless you have the appropriate skills and experience. Basically, if you have never done something before, don't start now! Ask for help.

Disclaimer

All information contained in this book, including suggested management strategies, has been developed by the authors through combining their clinical experience with multiple different widely accepted clinical guidelines, current at the time of printing. Best practice for any medical condition is constantly evolving. Just one new study can change best practice forever. In addition, individual patients often will not fit perfectly into a predetermined guideline. This book is intended as a guide only and medical practitioners must always rely on their own clinical experience and judgment in conjunction with their local clinical guidelines when managing patients. The authors accept no responsibility for any adverse outcomes, injury, negligence or damage to persons or property as a result of use of this book.

Who is Squid?

Doctor Lydia (Lyd the Squid) Lozzi (BSci, BMedBSurg (Hons), FACEM) always carried around a little book with a pink cover. This book had been handwritten as a resident to prepare for the step up to registrar and the night shifts that would follow. Over the years, the book was altered and added to. After about 10 years of doctors asking about that little pink book she kept referring to and could they have a copy, Squid decided it was time to share.

Luckily Squid has fabulous friends that are amazing emergency specialists who kindly agreed to help. The following FACEMs reviewed and contributed to this book.

Principal Reviewer

Nadia Bowman BSc, MBChB, FACEM

Specialist review panel

Associate Professor Mark Gillett MB BS, DipRACOG, FRACGP, FACEM, MClinEd, Grad Cert Sono

Dr Jennifer Martin OAM MB BS (Hons), Dip CH, FACEM

Dr Holly Smith MDCM, FRACP

Dr John Kennedy MBBS, MPHTM, FACEM

Dr Jo Oo MBBS, BSc (Med), GCertPH, FACEM

Dr Tom Harwood MBChB, FACEM

Dr Davina Julliard BSc, MBBS (Hons), MIPH, FACEM

Bibliography

Most sections in this book were derived from combining multiple resources and clinical experience. The following textbooks were used throughout this book: *Tintinalli's Emergency Medicine* by Judith Tintinalli et al., *The Emergency Medicine Manual* by Robert Dunn et al., *Textbook of Adult Emergency Medicine* by Peter Cameron et al. and *Textbook of Paediatric Emergency Medicine* by Peter Cameron et al. Online resources included: Therapeutic Guidelines, Life in the Fast Lane, Medscape, Orthobullets, Australian Resuscitation Council and the Royal Children's Hospital Clinical Guidelines.

Thank you to

Craig—Best most supportive husband

Annette, Andrei and Jan—Grandparents to my babies and babysitter extraordinaires without which I achieve nothing

Tanya Smith—Literally best word processer ever

Frederick, Giselle and Harvey—World's loveliest squirrels

Contents

Important phone numbers

Use this page to record phone numbers for your workplace that you may need in a hurry

- Medical teams

Gen med:

Resp:

Gastro:

Cardio:

Paeds:

- Surgical teams

General surgery:

Obstetrics and gynaecology:

Neuro surgery:

Theatres:

Orthopaedics:

ENT:

Plastics:

- Critical care

Intensive care unit (ICU):

Anaesthetist:

Poisons information: 13 11 26

- Allied health

Physiotherapist:

Social worker:

- Local police station
- Bloods and imaging

Radiology:

Pathology:

Blood bank:

- Other

Important drug doses for intubation and resuscitation

Drug	Adult dose	For example, 70–80 kg adult	Child
Thiopentone	1–5 mg/kg	200 mg (↓↓ dose if unstable, e.g. 50 mg)	2–5 mg/kg
Suxamethonium	1.5 mg/kg	100 mg	2 mg/kg
Propofol	1–2.5 mg/kg	150 mg (less if unstable)	1.5–2.5 mg/kg
Ketamine	1–2 mg/kg	100 mg	1–2 mg/kg
Vecuronium	0.2 mg/kg (IBW)	10 mg	0.1 mg/kg
Rocuronium (rapid sequence intubation [RSI] dose)	1.2 mg/kg (IBW)	75–100 mg	0.6–1.2 mg/kg
Adrenaline anaphylaxis		0.5 mL of 1 in 1000 = 0.5 mg IM *Infusion 0.05 microgram/kg/min*	0.01 mL/kg of 1 in 1000 = 0.01 mg/kg (10 microgram/kg) IM *Infusion 0.05 microgram/kg/min*
Adrenaline arrest		1 mg IV or IO (intraosseous)	0.01 mg/kg (10 microgram/kg) IV/IO
Atropine resus		1 mg	0.02 mg/kg min 0.1 mg
Amiodarone		300 mg	5 mg/kg
Glucose		25 mL of 50%	0.25 mg/kg 2.5 mL/kg of 10%
Defibrillation		200 J	4 J/kg
Calcium	0.1–0.2 mmol/kg $CaCl_2$ slow push	10 mL of 10% $CaCl_2$ (slow) 20 mL of 10% calcium gluconate	0.5 mL/kg 10% calcium gluconate
Magnesium	0.1 mmol/kg	5 mmol	25–50 mg/kg = 0.1–0.2 mmol/kg
$NaHCO_3^-$	1 mmol/kg	1 mL/kg of 8.4% $NaHCO_3^-$	1 mmol/kg

IBW = ideal body weight

Note: All doses IV unless otherwise stated.

General tip: In an unstable patient with poor circulatory flow and/or low blood pressure, decrease your induction agent dose but use the maximum dose of the paralysis agent.

Some common concentration calculations

$$\% = \text{g} / 100\ \text{mL}$$

$$\text{therefore } 1\% = 10\ \text{mg} / 1\ \text{mL}$$

$$1 \text{ in } 1000 = 1\ \text{g in } 1000\ \text{mL}$$

$$= 1000\ \text{mg in } 1000\ \text{mL}$$

$$= 1\ \text{mg in } 1\ \text{mL}$$

$$1 \text{ in } 10{,}000 = 1\ \text{mg in } 10\ \text{mL}$$

CHAPTER 1

Resuscitation and trauma

Resuscitation

Advanced life support (ALS)

(For paeds see p. 318)

- Check for **D**anger
- Check **R**esponse and **S**end for help
- **A**irway: Suction, Guedel, nasal pharyngeal aspirate (NPA), position (lift; thrust)
- **B**reathing: Is it normal?
- **C**irculation: 30 compressions to 2 breaths at 100 bpm (beats per minute)

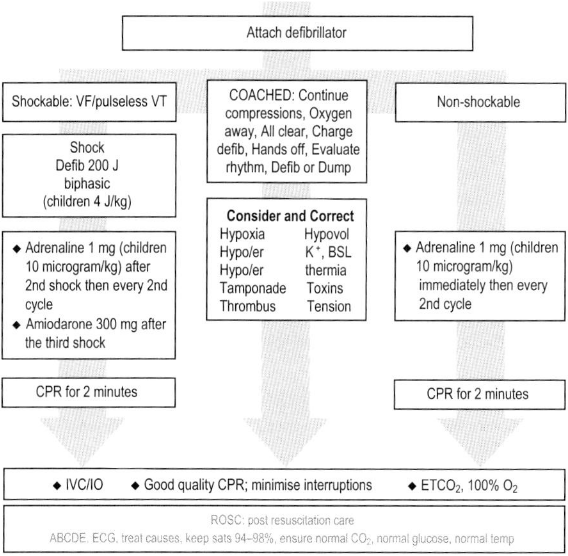

Attach defibrillator

Shockable: VF/pulseless VT	COACHED: Continue compressions, Oxygen away, All clear, Charge defib, Hands off, Evaluate rhythm, Defib or Dump	Non-shockable
Shock Defib 200 J biphasic (children 4 J/kg)		
◆ Adrenaline 1 mg (children 10 microgram/kg) after 2nd shock then every 2nd cycle ◆ Amiodarone 300 mg after the third shock	**Consider and Correct** Hypoxia — Hypovol Hypo/er — K^+, BSL Hypo/er — thermia Tamponade — Toxins Thrombus — Tension	◆ Adrenaline 1 mg (children 10 microgram/kg) immediately then every 2nd cycle
CPR for 2 minutes		CPR for 2 minutes

◆ IVC/IO ◆ Good quality CPR; minimise interruptions ◆ $ETCO_2$, 100% O_2

ROSC: post resuscitation care

ABCDE, ECG, treat causes, keep sats 94–98%, ensure normal CO_2, normal glucose, normal temp

Basic airway manoeuvres

(For paeds see p. 320)

- Indications: Improve oxygenation, open airway
- Contraindications: Awake patient, C-spine immobilisation/fracture (relative, airway comes first), traumatic head injury (NPA contraindicated only)
- Risks: Failure, worsening of spine injury, mucosa trauma, bleeding
- Preparation: Patient supine
  - Jaw thrust: Fingers mandible/jaw, thrusts jaw up without moving rest of head; preferred in suspected C-spine injury
  - Chin lift with head tilt: One hand on forehead pushing back and hand lifting chin up
- Procedure
  - Oropharyngeal airway (OPA)/Guedel: Measure from front incisors to angle of mandible. Insert upside down with tip facing palate then rotate on insertion 180 degrees. (The preferred method in children is to just insert directly without rotating.) If patient gags or cannot tolerate, remove by pulling out and down towards chin
  - NPA: Measure from nostril to ear lobe, lubricate, insert with bevel facing septum; this will follow normal curve on the right but on left will need to be rotated once it reaches nasopharynx. Insert until fully in nostril
  - Ventilate with bag valve mask (BVM). Always use two-person technique, one person bagging, one person holding mask (2 thumbs down, with jaw thrust). Use with OPA and 2 NPA if required

Laryngeal mask airways (LMAs)

- Choose size as per patient weight
- Fully deflate cuff
- Lubricate cuff (water-based lubricant)
- Insert index finger into slot formed behind flat cuff and junction tube
- Tilt head back
- Insert LMA by following normal curve of airway or insert upside down and rotate
- Inflate cuff; tube should rise slightly

- Or use appropriately sized i-gel—just lubricate and insert
  - Note: i-gel comes in protective cradle; can use cradle to lubricate tube and always rest i-gel in cradle. DON'T INSERT CRADLE. i-gel has non-inflatable cuff.
  - If meet early resistance, try jaw thrust or rotation technique.
  - Tubes have size and corresponding weight on them.
- Sizes

Age	Weight	Size	Cuff vol.
0 to 2 months	< 5 kg	1	4 mL
2 months to 1 year	5–10 kg	1.5	7 mL
1 to 6 years	10–20 kg	2	10 mL
6 to 11 years	20–30 kg	2.5	14 mL
11 years to adult	30–50 kg	3	20 mL
Adult	50–70 kg	4	30 mL
	70–100 kg	5	40 mL
	> 100 kg	6	50 mL

Intubation

(For additional information on paeditatric airways see p. 320)

- Indications: Create an airway, maintain an airway, protect an airway or provide ventilation
- Preparation: History (Hx), examination (Ex) and always use an intubation checklist

  Make your first attempt your BEST attempt

  - Hx: AMPLE (Allergies, Medications, Past medical history, Last eaten, Events leading), previous intubations, neck issues
  - Ex: Observe face shape, teeth, hair, neck, potential obstructions (foreign body [FB], burn), mouth opening, neck range of movement (ROM), level of consciousness
    - Vitals: Respiratory rate (RR), haemodynamics and reserve
    - Listen: Breathing, voice
    - Assess injuries: Face, swelling, subcutaneous emphysema, C–spine
  - 4 × 4 checklist
    - Monitoring: BP, electrocardiogram (ECG), oxygen saturation (sats), $ETCO_2$

        - Drugs: Induction, sedation, muscle relaxant, cardiovascular (metaraminol/adrenaline/atropine)
        - Equipment: Oxygen (pre-oxygenate—BVM, bilevel positive airway pressure [BiPAP] and apnoeic oxygen), fluids on pump set, blades (check ×2) and tubes, suction
        - Backup: Video blade, Bougie, LMA, cricothyroidotomy (cric) kit (if available, all of these need to be out and ready)
    - Tubes: Check cuff
        - Adults: Usually 7, 7.5 mm in females and 8, 8.5 mm in men
        - Children > 2 years: $(\frac{age}{4}) + 4$ if uncuffed or $(\frac{age}{4}) + 3.5$ cuffed
            - Usually use cuffed but can use uncuffed children < 10
            - Neonates usually use size 3
- Intubating
    - Vocalise to entire group the checklist and backup plan (such as two-person BVM, LMA, intubate with bougie and video). You must try these if available; however, let the group know 'YOU WILL proceed to emergency cricothyroidotomy if you can't intubate and can't ventilate'
    - Designated person to time attempts and length of desaturation: When things go wrong, often people lose track of time
    - Pre-oxygenation for at least 3 minutes for nitrogen washout
    - Optimise patient: Cardiovascular, vasoactive agents, fluid bolus
    - Optimise position: Ear to sternal notch, may need to ramp or towel under shoulders
    - May need C-spine immobilisation
    - Administer sedation: Decrease dose in compromised patients
    - Administer paralytic: Use maximum dose in compromised patients
    - Blade in left hand, insert tube in corner of mouth, right side
    - Visualise epiglottis then visualise arytenoids
    - Lift epiglottis and expose larynx, visualise cords. External laryngeal manipulation by intubator or an assistant may improve view; may need backwards, upwards, rightwards pressure (BURP)
    - Pass Bougie, railroad tube, may need to rotate tube to get past cords
    - Visualise tube passing through cords, remove Bougie; make sure you see the tube pass through the cords before you remove the laryngoscope

    - Connect to bag, inflate cuff
    - Check placement: Breath sounds, fogging, $ETCO_2$, chest x-ray (CXR)
    - Connect to ventilator
    - Ensure ongoing sedation
- Ventilate: Start O_2 100% and wean
    - Tidal vol. 6–8 mL/kg
    - Positive end-expiratory pressure (PEEP)
        - Start at 5 cm
        - ↑ in lung disease (causes ↓ BP, ↓ cerebral blood flow [CBF])
        - ↓ if unstable or ↑ intracranial pressure (ICP)
        - Inspiratory pressure < 30 cm. Peak inspiratory pressure more important than mean. May need to allow higher pressures in asthma
- Problems
    - CAN'T TUBE: Call for help
        - External laryngeal manipulation, Bougie, optimise position (should have been optimised on the first attempt). Don't keep trying if sats are falling. Don't repeat an attempt if you have not changed anything
        - LMA
        - Bag and mask, ALWAYS 2-person technique, use multiple adjuncts 2 × NPAs AND an OPA
        - Surgical airway—if you can't intubate and can't ventilate
    - Cricothyroidotomy—(increased risks in < 10 year olds but can still do in younger patients if absolutely needed) **Scalpel—finger—Bougie** (see p. 40)
    - Needle cricothyroidotomy (see p. 38)
        - In a child < 10 years old, preferred
    - Unable to ventilate once intubated: DOPE
        - **D**isconnect: Go back to bagging, the ventilator may be causing the issue
        - **O**bstructed: Check for blockages or kinking of the tube; is their mucus plugging?
        - **P**neumothorax
        - **E**quipment failure: CHECK ALL EQUIPMENT from the patient to the wall; if in doubt, replace equipment

Rapid sequence intubation (RSI) drugs

- Induction
  - Ketamine 1–2 mg/kg
  - Thiopentone 3–5 mg/kg (don't use in patient with porphyria)
    - 1–2 mg/kg if ↓ level of consciousness or hypotensive, even less if very unstable
    - 200 mg for normal, stable 70–80 kg adult
  - Propofol 1–2 mg/kg
    - NOT in egg allergy
- Muscle relaxants
  - Rocuronium 1.2 mg/kg (preferred in children)
  - Suxamethonium 1–2 mg/kg (see Precautions below)
- Infusions
  - Midazolam/morphine 1 mg/mL of each in 50 mL; start at 3–5 mL/hr titrate up/down
  - Propofol 1–3 mg/kg/hr
  - Vecuronium 0.1–0.15 mg/kg or stat dose 10 mg vecuronium lasts approximately 1 hour
  - Adrenaline or noradrenaline: 0.05 microgram/kg/min, start at 1 microgram/min
    - 'Quick and easy adrenaline infusion': 1 mg adrenaline in 1 L normal saline = 1 microgram/mL
    - Usual infusion: 6 mg in 100 mL normal saline = 60 microgram/mL
  - Metaraminol: 10 mg in 50 mL normal saline = 200 microgram/mL, start at 1 mL/hr
- Rescue drugs
  - Metaraminol 0.5–1 mg intravenous (IV) boluses for hypotension
  - Adrenaline 50 microgram IV or 0.05 microgram/kg/min infusion for hypotension
  - Atropine 20 microgram/kg IV max. 1.2 mg for severe bradycardia
  - Sugammadex 16 mg/kg for emergency reversal of rocuronium
- Precautions
  - Suxamethonium
    - DON'T use in ↑ K^+, non-acute burns, nerve damage, neuromuscular disease

        - Can lead to ↑ intraocular pressure (IOP), ↑ ICP, ↑ intragastric pressure, muscle pain. 2nd dose brady
        - Children especially susceptible to bradycardia; however, DON'T need to pre-treat for prevention
    - Malignant hyperthermia
        - Treat with IV dantrolene 2.5 mg/kg IV bolus. Repeat 1 mg/kg boluses as required to max. 10 mg/kg total

Extubation in emergency department (ED)

- Indications: Resolution of causative issue leading to intubation, normal vitals (RR < 30, sBP > 100, pulse rate [PR] < 120, sats > 95%), not needing ventilator support (pressure support [PS] ≤ 5, PEEP ≤ 5, FiO_2 ≤ 30%), sedatives off, awake and compliant
- Contraindications: Difficult airway on intubation, non-compliant patient, resources unavailable/other departmental issues requiring resources
- Consent: Obviously can't get formal consent but must be able to explain procedure to cooperative patient
    - Risks: Failure requiring re-intubation, aspiration
- Preparation
    - Turn off sedatives (can keep low dose fentanyl)
    - Allow full return to consciousness
    - Assess if patient can: Raise arms for 15 seconds, raise head off bed, cough
    - Ventilator settings: PS 5, PEEP ≤ 5, FiO_2 ≤ 30%
    - Sit patient at ≥ 45 degrees and observe for 30 minutes
    - Ensure vitals stable: If PR > 120, sBP > 200, sats decrease, significant anxiety—DON'T PROCEED
- Procedure
    - Patient sitting up
    - Suction endotracheal tube (ETT) and oropharynx
    - Deflate cuff (must have a leak)
    - Patient cough—pull tube on cough
    - Suction oropharynx
    - Place mask with neb of normal saline
    - Encourage patient to cough up secretions
- After care: Monitor in resus room

Tracheotomy (trachy) emergencies

- Components to trachy
  - Outer tube
  - Inner tube (can remove)
  - Flange—plastic plate that secures to patient
  - Outer diameter connecter
  - +/– cuff, air inlet valve, pilot cuff, fenestrations, speaking valve, cork, extra length
- Potential complications
  - Complications of insertion
  - Haemorrhage
  - Occlusion (blood, secretions, crust)
  - Granulation tissue (obstruct, bleed)
  - Accidental dislodgement
  - Airway stenosis
  - Tracheomalacia
- Preparation: Emergency equipment to patient bedside
  - Difficult airway trolley
  - Spare trachy tubes (same internal and external diameter, length and curve as patient's)—patients often have a spare with them
  - Hooks
  - Dilators
  - Suction
  - Resus bag with straight attachment
  - 10 mL syringe
- Managing respiratory distress in trachy patient
  - Differential diagnosis: DOPES—Displacement, Obstruction, Pneumothorax/pulmonary embolism (PE)/pulmonary oedema, Equipment failure, Stacked breaths/bronchoconstriction
  - Assess: MASH—Movement of chest, Arterial sats and $ETCO_2$, Skin colour, Haemodynamics
  - Ask patient: Is it cuffed (will have pilot tube), what is outer diameter (need smaller tube than that), duration (only change if more than 7 days old), indication for placement
  - Do: High-flow oxygen, suction (if can't—likely blocked or displaced), is there $ETCO_2$, remove/replace inner tube

  - If unsure if total laryngectomy or not, place O_2 over trachy and also mouth
  - Consult with urgency if needed: ICU; respiratory; ear, nose and throat (ENT)
- Managing bleeding
  - Differential diagnosis: Early complication (Cx) (suction/manipulation, bleed from surgical site), late Cx (granulation, infection, fistula, bleeding diathesis, haemoptysis)
  - Do: Airway, breathing, circulation (ABC); clear clots/suction; finger pressure to bleeding if possible or root of neck; inflate trachy cuff; blood products
- Consult urgent: ENT

Shock

- Signs and symptoms: Change in mental state, acidosis, ↓ urine output (UO), ↑ PR, ↓ BP, ↓ capillary return (CR), pale, cold
- Overall management
  - **A**irway: Secure
  - **B**reathing: O_2, +/– ventilate
  - **C**irculation: Control bleed, IV lines, large bore
  - Fluids: Bolus (may need cautious 300–500 mL bolus in cardiogenic shock), +/– vasoactives/inotropes
  - Monitor: Sats, BP, pulse, blood sugar level (BSL), UO, temperature, ECG
  - Investigate
- **Hypovolaemic**: e.g. blood loss, dehydration (see Trauma for MTP, p. 27)
  - *Signs and symptoms*: ↓ skin turgor, dry mucous membrane, ↓ jugular venous pressure (JVP), bleeding
  - ABC
  - Large-bore IV access
  - Fluids: Warm fluids, normal saline bolus 500 mL to 1 L, 20 mL/kg for children. Can repeat. If blood loss, need early use of blood products, tranexamic acid (TXA)
  - Warm blood: Cross-match or O– (1 × red blood cells [RBC] / 1 × fresh frozen plasma [FFP] / 1 × platelets [PLT])
  - Treat cause: e.g. operating theatre (OT), embolisation
    - Titrate to BP > 90/60
    - Use minimum volume resus in abdominal aortic aneurysm (AAA), ectopic, penetrating trauma

- **Cardiogenic**: e.g. acute myocardial infarction (AMI), arrhythmia, cardiomyopathy, valve rupture
  - *Signs and symptoms*: ↑↓ PR, ↑ JVP, murmur, acute pulmonary oedema (APO), abnormal ECG
  - ABC
  - Can trial fluid bolus but with caution, 250 mL normal saline IV
  - Dobutamine 2.5–10 microgram/kg/min IV; need central access
  - Avoid adrenaline (consider if BP ↓↓)
  - Treat cause: e.g. antiarrhythmic, PCI
  - In AMI if BP high enough consider glyceryl trinitrate (GTN). CAUTION with GTN in posterior AMI
  - Milrinone
- Distributive
  - Septic
    - *Signs and symptoms*: Fever, peripherally vasodilated, infection source
    - ABC
    - Fluids, large IVC, venous gas lactate, cultures—investigations
    - Inotropes: Noradrenaline 0.05 microgram/kg/min can start at 1 microgram/min. Central access preferred but can give peripherally to start
    - Aim for euglycaemia
    - Monitor: BPs, arterial line, central venous pressures (CVPs)—filling, central line, UO, BSL
    - Treat source quickly: Empiric antibiotics (AB) in under 1 hour, OT/debride
    - +/– e.g. flucloxacillin 2 g (50 mg/kg) 6-hourly AND gentamicin 5 mg/kg, (up to 7.5 mg/kg in child)
- Anaphylactic/anaphylaxis
  - *Signs and symptoms*: Generalised urticarial rash, wheeze, angio-oedema, hypotension, abdomen pain, diarrhoea/vomiting
  - *Life-threatening if*: Airway swelling, hoarse voice, stridor, increased RR, fatigue, cyanosis, pallor, hypotensive and altered level of consciousness
  - *Causes of arrest in anaphylaxis*: Bronchospasm, mucous plug, hypoxia and meds (e.g. salbutamol) precipitating arrhythmia, dynamic hyperinflation, tension pneumothorax

- *Management*
  - Stop precipitant, lay patient flat
  - Intramuscular (IM) adrenaline: IM lateral thigh (use 1 in 1000)
    - Dose by weight: 10 microgram/kg (= 0.01 mg/kg = 0.01 mL/kg of 1 in 1000)
    - Max. dose/adult dose: 500 microgram–1 mg (= 0.5–1 mL of 1 in 1000)
    - Pregnant women use 300 microgram
    - Children: 500 microgram (> 12 years), 0.5 mL 1 in 1000; 300 microgram (6–12 years), 0.3 mL 1 in 1000; 150 microgram (< 6 years), 0.15 mL 1 in 1000
  - IV access or IO if cannot get IV
  - Protect airway, 100% O_2
  - If requires intubation, likely to be difficult—get help, anaesthetics, airway plan, be ready to do surgical airway if required
  - Steroids—IV/IM preferred as decreased absorption in anaphylaxis
    - Hydrocortisone IV/IM
    - 200 mg in adult, children 4 mg/kg
    - Or by age: 200 mg if > 12 years old, 100 mg if 6–12 years old, 50 mg if 6 months–6 years old, 25 mg if under 6 months old
  - If low BP give 20 mL/kg up to 1 L IV bolus normal saline
  - Inadequate response
    - Repeat adrenaline IM
    - Adrenaline IV bolus: 50 microgram in an adult, 1 microgram/kg in a child
    - Adrenaline infusion: 0.05 microgram/kg/min titrate
    - Repeat fluid bolus
    - Atropine if ↓ PR: 0.02 mg/kg IV
    - Consider glucagon if beta blocked (1–2 mg IV/IM)
  - Bronchospasm: Salbutamol nebuliser, adrenaline nebuliser
  - If arrest:
    - Adrenaline 1 mg q2min (every 2 minutes) IV
    - Fluid bolus 20 mg/kg normal saline as a push IV

   - Post resuscitation care
     - Monitor post 4–24 hours
     - Follow-up
     - EpiPen
- **Neurogenic**
  - *Signs and symptoms*: Cord cut >T6, flaccid, ↓ PR, priapism, hypotension
  - ABC
  - Look for other causes ↓ BP; e.g. blood loss
  - Don't overhydrate with IV fluids
  - Treat ↓ BP with pressors
- Obstructive
  - *Signs and symptoms*: PE, tamponade, tension
  - ABC
  - Treat cause; e.g. pericardiocentesis, needle thoracotomy, thrombolysis/embolectomy

Inotropes

Note: Always use your hospital's protocols if available

- Digoxin
  - Increased intracellular calcium—inotropic, increased automaticity, slows atrioventricular (AV) conduction
- Dopamine (DA) > β > α dose dependent
  - Start at 5 microgram/kg/min titrate to 2–30 microgram/kg/min
- Dobutamine $\beta_1 > \beta_2$
  - Start at 5 microgram/kg/min titrate to 2–10 microgram/kg/min
- Noradrenaline $\alpha > \beta_1$
  - Start dose = 0.05 microgram/kg/min or 1 microgram/min, titrate to 1–20 microgram/min
  - To make: 6 mg of noradrenaline (NAd) in 100 mL of normal saline = 60 microgram/mL (i.e. 1 microgram/kg/mL for a 60 kg adult)
  - Starting infusion rate: 0.05 mL/min or 3 mL/hr
- Adrenaline α and $\beta_1 > \beta_2$
  - Start dose = 0.05 microgram/kg/min or 1 microgram/min, titrate to 1–20 microgram/min

  - To make: 6 mg of adrenaline (Ad) in 100 mL of normal saline = 60 microgram/mL (i.e. 1 microgram/kg/mL for a 60 kg adult)
  - Starting infusion rate: 0.05 mL/min or 3 mL/hr
  - *ALTERNATIVE IF IN A HURRY*: Take any vial of adrenaline (= 1 mg) put it in 1 L normal saline = 1 microgram/mL solution, start at 1 mL/min or run wide open or bolus
- Isoprenaline β_1 and β_2
  - Start dose = 0.05 microgram/kg/min, titrate to 1–20 microgram/min
- Milrinone
  - Phosphodiesterase inhibitor
  - 0.5 microgram/kg/min
- Metaraminol
  - 10 mg in 50 mL normal saline = 200 microgram/mL, start at 1 mL/hr
  - 0.5–1 mg boluses
- Levosimendan (currently unavailable in Australia)—binds troponin c
  - Doesn't ↑ heart O_2 consumption; use in acute heart failure
  - 0.5 microgram/kg/min

Electrocution

- High risk
  - High volt, > 1000 (Australian household voltage 230)
  - High amp, 100 mA–1 A can induce ventricular fibrillation (VF)/respiratory arrest, > 2 A can cause burns, > 10 A can cause asystole
  - Low resistance (e.g. wet skin) produces higher current
  - Current: AC causes tetanic contraction; i.e. more dangerous than DC
  - Pathway across heart (e.g. hand–hand)
  - Exposure duration (increased with AC current)
- Vessels, heart, nerves most at risk
- Types of injuries
  - Disrupted cell function—muscle, respiratory, heart cells
  - Blunt trauma
  - Blast trauma
  - Thermal burns

- Look for and consider:
  - Arrhythmia (delayed arrhythmia is rare), myocardial necrosis
  - Vascular injury, compartment syndrome
  - Burns, entry and exit wounds
  - Seizure
  - Organ injury—colon, pancreas, gall bladder, small intestine
  - Spinal injury
  - Blast injury—check tympanic membrane
- Management
  - First responder must avoid danger
  - ABC/cardiopulmonary resuscitation (CPR)—prolonged resuscitation
  - Always assume a spinal cord injury
  - Defibrillator for VF; asystole may spontaneously resolve
  - Monitor/ECG, monitor fetal heart rate (HR) with cardiotocograph (CTG) if pregnant
  - Check creatine kinase (CK)
  - Admit and monitor if: High volt, ECG changes, loss of consciousness (LOC)/seizure, previous cardiac disease, documented arrhythmia, burns
  - Treat burns, and investigate for and treat deep tissue injury
  - In patients with low voltage exposure (e.g. household shock) and normal Ex and normal ECG—no further investigations are required

Burns

- Initial management
  - Cool tap water 20 minutes (beware of inducing hypothermia)
  - Burns sheet/cling film
  - Airway: Intubate early if concerns of airway involvement
- Assess extent: Total burn surface area (TBSA)
  - Patient palm = 1% TBSA OR burns charts
  - Rule of 9s (Table 1.1)
  - Depth
    - Superficial; e.g. sunburn = erythema, pain, bright red, normal CR
      - Usually no dressing; topical treatments and analgesia as required

Table 1.1 Rule of 9s

Body part	Adult (%)	Child (%)	Baby (%)
Entire head	9	14	18
Whole arm	9	9	9
Both arms	18	18	18
Anterior leg	9	8	7
Whole leg	18	16	14
Both legs	36	32	28
Entire back	18	18	18
Entire thorax and abdomen	18	18	18
Perineum	1	1	1

    - Partial: Superficial = very painful, ooze, hair intact, CR normal, blanching, blisters
        - Dress with antibiotic-impregnated gauze
    - Partial: Deep = variable pain, little ooze, hairs come out, absent CR, does not bleed with pin prick, red/blotchy/dry
        - Dress with silver sulfadiazine (except the face) dressing daily; specialist review
    - Full thickness = absent pain, dry, hair follicles and sweat glands destroyed, absent CR, absent sensation, no blisters, no bleed on pin prick, dry/pearly/leathery white
        - Need debride and graft
- Analgesia: Paracetamol, N_2O, morphine, intranasal or IV fentanyl
- Fluids
    - Bolus fluids if in shock use normal saline—not included in Parkland formula
    - Parkland formula if > 20% TBSA burn in adult or > 10% in children; partial or full-thickness burns
        - 2–4 mL/kg × % TBSA over 24 hours (maximum TBSA to be used is 50%)
        - + maintenance (4 mL/kg 1st 10 kg, 2 mL/kg 2nd 10 kg, 1 mL/kg remainder = volume to give per hour, max. 100 mL/hr)
        - Give 50% over the first 8 hours, 50% over the next 16 hours
        - Titrate to UO aim 0.5–1 mL/kg/hr

    - ○ Strict input/output chart
    - ○ Can use normal saline or Hartmann's
- When to admit or transfer to specialist
  - Discharge likely in mild burns
    - Partial thickness < 15% in adult, < 5% in child
    - Full thickness < 2%
  - Admit patients with moderate burns
    - Partial thickness 15–20% adult, 5–10% in child
    - Full thickness 2–5%
  - Transfer to burns unit for severe burns
    - Partial thickness > 20% adult, > 10% children
    - Full thickness > 5%
    - Special circumstances: inhalation burns, electrical burns, chemical burns, burns and significant injury
    - Special areas: Face, hands, feet, perineum, ears
- **Escharotomy**
  - Full-thickness burns result in eschar that is inelastic and can result in compartment syndrome. Full- and partial-thickness circumferential extremity burns are most likely to impede blood flow. Chest wall burns can restrict ventilation
  - Clinical assessment of tight compartments can be aided by cap refill, Doppler, pulse oximeter, direct measurement of compartment pressures
  - When required, escharotomy is usually performed within 2–6 hours of burn
  - Technique: Limbs
    - No anaesthesia required for full-thickness burns, may be required for partial
    - Sterile conditions
    - Lateral and medial aspects of limbs
    - Careful to avoid obvious nerves and vessels—ulnar N (incision should pass in front of medial epicondyle), radial N, peroneal N (incision should not pass over neck of fibula), posterior tibia A (incision pass in front of knee), long saphenous V and saphenous N (incision should pass behind medial malleolus)
    - Incise approx. 1 cm proximal and 1 cm distal to burned area

    - Carry incision through full thickness of skin only to expose fat
    - In feet extend to proximal big toe medially and 5th toe laterally
    - In hands extend to thenar and hypothenar eminences
    - Can check Dopplers, vascular and O_2 to indicate adequate release
  - Technique: Chest
    - Make incisions along the anterior axillary lines bilaterally starting from just below the clavicles and continuing to the upper abdomen/lower costal margin
    - Join these two incisions superiorly with a transverse slightly convex incision just below the clavicles, and inferiorly following the lower costal margin
  - Neck: Incise laterally and posteriorly to avoid carotid and jugular vessels
  - Penis: Incise midlaterally to avoid dorsal penile vessels
  - Complications: Bleeding, infection, damage to underlying structures. Complications of inadequate or no decompression include muscle necrosis, nerve injury, amputation limb, rhabdomyolysis and multi-organ failure
- **Chemical burns**
  - Acid/alkali
    - Dilute with water, remove clothes, adsorbed diphtheria and tetanus (ADT) vaccination
  - Cement
    - Irrigate, remove cement dust
  - Bitumen
    - Soak in ice water, don't remove clothes or tar
    - Split tar if circumferential
    - Dress with tulle gras
  - Hydrofluoric acid (see also Toxicology, p. 231)
    - Irrigate with water +++
    - Don't use local anaesthetics
    - Neutralise with Ca gluconate, topical, gel, IV, intraarterial (IA)

Drowning

- Complications of drowning: Hypoxia, aspiration, pulmonary oedema, electrolyte abnormalities, hypothermia, associated trauma

- Pulmonary oedema may be delayed so observe for 4+ hours if suspected
- Management
  - History: Important in assessment of patient and prognosis
    - Precipitating event: Syncope, seizure, trauma, drugs and alcohol
    - Immersion: Type of water, temperature, contaminants, time
    - Pre-hospital: When were they found and removed, resuscitation commenced, vitals with ambulance
    - Previous history (PHx): Non-accidental injury (NAI) concerns, comorbidities
  - Examination
    - Vitals, ABC
    - Look for causes or precipitating event
    - Look for trauma
    - Assess neuro category: A = awake, B = obtunded, C = coma, C1 = flex to pain, C2 = extend to pain, C3 = flaccid
  - Investigations
    - Venous blood gases (VBG); electrolytes, urea and creatinine (EUC); CXR
    - ECG
    - Osmolarity, alcohol (EtOH), coagulation profile (coags)
    - C-spine imaging, computed tomography of the brain (CTB), skeletal survey
  - Management
    - Advanced cardiac life support (ACLS), CPR, keep C-spine immobilised if suspicion of injury
    - A/B: Oxygen, continuous positive airway pressure (CPAP), ETT, titrate PEEP to sats > 95%, lowest FiO_2
    - C: IV fluids with care, monitor electrolytes
    - Temperature: Avoid hyperthermia. Target temperature < 36°C equivocal
    - If hypothermic aim to increase temp with warm fluids, warm blankets, warm humidified O_2, warm bladder irrigation etc. while continuing resus attempts as per hypothermic ALS arrest protocols—see below
    - Aim normal glucose

    - IV antibiotics only if contaminated water
    - No role for steroids
  - Prognosis
    - Poor prognosis = Orlanski scale > 3
      - Age < 3
      - Submersion > 5 minutes
      - Coma on arrival in ED
      - Resuscitation not started within 10 minutes
      - pH < 7.10 on arrival
  - Good prognosis
    - Submerged < 6 minutes
    - Time to first spontaneous breath < 30 minutes
    - Spontaneous respiration and heartbeat on arrival to ED
  - **Immersion syndrome:** sudden death/cardiac arrest, vagally mediated on cold water immersion

Hypothermia

- Definition = core temperature < 35°C
- Classification
  - Mild = 32–35°C: Normal BP, shiver, increased respiratory stimulation
  - Moderate = 28–32°C: Stupor, decreased shiver, arrhythmia, decreased PR and cardiac output, decreased level of consciousness, decreased oxygen requirements
  - Severe = < 28°C: Decreased reflexes, decreased CBF, acid–base abnormal, decreased BP, flat ECG, can look clinically dead
- Investigations
  - Full blood count (FBC), EUC, coags, VBG
  - Glucose, CK, lipase
  - ECG—bradycardia, blocks, conduction abnormalities, arrhythmia, Osborn J waves, ectopics, asystole; atrial fibrillation (AF) considered 'normal' in hypothermia
- General management
  - ABC, rewarm, handle gently, indwelling catheter (IDC)/ nasogastric tube (NGT), IV medications, monitor core temperature, monitor ECG, fluids
  - Increased resuscitation times
  - Drug intervals in resuscitation to be doubled until temp > 30°C

- Rewarming
  - Passive warming: Remove wet clothes, warm environment
  - Active warming: Warm blanket, radiant heat, Bair Hugger
  - Internal warming: Warm humidified oxygen, blood warmer
  - Invasive: Most commonly warm bladder irrigation with three-way catheter, abdominal or thoracic lavage, dialysis, ECMO, bypass; e.g. 250 mL aliquots of fluid warm up to 42°C in bladder/IDC or stomach/NGT with 15 minutes dwell time.
- Other treatments
  - Treating arrhythmia VT/VF: Give up to 3 defibrillations then wait for temperature to be > 30°C before shocking again

Hyperthermia

- Classification of heatstroke
  - Classic: Passive exposure, heatwave, skin is hot and dry
  - Exertional: Strenuous exercise, sweating, more rhabdomyolysis and disseminated intravascular coagulation (DIC)
- Differential diagnosis of the hot and altered patient
  - Sepsis, encephalitis
  - Hyperthyroidism, thyroid storm
  - Drugs: Overdose (OD) of amphetamines, cocaine, aspirin, anticholinergics or withdrawal (e.g. delirium tremens)
  - Serotonin syndrome, neuroleptic malignant syndrome
- Complications of hyperthermia
  - Cardiac: Tachycardia/arrhythmia, hypovolaemic +/– shock
  - Neurological: Delirium, seizure, coma
  - Rhabdomyolysis: With hyperkalaemia and acute kidney injury
  - Haematological: Exertional petechiae, DIC
  - Multi-organ failure
- Investigations
  - EUC, FBC, glucose
  - VBG (increased lactate, respiratory alkalosis, metabolic acidosis)
  - CK, liver function test (LFT) (increased aspartate transaminase [AST], lactate dehydrogenase [LDH]), coags

- ECG (increased QT, tachycardia, AF, SVT, right bundle branch block [RBBB], ST changes)
- Urine myoglobin, increased urate

- Cooling
  - Aim < 39°C
  - Remove from heat, remove clothes
  - Evaporative: Spray with water, use fan
  - Immersion: Ice water, ice pack, wet sheet
  - Internal: Cold IV fluids (e.g. 4°C), lavage, ECMO, bypass
- Management
  - ABC avoid suxamethonium
  - Careful use of IV fluids (can cause APO)
  - Monitor ECG, core temp
  - Sedatives: benzodiazepines
  - Paralysis, ETT if needed
  - If need pressors consider dopamine (adrenaline and noradrenaline vasoconstrict)
  - Aim urine output > 50 mL/hr, alkalise urine if severe
  - Dialysis

Trauma

General approach to trauma

- Preparation
  - People
    - Consider activating trauma team—what are your ED's criteria?
    - Gather your team and assign roles
    - Notify radiology, theatres, ICU, blood bank as required
    - Do you need security?
    - Consider the rest of the department and keep it running
  - Place
    - Resuscitation bay ideally
    - Prepare the space
    - Bring in the equipment you need
    - Remove the stuff you don't need

- Equipment
  - Check airway and breathing equipment (ETT, blades, backup plan, Bougie, airway adjuncts, video blade, suction, oxygen)
  - Vascular access, IVC equipment, blood tubes, blood alcohol kit if needed, intraosseous kit on standby, rapid infusers, blood warmer
  - Chest tubes, thoracotomy tray
  - Pelvic binders, femoral splints
  - Warming of patient: Bair Hugger
  - Spine board, C-spine collars
  - Monitors: Sats, ECG, BP, $ETCO_2$
  - ECG machine available
  - Ultrasound machine available
- Medications
  - RSI: Sedation, paralytic
  - Fluids: Warmed
  - Blood products on hand: Warmed
  - Analgesia
  - Inotropes
  - Antibiotics

- Patient arrival
  - Transfer patient from ambulance stretcher with spinal precautions
  - Handover from ambulance
    - Best done pre transfer of patient
    - Done during or post transfer when patient is unstable
  - Obtain vital signs, attach monitors, gain access to patient—remove clothing
- Primary survey (control catastrophic bleeding immediately)—ABCDEFG
  - **A**irway
    - Look for obstruction, foreign body, oedema
    - Protect, establish airway
  - **B**reathing
    - Breath sounds, asymmetry
    - Shortness of breath (SOB)
    - Hyperresonance, dullness

- **C**irculation
    - Control external bleeding; e.g. tourniquet, pressure
    - Cardiac tamponade
    - Hypovolaemia
- **D**isability: Neurological examination
    - Level of consciousness
    - Pupils
    - Grossly abnormal neurology
    - Evidence of head or spinal cord injury
- **E**xposure: While preventing hypothermia
    - Wounds, bleeding, bruising, obvious fractures
    - Abdominal examination
- **F**AST scan: eFAST
- **G**lucose: DON'T EVER FORGET GLUCOSE

- Secondary survey
    - Head to toe examination
        - Head, face: Look in mouth for injury, missing teeth, look in ears, eyes, look under hair for injury/lacerations/haematoma, look at nose, check for septal haematoma if suspected nasal fracture
        - Neck: Look for injury, hard and soft signs, subcutaneous emphysema
        - Chest: Examine lungs, look for rib fractures, could there be flail chest, air leaks
        - Upper limbs: Injury, fractures, movement, gross sensation
        - Abdominal examination
        - Lower limbs: Injury, fractures, movement, gross sensation
        - Log roll: Spinal injury, rectal and perineal examination (not if unstable or pelvic fractures)
    - History: If able obtain from patient, responders, ambulance, police, family
        - AMPLE history
    - Investigations
        - X-ray: Chest, pelvis in resus room
        - CT head, neck, chest, abdomen, pelvis
        - CT aortogram, CT angiography

- Management
  - Team approach
  - ABCD in addressing injuries
  - Manage life-threatening injuries as found
  - Aim for definitive care—theatre
  - Involve early ICU, anaesthetics, surgeons
  - May need massive transfusion protocol
    - Early use of blood products
  - Consider need for antibiotics
  - ADT
  - Consider need for support for family—social worker
- Observation
  - Most trauma patients will need period of observation with serial examinations
  - Many significant diagnoses can be delayed; e.g. traumatic pancreatitis and oesophageal rupture post motor vehicle crash (MVC)
  - The more significant the trauma or potential for delayed diagnosis, the longer the observation period
  - Check local policies and consider admission to short stay if available

Head injury

- Assessment
  - History and examination used to guide decision whether to investigate with imaging (usually CTB)
  - In adults—Canadian Head Injury Guidelines (used in patients with head injury + LOC and/or amnesia of event and/or witnessed disorientation).
    - Excludes: Glasgow Coma Scale (GCS) < 13, age < 16 years, focal neurology, seizure, anticoagulation or bleeding diathesis
    - High risk: GCS not 15 within 2 hours, open or depressed skull fracture, basilar fracture, vomited twice or more, age 65 or over
    - Medium risk: Amnesia > 30 minutes, severe mechanisms (assault, fall more than 3 feet, ejected from vehicle, pedestrian versus car)
    - Note: NOT sensitive if EtOH intoxication

  - In children—Paediatric Emergency Care Applied Research Network (PECARN) clinical decision rule
    - Excludes GCS < 14, age > 18, trivial injury, penetrating injury, brain pathology, focal neurology, bleeding diathesis
    - Children < 2 years old: Skull fracture, abnormal mental state/GCS = 14, agitated, severe mechanisms, LOC 5 sec or more, non-frontal haematoma, drowsiness, agitated/not acting normal (as per parent)
    - Children > 2 years old: base of skull (BOS) fracture, agitated, vomiting, abnormal mental state/GCS = 14, severe injury, LOC, severe headache,
  - Note: Vomiting is the least sensitive of these factors
  - Multiple guidelines exist. Clinical guidelines assist in decision-making but always use clinical judgement in the context of individual cases
- Grading of head injury
  - Mild GCS = 13–15
  - Moderate GCS = 9–12
  - Severe GCS < 8
- Management of a diagnosed moderate or severe head injury
  - Prevent secondary injury
    - Protect the airway
    - Tape ETT, don't tie it
    - Avoid hyper and hypoxia, aim normocarbia, aim pCO_2 35 mmHg
    - Maintain cerebral perfusion, systolic BP (sBP) > 90
    - Use saline and vasopressors, treat anaemia; DON'T use albumin
    - Head of bed up to 30 degrees
    - ICP monitor GCS < 8 with abnormal CT result
    - Tight glycaemic control
  - Avoid hyperthermia; cool if temp > 39°C
  - Protect C-spine
  - Sedation and analgesia
  - Second line therapies
    - Mannitol 0.25–1 g/kg IV
    - Hypertonic saline (3%) 250 mL over 30 minutes for adults (3 mL/kg)

- Treat seizure
  - Unclear benefit/harm of prophylactic antiseizure meds
  - Phenytoin 20 mg/kg IV over 1 hour
  - Levetiracetam (Keppra) can also be used
- Rescue therapies—other therapies not working
  - Barbiturates
  - Therapeutic hypothermia
  - Aggressive hyperventilation—only if coning
- DON'T use steroids
- Treat other injury
  - Antibiotics for compound fracture
  - ADT if open wounds
- Reverse anticoagulation (see p. 180)
- **Emergency craniotomy (see Procedures, p. 48)**

- Management of mild/minor head injuries, not requiring CT scan
  - Observe 4–6 hours
  - CTB if:
    - Deterioration GCS
    - Focal neurological signs develop
    - Abnormal alertness/behaviour/cognition
    - Vomiting develops
    - Severe headache develops
  - Discharge with head injury advice
    - Avoid aspirin and nonsteroidal anti-inflammatory drugs (NSAIDs)
    - Avoid contact sports > 1 week
    - If concussion suspected see below
- Concussion
  - Signs of concussion (seen at time of injury or after)
    - LOC, slow to respond or get up from ground after event, confusion, looking dazed, more irritable or emotional, unsteady/incoordination, seizure
  - Symptoms of concussion
    - Headache, dizziness, confusion, decreased LOC, problems with vision, photophobia/photophonia, fatigue

- Management
  - Variations in practice; use your local guidelines and concussion assessment tools
  - Education (if possible give a patient handout; can find online)
  - Patient must be removed from contact sports (minimum 1 week for adults, 2 weeks for children; varies depending on age and sport)
  - Need follow-up (usually with local medical officer [LMO] but sometimes teams have their own sports doctor or speciality clinics available)
  - Graduated return to physical and cognitive (e.g. work, school, crosswords, TV, iPad, phone) activities
    - Early gentle physical activities shown beneficial in recent study; any activity that causes symptoms should be ceased

Massive transfusion protocol (MTP)

- Patients at increased risk of needing massive transfusion
  - sBP < 90, PR > 120, penetrating mechanism, positive FAST ultrasound (US), extremity or pelvic fractures
- Massive transfusion considered if you need to, or will likely need to, replace 1 blood volume in 24 hours or > 50% of blood volume in 4 hours; in children blood volume = 80 mL/kg
- Goals of MTP
  - Early recognition
  - Maintain tissue perfusion
  - Arrest bleeding
  - Judicious use of blood products
  - Use blood product ratios initially 1 : 1 : 1 (packed RBC:PLT:FFP)
  - Adjust blood products with specialist haematologist input and targeted end points
  - Urgent definitive treatment
- End points
  - Temperature > 35°C
  - pH > 7.2
  - Lactate < 4 mmol/L
  - Base excess < –6 mmol/L
  - Ionised calcium (iCa) > 1 mmol/L

  - Fibrinogen > 1 g/L (give cryoprecipitate 8 units to correct)
  - Platelets > 50 or > 100 ($\times 10^9$/L) in head injury (give platelets 4 units to correct)
  - PT/APTT < 1.5 × normal
  - International normalised ratio (INR) < 1.5 (give FFP to correct)
- Other elements of care
  - Give oxygen
  - Aggressively warm to keep normothermic
  - Prevent acidosis
  - Beware lethal triad—hypothermia, acidosis, coagulopathy
  - Tranexamic acid 1 g (10 mg/kg) over 10 minutes then 1 g over 8 hours
- Complications
  - Volume overload
  - Over transfusion
  - Hypothermia
  - Hyperkalaemia
  - Hypocalcaemia
  - Transfusion-related acute lung injury (TRALI)
  - Dilutional coagulopathy
  - Disease transmission (very rare)

Spine injuries

- Imaging rules
  - NEXUS: DON'T image if ALL of the following:
    - **N**o focal neurology
    - **E**TOH and/or drugs not used
    - e**X**treme distracting injury not present
    - **U**naltered mentation
    - **S**pine not tender midline
  - Canadian C-spine: <u>a rhyme</u> to remember it by (Disclaimer: I didn't make this rhyme up!)
    - *Exclusions*: unstable patient, penetrating injury, injury > 48 hours ago, non-traumatic injury, GCS < 15
    - *High risk*: Need imaging
      - <u>Fast drive</u> = serious mechanism (fall > 1 m, axial load, high speed, bicycle, rollover or ejected from vehicle, motorised recreational vehicle)

- Age over 65
- Sensation deprived (altered sensation)

○ *Low risk*: Don't image if all of the following apply and no high risk

- Slow wreck = simple rear collision
- Slow neck = neck pain is delayed
- Sitting down = sitting in ED
- Walking around = walked post injury
- C-spine fine = non-tender C-spine
- Let them move and image if they whine = ask patient to gently move their neck and if there is pain, perform imaging

• X-rays

■ If clinical concern, should consider performing CT instead; consider radiation risk versus missing injury with plain x-ray

■ Lateral:

○ Need to see on image down to C7–T1 junction

○ Check alignment (anterior longitudinal ligament line, posterior longitudinal ligament line, spinolaminar line, spinous processes)

○ Soft tissues (> 7 mm at C2 [30% of vertebral body], > 2 cm C6 [100% of vertebral body])

■ Anteroposterior (AP):

○ Look for angulation

○ Look at spinous processes: straight line

■ Peg view: Dens should be centred between lateral masses; lateral mass C1 should be directly over lateral portions of C2

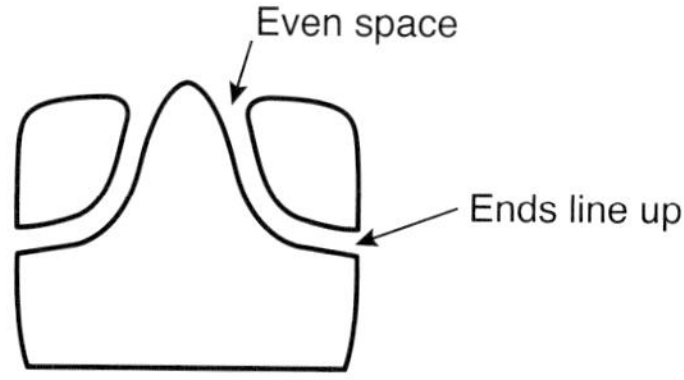

- Management
  - Avoid further injury
  - Immobilise
  - Consult with spine specialty
  - Treat other injuries
  - Identify spinal shock
    - SCI/spine concussion
    - Flaccid areflexia, loss sensation and flaccid paralysis below level of injury
    - Flaccid bladder, decreased rectal tone
    - Transient (days to months)
  - Identify and treat neurogenic shock
    - Lesions above T6 result in loss of vascular tone
    - Hypotension, bradycardia (a hypovolaemic patient is usually tachycardic)
    - Peripheral vasodilation
    - Poikilothermia—inability to regulate core body temperature
    - Ensure other injuries have been excluded; consider blood loss
    - Treat with fluids, IV saline
    - Vasopressors when adequately filled and definitely not due to blood loss

Spinal fracture and cord injury

- Types
  - Minor
    - Direct blunt trauma to posterior, spines: isolated fracture, transverse and spinous processes stable
  - Major
    - Compression or wedge #
      - Axial load + flexion, affect anterior column
      - Usually stable
    - Burst fracture
      - Axial load, affect anterior and middle column with retropulsion of bone and disc into canal
      - Can affect cord; unstable fracture

- Jefferson fracture
  - Compression of C1, usually from vertical compression
  - Unstable
- Chance fracture
  - Horizontal fracture through vertebral body of thoracolumbar spine
  - For example, from lap belt injury
  - Associated with other significant injury, 65% intestinal injury
- Flexion: distraction
  - Seatbelt/lap belt = axis of rotation during distraction; affect posterior and mid-column
  - Unstable fracture
- Translational
  - Most damaging, all 3 columns fail
  - Unstable

- Spinal cord syndromes
  - Anterior cord (anterior cord compression/thrombosis; flex C-spine): paralysis below lesion, loss pain and temp, preserved proprioception. Poor prognosis
  - Central cord (hyperextension, disrupted blood flow to spinal cord, C-spine stenosis, usually elderly): quadriparesis upper limb > lower, pain and temperature sensory loss greater in upper limb. Good prognosis
  - Brown-Séquard (transverse hemisection cord, unilateral cord compressed): ipsilateral spastic paresis/loss proprioception; contralateral pain and temp loss. Moderate prognosis
  - Cauda equina (peripheral nerve injury): variable motor and sensory ↓ lower limbs, sciatica, bladder/bowel dysfunction, loss saddle sensation, decreased or lost ankle reflex
- Management: ABCD
  - Airway: ≥ C5 injury likely to need semi-urgent/urgent intubation
    - C3–4–5 diaphragm, difficult intubation!
  - Hypotension: Query neurogenic shock (see previous section, management of spine injuries, p. 30). Cervical and thoracic injuries lead to ↓ BP due to ↓ α tone, T1–T4 lead to ↓ HR due to ↓ sympathetics, unopposed vagus nerve
  - MUST CONSIDER/EXCLUDE BLEEDING! Need CXR, fast US, pelvic x-ray, +/– CT abdomen to look for bleeding

  - Neuro examination
    - Detailed neuro examination after explored/excluded other injuries
    - Imaging: x-rays, CT, MRI
  - Determine if the injury is unstable and if neuro deficit complete or incomplete; neurosurgical review
- Autonomic dysreflexia
  - Injuries at or above T6 at risk
  - Noxious stimulus below injury level
    - unopposed sympathetic outflow
    - ↑ BP, vasoconstriction, piloerection, pallor (below SCI)
    - carotid/aortic baroreceptor ↑ parasympathetic
    - ↓ PR, sweating and vasodilation (above SCI)
    - Note: BP 130–150 may be significantly high as T6 + SCI patient may normally be 90–110 sBP
    - headache, anxiety
  - Management
    - Monitor BP, sit patient up, lower legs, remove constrictive clothing and TEDs
    - Antihypertensives if > 150 systolic
      - DON'T use if patient on Viagra
      - GTN infusion/sublingual (SL), tablet, spray
      - Nifedipine 10 mg orally (PO)
      - Clonidine: 75–300 microgram IV
      - Sodium nitroprusside (SNP): 0.3 microgram/kg/min IV infusion (IVI) for 10 minutes then titrate up or down
    - Look for cause
      - Check bladder, unblock IDC or insert IDC, urine MSU
      - Check for faecal impaction
    - MUST treat BP first
    - When inserting or unblocking an IDC or performing a PR must use lidocaine (lignocaine) and monitor BP carefully
    - Monitor

Penetrating neck trauma

- Zones of injury and associated structures
    - Zone 1
        - Landmarks: Clavicles to cricoid
        - Structures: Vertebral and carotid arteries, subclavian artery and vein, spinal cord, thoracic vessels and duct, lung, oesophagus, trachea
    - Zone 2
        - Landmarks: Cricoid to mandible
        - Structures: Vertebral and carotid arteries, spinal cord, larynx, jugular vein, oesophagus, trachea, cranial nerves
    - Zone 3
        - Landmarks: Mandible to base of skull
        - Structures: Vertebral and carotid arteries, spinal cord, pharynx, cranial nerves
- Signs of concerning injury
    - Signs of vascular injury
        - Hard signs: Shock unresponsive to initial fluid bolus, active arterial bleed, pulsatile expanding haematoma, pulse defect, thrill or bruit
        - Soft signs: Decreased BP in the field, history of arterial bleeding, non-pulsatile expanding haematoma, proximity wounds
    - Signs of laryngotracheal injury
        - Hard signs: Stridor, haemoptysis, dysphonia, air/bubbling wound, airway obstruction
        - Soft signs: Hoarse voice, tender neck, subcutaneous emphysema, cervical haematoma, tracheal deviation, laryngeal oedema, restricted vocal cord mobility
    - Signs of pharyngo-oesophageal injury
        - Odynophagia, dysphagia, subcutaneous emphysema, haematemesis, blood in mouth, saliva in wound, severe neck tenderness, prevertebral air, trans midline trajectory
- Assessment
    - Assess for the above hard and soft signs
    - Identify if platysma is penetrated
        - Assume serious injury if penetrated and obtain surgical review

  - If no hard signs but suspect injury and patient stable: CT angiography
- Management
  - Urgent surgical review and theatre if hard signs.
    - May consider imaging first in stable patients
  - Early airway intervention if concerns of obstruction or stridor
    - Proceed with caution, ENT/surgical team present if possible
    - Most experienced person should perform the intubation
    - Optimise the patient position, haemodynamics and pre-oxygenation first where possible
    - BVM/positive pressures pre-ETT may worsen subcutaneous emphysema and increase difficulty of intubation
  - Always consider spinal injury—treat the neck with care and sandbags but don't collar
  - Control local bleeding with pressure
  - Patient may need massive transfusion protocol

Thoracic trauma

- Haemothorax classification
  - Mild ≤ 350 mL
    - Small effusion on erect CXR
  - Moderate = 350–1500 mL
    - Moderate effusion on erect CXR, diffuse effusion on supine CXR
  - Large ≥ 1500 mL
- Assessment
  - Decreased breath sounds
  - Dull to percussion
  - Ultrasound is 90% sensitive and 95% specific
  - CT
- Management
  - Note: Several guidelines available. Check what your hospital guidelines are
  - Tube thoracostomy for traumatic haemothorax
  - Proceed to urgent thoracotomy in OT if:
    - Stable patient with intercostal catheter blood loss of > 1500 mL total or > 200 mL/hr

    - Unstable patient with blood loss from intercostal catheter < 100 mL/hr, > 1000 mL in total
  - Patient may require massive transfusion protocol

Pelvic trauma

- Classification
  - AP compression fracture
    - Pubic symphysis diastasis or vertical fracture pubic rami
    - 25% of pelvic fractures
  - Lateral compression fracture
    - Transverse fracture of pubic rami
    - Most common—60% of pelvic fractures
  - Vertical shear
    - Vertical fracture pubic rami
    - 5% of pelvic fractures
    - Mechanism; e.g. jump from height
    - Highest risk of severe bleeding (70%)
- Associated injuries
  - Haemorrhage
    - From fractured bone surfaces
    - From pelvic venous plexus (about 90%)
    - From pelvic arterial injury (about 10%)
    - From extra pelvic sources
  - Sacral plexus
  - Bladder
  - Bowel/intestines
  - Urethra
  - Rectum
  - Vaginal tears
- Signs of pelvic fracture
  - Pelvic examination
    - Look for bruising, deformity, asymmetry, wounds
    - Compress iliac crests—is there pain or instability?
    - Do Not Rock the Pelvis

    - Rectal examination
        - Palpate for rectal injury (blood, wounds etc.)
        - Palpate for bony fragments—be careful as can be sharp
        - Sphincter function
        - Boggy or high-riding prostate
    - Perineum and genitals
        - Scrotal or perineal haematoma
        - Vaginal exam for tears
        - Blood at meatus
    - Abdominal examination
    - Leg length discrepancy without leg fractures

A normal examination in an alert patient without distracting injuries essentially rules out significant pelvic injury

- Investigations
    - Bloods: VBG (look for Hb and signs of shock pH, lactate), group and hold (G&H), FBC, coags, βhCG in women of childbearing age
    - eFAST scan (extended focused assessment with sonography for trauma)
    - Imaging
        - Pelvic x-ray: Normal x-ray does not rule out pelvic fracture but makes pelvic fracture as cause of haemodynamic instability very unlikely
        - CT abdomen and pelvis: In stable patients or those that might have radiological intervention
        - Angiography: To guide embolisation
- Management
    - Team approach ABCDEFG
    - Resuscitation if required, consider massive transfusion protocol
    - Stabilise pelvis
        - Pelvic binder
    - Assess for other injuries including spine
    - Aim for definitive care
        - Surgery
        - CT embolisation

Analgesia

(For paeds see p. 354)

- Reassurance, ice packs, splint, elevation
- O_2/oxygen
- Inhaled methoxyflurane (dose = 3 mL, can repeat once at 20 minutes)
- Simple analgesics
  - Paracetamol 1 g four times a day (QID)
  - NSAIDs: Ibuprofen 400 mg three times a day (TDS)
  - Indomethacin 50 mg QID PO, 100 mg twice a day (BD) PR
- Opiates: oral
  - Oxycodone IR (endone) 5 mg QID
  - Oxycodone SR (oxycontin) 10 mg BD titrate ↑
- Opiates: IV/IN
  - Morphine 2.5–5 mg IV then titrate ↑↓
  - Fentanyl 50–100 microgram IV then titrate ↑↓
  - Intranasal fentanyl 1.5 microgram/kg max. 75 microgram
- Ketamine
  - 0.1–0.3 mg/kg IV, 0.1 mg/kg/hr infusion IV
  - 0.5 mg/kg IM
  - New studies suggest intranasal effective for analgesia
- Midazolam for sedation 1–2.5 mg IV then titrate
- Nerve blocks (see Procedures, pp. 59–67)
- Neuropathic pain: Aspirin, paracetamol, NSAIDs
  - TCAs; e.g. amitriptyline 10–25 mg at night (nocte) ↑ to 75–100 mg OR
  - Gabapentin 300 mg PO ↑ to max. 2.4 g/day OR
  - Pregabalin 75 mg PO ↑ up to 300 mg/day

CHAPTER 2

Procedures and ultrasound

Perimortem C-section

- Pregnant patients place in LEFT LATERAL TILT with wedge under RIGHT hip
- Indications: Pregnancy and fundus > umbilicus, arrested (consider in peri-arrest), best if within 5 minutes but no absolute timeframe
- Splash with iodine/antiseptic
- Vertical incision xiphoid to symphysis pubis down to fascia
- Blunt dissect with fingers to muscle
- Enter peritoneum, use retractors superior and inferior
- Vertical incision uterus midline (start lower half to avoid placenta), suction fluid
- Place hand in at level of symphysis pubis, remove baby's head (or bum if breech), assistant pushes fundus, deliver baby
- Double clamp cord and cut between
- Clean out uterus with sponges
- Close uterus, close fascia, close skin

Needle cricothyroidotomy

- Indications: Can't intubate, can't ventilate, occasionally performed semi-electively if difficult intubation. Preferred to surgical cricothyroidotomy in children < 10 years old
- Contraindications (relative as usually procedure of last resort): Local infection, non-identifiable anatomy, previous failed attempts
- Consent: Not usually needed as urgent procedure
  - Risks: Failure (kinking, blood or vomit in airway, difficult anatomy), cannula obstruction, dislodgment, injury to local structures, surgical emphysema
- Preparation
  - 5 mL syringe containing 1–2 mL saline connected to a 14 G cannula
  - Oxygen tubing that will attach to cannula
- Procedure
  - Extend patient's neck to optimise identification of anatomy. Usually stand on the patient's left side
  - Identify cricothyroid membrane and stabilise with non-dominant hand (see Fig. 2.1)

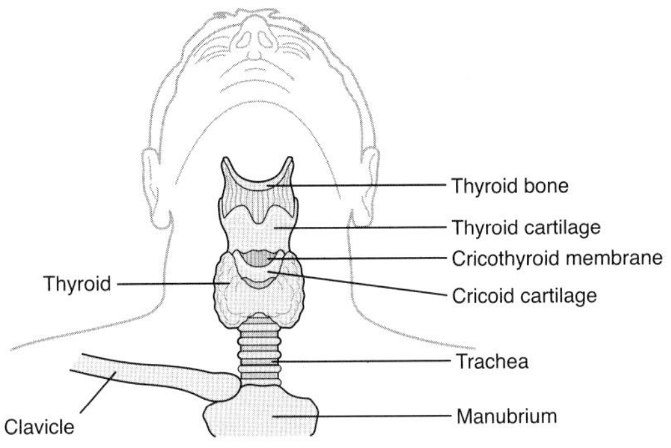

Figure 2.1 Anatomy of the neck

    - Using non-dominant hand, stabilise trachea with thumb and middle fingers while palpating membrane with index finger
    - Using dominant hand, insert needle at 45 degrees caudal direction, continuously aspirating until free aspiration of air up entire barrel of syringe. Should not recoil
    - Stabilise cannula hub in non-dominant hand and stabilise the trocar in dominant hand while resting on patient
    - Advance cannula over trocar with non-dominant hand
    - Remove trocar
    - Reattach a 5 mL syringe with 1–2 mL water and confirm aspiration of air up entire barrel without recoil
    - Secure cannula
    - Attach to jet oxygen
- Flow rates jet oxygen
    - Use I:E ratio of 1:4 to 1:5, with a breath rate of 10–12/min for most children
    - Change the ratio to 1:2 to 1:3 with a breath rate of 15–20/min in the setting of increased intracranial pressure to improve CO_2 elimination
    - With partial or complete upper airway obstruction, use the ratio of 1:8 to 1:10 with a breath rate of 5–6/min to reduce the risk of pulmonary barotrauma

    - Adjust these ratios based on clinical monitoring, blood gas measurements and chest radiography
- After care: Definitive airway as soon as possible

Surgical airway

- Indications: Can't intubate, can't ventilate, maxillofacial injuries
- Contraindications: Ability to secure airway in less invasive means, airway trauma rendering access futile (e.g. tracheal transection). Relative contraindication: child < 10 years old, preferred procedure is needle cricothyroidotomy due to potential complications
- Consent: Emergency procedure, no explanation
    - Risks: Failure of procedure, bleeding, infection, damage to local structures (larynx, vessels, nerves, oesophagus, cartilage), cricoid fracture, fistula, scarring, hypoxia, death
- Preparation
    - Scalpel, Bougie, 6.0 ETT, artery forceps
- Procedure: Remember '**scalpel—finger—Bougie**'
    - Splash antiseptic
    - Keep oxygen on if possible
    - Extend neck to make anatomy more visible (see Fig. 2.1, p. 39)
    - Stabilise thyroid cartilage with non-dominant hand
    - Dominant hand holds scalpel and rests on patient's sternum
    - Locate membrane with index finger of dominant hand
    - Vertical incision over membrane between thyroid cartilage (superior) and cricoid cartilage (inferior) approx. 4 cm; larger if can't see anatomy (may need to go from mandible to sternum)
    - Palpate cricothyroid membrane, blunt dissect with fingers (can use artery forceps) until membrane readily palpable. Ignore bleeding until airway secure (unless massive)
    - Horizontal incision through membrane then turn blade through 180 degrees
    - Dilate with gloved little finger and palpate trachea, ideally posterior wall
    - Pass Bougie alongside little finger into trachea
    - Confirm Bougie position with little finger
    - Bougie usually holds up at carina—don't force
    - Railroad ETT (ensure balloon fully deflated), twist as it passes skin

- Only advance ETT until balloon just out of sight but in the trachea
- Remove Bougie while holding ETT firm
- Connect to BVM with ETCOs
- Confirm placement, secure

Emergency thoracentesis/finger thoracostomy

- Indications: Tension pneumothorax or haemothorax
- Contraindications: None, it's an emergency!
- Consent: No consent needed
  - Risks: Failure, bleeding, malposition, damage to structures
  - Needle versus finger
    - Needle: Will often fail, often doesn't reach pleura, cause a pneumothorax if there wasn't one, cannula can kink, axillary needle better than anterior chest wall
    - Finger in axilla: Thinner chest wall, no major blood vessels nearby, no kinking, if patient deteriorates can re-finger
- Preparation: Scalpel, Kelly clamp, and finger or large-bore long IV cannula
- Procedure
  - 5th intercostal (IC) space mid-axillary line
  - Scalpel over rib (avoid neurovascular bundle just below rib), blunt dissect to pleura, finger in hole

    OR
  - Using large-bore long IV at same space as above or 2nd IC space mid-clavicular line
    - Insert the cannula with a syringe attached
    - Aspirate air then advance cannula
- After care: Definitive treatment—needs formal chest drain

Resuscitative thoracotomy

- Aim
  - Relieve tamponade
  - Control bleeding
  - Cross clamp hilum, cross clamp aorta
  - Restore circulation

- Indications
  - Stab wound to the heart with tamponade
  - Penetrating chest trauma and signs of life within the last 10 minutes
  - Blunt trauma with evidence of tamponade
- Contraindications
  - No signs of life for > 10 minutes
  - Blunt trauma without likely tamponade
- Procedure: Two-person approach (various other approaches)
  - DO PERIMORTEM C-SECTION FIRST IF APPLICABLE
  - Obtain handover: Injuries, signs of life, what's been done
  - Cease CPR
  - Rapidly place ETT, 3–4 cm too far and therefore down right main bronchus
  - Splash skin prep
  - Bilateral finger thoracostomies 5th intercostal space
    - Count down the spaces with the assistant
  - Cut through all layers leaving only sternal bridge
  - Wire/cut/saw sternum
  - Use retractors
  - Open pericardium to relieve tamponade
  - Inspect for tears or bleeding
  - Repair (staples, sutures) or occlude (with direct pressure, finger)
  - Consider aortic cross-clamping usually at level of diaphragm
  - Cardiac massage, flick heart
  - IF RETURN OF SPONTANEOUS CIRCULATION (ROSC) AT ANY POINT IN PROCEDURE: CEASE PROCEDURE
  - URGENT OPERATION

Rapid infusion kits

- Indications: Rapid IV fluid and blood product administration
- Contraindications: Relative—coagulopathy, infection over site, uncooperative patient
- Consent: Often not necessary, usually inserted urgently
  - Risks: Infection, thrombosis, failure to remove dilator
  - Benefits: Rapid delivery of large amount of fluid/products

- Preparation: Kit (venous catheter—short and wide bore, dilator preloaded on catheter, guidewire, scalpel), skin prep
- Procedure
  - Obtain IV access with standard pink 20 G cannula. Best in cubital fossa because you need at least 5 cm of straight vein
  - Insert wire from kit approx. 10 cm (don't force)
  - Remove IV cannula leaving wire in situ
  - Cut down onto the wire with the scalpel. Ensure 3–4 mm or line won't feed
  - Railroad the rapid infuser cannula, which at this stage is together with the dilator. Push the whole unit in (dilator and cannula) to the hub. Will need twisting action
  - Remove dilator and guidewire together
  - Connect
  - Usually messy, have lots of gauze

Intraosseous access

- Indications: Can't get an IV in trauma, burns, shock. Life-threatening situation and can't get an IV in max. 90 sec. Any situation where blood sample and/or IV access is urgently needed and IV cannula difficult and time consuming
- Note: Preferred access in paediatric cardiac arrest. In a newborn the umbilical vein is preferred
- Contraindications: Osteogenesis imperfecta, osteopetrosis
- Use another site if: Fracture (absolute contraindication on that limb), vascular injury, prior attempt, overlying infection
- Consent: Don't need consent in life-threatening or urgent situation. Explain procedure if time enables
  - Risks: Failure to perform, local pain with infusion, incorrect placement including through and through bone penetration, extravasation (usually due to incorrect placement), tissue necrosis secondary to extravasation, compartment syndrome, infection, osteomyelitis, haematoma, injury of growth plate, fat micro-emboli (not clinically significant)
- Preparation: Alcohol swabs, EZ-IO device power driver, EZ connect IV tubing—primed, 10 mL syringe × 3, sterile saline flush, dressing, 2% lidocaine (lignocaine) for infusion if needed for pain, infusion fluid
  - IO needle set:
    - 45 mm (yellow) for humerus insertion or excessive tissue
    - 35 mm (blue) > 40 kg
    - 15 mm (pink) 3–39 kg

- Procedure
  - Choose site
    - Proximal humerus: 1 cm above surgical neck (slide thumb up anterior humerus shaft until you feel greater tubercle). Patient with palm down on their abdomen, elbow adducted
    - Proximal tibia: 2–3 cm below tibial tuberosity and slightly medial
    - Distal tibia: 3 cm above most prominent part of medial malleolus
    - Femoral: Anterior lateral. 3 cm above lateral condyle
    - Iliac crest
  - Clean site
  - Connect needle to driver
  - Stabilise site
  - Needle perpendicular to bone. Puncture skin with needle until needle touches bone. Ensure one black line still visible; if not use larger needle
  - Squeeze driver's trigger and apply gentle downward pressure to penetrate bone
  - Release trigger once a give/pop is felt
  - Stabilise catheter hub and remove driver
  - Remove stylet by turning anticlockwise
  - Secure site
  - Aspirate sample (does not always aspirate)
  - Connect primed tuning
  - Flush with normal saline or in a conscious patient 2 mL/40 mg of 2% lidocaine (lignocaine) (DON'T EXCEED 3 mg/kg)
  - Start infusion using pressure delivery system
  - Document time and date of placement
- After care: Monitor for complications. Serial checks or extravasation, erythema, swelling (remove if seen). Attempt to gain IV access within 3–4 hours and remove IO once obtained
- Removal: Disconnect infusion. Attach 10 mL Luer-lock syringe to catheter hub. Rotate clockwise while pulling straight back. Dispose of catheter and apply simple dressing

Umbilical vein catheterisation in newborn resuscitation setting

- Indications: Vascular access in emergency resuscitation of newborn. Umbilical veins remain patent up to approx. 1 week of age

- Contraindications: Infection (omphalitis, peritonitis, necrotising enterocolitis), abdominal surgery incision above umbilicus, abdominal wall defect
- Consent: Not required in resuscitation
  - Risks: Infection, thromboembolism, thrombophlebitis, blood loss, migration of catheter fragment, false lumen, air embolism
- Preparation: 3.5 or 5 French catheter (specific umbilical veins catheters [UVCs]), UVC insertion tray (scalpel, cotton umbilical tape, 3-way tap), Normal saline flush, skin prep
- Note: No need for sterile gown/gloves in resuscitation setting
- Procedure
  - Prepare the catheter
    - Attach 3-way tap
    - Attach saline flush to 3-way tap
    - Flush catheter and flush side ports of 3-way tap
  - Prepare infant
    - Clean cord with skin prep
    - Tie cord with umbilical tape from tray
    - Cut cord with scalpel below cord clamp approx. 1–2 cm from skin
  - Identify umbilical vein: Larger thin-walled vessel. (There are 2 arteries which are thick walled and 1 thin-walled vein)
  - Insert catheter about 3–4 cm until free flow of blood; never force insertion
  - Administer resuscitation medications and/or fluids
  - Check cord tie
  - Secure with transparent dressing
- After care: Continued check for dislodgment; temporary, need specialist help

Pericardiocentesis

- Indications: Urgent—pericardial effusion and compromised patient; i.e. suspect tamponade
- Contraindications: ACD
- Consent: Explain procedure if not urgent (we probably wouldn't be doing this in ED if it wasn't urgent)
  - Risks: Myocardial perforation, bleeding, pneumothorax, arrhythmia, APO

- Preparation: Long 18–22 G needle attached to syringe—can use spinal needle. Sit patient at 45 degrees. Patient monitored. Use ultrasound (US) (can be difficult to visualise needle tip), local anaesthetic (LA) with syringe and needle, scalpel, antiseptic, sterile gloves and gown, drapes, alligator clip connector for connection to V1 of ECG (don't need if US available)
- Procedure
  - LA if time
  - Subxiphoid approach. Identify effusion with US
  - Insert needle between xiphisternum and left costal margin
  - Direct towards left shoulder, at 45-degree angle to skin using real-time US if available
  - Continual aspiration as needle approaches right ventricle (RV)
  - If using ECG connection, look for ST elevation and withdraw if seen
  - Once pericardial fluid aspirated either remove as much as possible or insert cannula via Seldinger and attach to 3-way tap, or pigtail catheter
- After care: Monitoring, confirm on US relief of tamponade, CXR to look for pneumothorax, refer to cardiology/cardiothoracics

Electrical cardioversion

(Note: Not the same as defibrillation which is used in ALS)

- Indications
  - Broad or narrow complex tachycardia (rate > 150) with signs of haemodynamic compromise; e.g. chest pain, hypotension, reduced level of consciousness
  - VT with pulse (note: In pulseless VT use ALS algorithm)
  - AF or atrial flutter (only do in ED if duration of arrhythmia is < 48 hours)
- Contraindications: Absent central pulse (use ALS algorithm), AF/flutter of uncertain duration (can consider if patient shocked), dysrhythmias of enhanced automaticity (e.g. digoxin toxicity and catecholamine induced), multifocal atrial tachycardia
- Consent: Must sign consent form. Consent also for sedation
  - Risks: Pain, arrhythmia (VF if not synchronised), burns, electrical injury to healthcare worker, thoracic/vertebral fracture, myocardial injury, skeletal muscle injury
- Preparation
  - Resus bay ready, 2× IVC, fluids on a pump set, oxygen, intubation equipment checked and ready

    - Equipment: Defibrillator with adhesive pads, monitoring (ECG, sats, BP, +/– $ETCO_2$)
    - Staff required: Doctor for sedation, doctor for direct current cardioversion (DCCV), nurse
    - Procedural sedation (see p. 49) and Analgesia (see p. 37)
    - Check AMPLE and anaesthetic Hx
    - Pad position: AP or sterno-apical
- Procedure
    - Connect defib and 3-lead ECG
    - Select synchronised mode on defibrillator (may need to be re-done after each shock)
    - Select energy (VT 100–150 J, flutter 50 J)
    - Procedural sedation (see p. 49) and Analgesia (see p. 37)
    - Safety check: Oxygen away, all clear from bed, deliver shock
    - Reassess patient: ABC (vitals), 12-lead ECG
- After care
    - Consult with cardiology if required
    - Ensure back to baseline after sedation (see Procedural sedation, p. 49)

Transcutaneous pacing

- Indications: Bradyarrhythmia with signs of hemodynamic compromise, complete heart block, overdrive pacing
- Contraindications: Asymptomatic, stable patients
- Consent: Verbal consent, not needed if life-threatening condition
    - Risks: Pain, failure to pace or capture, patient can't tolerate, respiratory alkalosis
- Preparation: May be preparing while putting on pads if patient severely compromised
    - Resus bay, monitoring, 2× IVC, fluids on a pump set
    - Equipment: Defibrillator capable of pacing with adhesive pads, monitoring (ECG, sats, BP, +/– $ETCO_2$)
    - Sedation/analgesia, will likely need IV opiates as painful
    - Pad position: AP or sterno-apical
- Procedure
    - Select pacing mode: Demand mode if organised rhythm, select rate (e.g. 80 bpm), select energy (usually start 0–50 mA), titrate

up by 10 mA until electrical and mechanical capture. Set at 10% or 20 mA over capture

- If severe/asystole can start at 200 mA and titrate down
- Temporising measure until definitive treatment available: Pacemaker

- After care
  - Temporising measure until definitive treatment available
  - Urgent cardiology consult: Permanent pacemaker (PPM)
  - Patient will need critical care unit (CCU)/intensive care unit (ICU)

Emergency craniotomy

- Indications: Deteriorating neurology and can't access surgery within 2 hours and pupils dilated or unequal
- Contraindications: GCS > 8, neurosurgical intervention available in a reasonable timeframe
  - No imaging: Relative contraindication. If CT not available and there is a very high clinical suspicion (e.g. palpable fracture) and clearly clinical urgency, this may be acceptable
- Steps
  - Have patient supine, optimise ABC, protect C-spine
  - Where at all possible neurosurgical consult pre and during procedure
  - Confirm location on CT
  - Mark position (see usual locations below) using CT to guide location. Need to be in centre of haematoma
  - Incise skin to bone with scalpel, control local bleeding
  - Drill perpendicular to skull with assistant holding head still
  - Drill until through bone; blood should escape
  - Do not tamponade blood oozing from wound. Control bleeding from skin edges
- Temporal (75% of extradural haematomas)
  - 2 fingers anteriorly and 2 fingers superior to external auditory canal
- Frontal
  - 4 fingers anteriorly and 4 fingers above external auditory canal

- Parietal
  - 4 fingers posterior and 4 fingers superior to external auditory canal
- Consider having a guide for burr holes open on the computer.

This guide adapted from Wilson MH, Wise D, Davies G, et al. Emergency burr holes: 'How to do it'. Scand J Trauma Resusc Emerg Med 2012;20:24.

Procedural sedation

- Prepare
  - History and examination
    - AMPLE history (allergies, meds, PHx, last ate/drank, events)
      - PHx: Particularly cardiac and respiratory disorders, previous intubations, airway or neck problems
    - Exam: Assess patient airway, Any positive predictors of difficult intubation, vital signs, signs of heart or lung disease
  - Consent and explanation
  - Check resuscitation trolley, perform airway checklist, size OPA/NPA
  - Apply monitor: Saturations, ECG are minimum, consider $ETCO_2$
  - IV fluids on a pump set
  - Pre-oxygenate
  - **If risk factors for sedation or significant comorbidities, DON'T DO IT**
- Drugs
  - Nitrous oxide 30–70% in O_2
    - NEVER in pneumothorax, eye operation, perforations, ↑ ICP, age < 1 year
    - NEVER give more than 70%
    - Give 100% oxygen for 3 minutes postprocedure
  - Midazolam 0.02–0.1 mg/kg IV, max. 5 mg; give slowly and in small increments
  - Fentanyl 2–3 microgram/kg IV
  - Ketamine 0.5–1 mg/kg IV (3 mg/kg IM)
    - Can use with atropine especially in children
    - Consider midazolam if emergence problems
    - Recovery in dark place

    - Propofol 0.2–0.5 mg/kg IV
        - NOT in egg allergy
- Postprocedure, give O_2, monitor until back to baseline

Intercostal catheter insertion

- Indications: Pneumothorax, haemothorax, haemopneumothorax, hydrothorax, chylothorax, empyema, pleural effusion. To be considered in patients at high risk of pneumothorax who are about to be air transported or positive pressure ventilated, especially if monitoring or access to patient may be difficult (e.g. a prone surgical procedure)
    - For pneumothorax: Usually do intercostal catheter (ICC) in secondary/traumatic especially if over 50, or if primary where patient is unstable or other methods have failed
- Contraindications
    - Absolute: Need for urgent thoracotomy
    - Relative: Coagulopathy, pulmonary bullae, adhesions, loculated effusion/empyema and overlying infection
- Consent: Explain procedure
    - Risks: Bleed, fistula, surgical emphysema, misplacement, infection, organ damage (lung, neurovascular, heart, stomach, liver, spleen), re-expansion pulmonary oedema, pain, allergic/ reaction to meds given, pain, failure of procedure
    - How we will reduce the risks: Careful placement
- Preparation: Chest tube, underwater seal, sterile gloves, surgical drapes, LA, syringe and needle for LA, blade, Kelly clamps, suture equipment and suture material, gauze, dressing, drape, sterile gloves, skin prep
    - Tube size: 28–32F adult, 12–28F child, 12–16F infant, 10–12F neonate
    - Patient on monitoring. Give analgesia. IV access
    - Position of patient usually at 45 degrees elevation, arm abducted and externally rotated
    - May need procedural sedation
- Procedure
    - Identify insertion site: 5th intercostal space, mid to anterior axillary line. Within triangle of safety—between border of pectoralis major (anteriorly), border of latissimus dorsi (posteriorly) and 5th intercostal space (inferiorly) which in men is in line with nipple

  - Aseptic technique, prep area, drape
  - Liberal use of LA at skin down to pleura (without exceeding toxic dose)
  - Incision with scalpel along rib approx. 4 cm (recall neurovascular bundle sits just below rib)
  - Blunt dissect to pleura across top of 5th rib
  - Enter pleural space
  - Insert finger, run ICC along finger 3–4 cm past last drain hole
  - Don't leave end open to air—either clamp or connect while securing
  - Connect to drain
  - Ensure bubble and swing of drain, fog of tube
  - Suture and secure, apply dressing
- After care: CXR, confirm placement, monitor of ongoing bubble and swing. Ensure analgesia. Consider suction with admitting team

Pigtail catheter insertion

- Patient on monitoring. Give analgesia. IV access
- Position of patient usually at 45 degrees elevation, arm abducted and externally rotated
- If pleural effusion can do posteriorly and with US guidance
- Usually don't need procedural sedation
- Identify insertion site: Axillary or posterior
- LA use
- Seldinger technique: Insert needle, aspirate air or fluid, insert wire and remove needle. Make small scalpel incision and dilate with dilator. Remove dilator
- Insert pigtail with stiffener over guidewire
- Always control wire
- Remove wire and stiffener together
- Attach 3-way tap or underwater seal drain
- Repeat CXR

Aspiration of pneumothorax

- Considered in: Small primary, iatrogenic, small secondary and age < 50
- Patient on monitoring. Give analgesia. IV access

- Position of patient usually at 45 degrees elevation, arm abducted and externally rotated
- Usually don't need procedural sedation
- Ideally use US
- Identify insertion site: 5th intercostal space, mid to anterior axillary line. Within triangle of safety, can do 2nd IC space mid-clavicular line
- 26 G IV cannula with 3-way tap and syringe
- Aspirate
- Repeat CXR

Lateral canthotomy and cantholysis

- Indications: Retrobulbar haemorrhage with acute loss of visual acuity, relative afferent pupillary defect (RAPD), increased IOP and proptosis. In unconscious or uncooperative and IOP > 40 especially with RAPD, consider if retrobulbar haemorrhage and severe eye pain, optic nerve pallor
- Contraindications: Suspected globe rupture
- Consent: Explain procedure. Sight saving time-critical procedure. Consent not always needed, often not time for detailed explanation
    - Risks: Iatrogenic injury to globe or lateral rectus, injury of adjacent structures, lacrimal gland or artery injury, bleeding, infection, ectropion
- Preparation: LA (lidocaine [lignocaine] 1% with adrenaline), sterile gloves, sterile drapes, normal saline for irrigation, forceps, suture scissors
- Position patient supine with head of bed 10–15 degrees. Patient must be cooperative; sedation may be required. Taping or assistant holding head may be required
- Procedure
    - Inject 1% lidocaine (lignocaine) with adrenaline 1 mL into lateral canthus. Direct needle tip towards lateral orbital rim and begin injecting when needle touches bone
    - Irrigate eye with saline
    - Crush lateral canthus with clamp to de-vascularise. Clamp for 1 minute
    - Incise skin overlying lateral canthus towards lateral orbital rim with scissors
    - Retract lower lid
    - Incise inferior lateral canthus ligament—feels like guitar string, eye should pop forward

  - If no decrease in IOP divide superior lateral canthus ligament (rarely needed)
- After care: Repeated eye observations. Repeat IOP measurements. Ophthalmologist review urgently

Shoulder reduction

- Indications: 1st dislocation of shoulder proven on x-ray, recurrent dislocated shoulder with consistent clinical findings
- Contraindications: Subclavicular or intrathoracic dislocation of shoulder should be done in OT, subacute dislocation—has been dislocated more than 4 weeks (risk of severe vascular injury on relocation), fracture of femoral neck suspected, inferior dislocation with buttonhole deformity. Major arterial injury (urgent angiography). Any significant nerve injury (e.g. brachial plexus) or avulsion of greater tuberosity or concern of vascular injury. Prompt atraumatic reduction is needed and avoidance of multiple attempts
- Consent: Explain procedure
  - Risks: Procedure failure, nerve injury, vascular injury, worsening or causing a fracture, ligamentous injury
- Preparation
  - Always check neurovascular status first. Check axillary nerve and other major nerves: motor and sensory
  - Prepare for procedural sedation if required (see p. 49)
  - Provide analgesia
- Procedure: Many reduction methods
  - Cunningham: Patient sits up, straight back, chest out and relaxed opposite operator, elbow at 90 degrees with patient's palm on operator's shoulder. Operator rests their arm at patient's elbow placing some mild traction then massages patient's traps, biceps and deltoid muscles
  - Scapular rotation: Arm 90 degrees at the shoulder, slight traction. Using thumbs push inferior tip of scapular medially, +/– slight external rotation of humerus and elbow flexion to 90 degrees
  - Stimpson: Patient prone, hanging arm down, attach weight or have patient hold a weight in hand; +/– scapular rotation
  - Milch: Thumb on humeral head, hand on shoulder. Abduct arm gently until above head
  - Traction: Counter-traction (preferred in posterior dislocation)
  - Spaso: Patient supine, patient palm up. Traction and vertical lift
  - Hippocratic: Patient supine, arm abducted and elbow flex 90 degrees, pull arm down with traction +/– rotation shoulder

- After care: Place in shoulder immobiliser, recheck neurovascular status, observe as per procedural sedation if given.
- Discharge advice: Can take out of immobiliser for shower and bed, warn of risk of recurrence, follow-up with orthopaedics (ortho)

Hip reduction—posterior dislocations

- Indications: Usually only considered suitable for reduction in ED if posterior dislocation and no complications. Consult ortho first
- Contraindications: Associated fracture, neurovascular injury, open dislocations, chronic dislocation
- Consent: Explain procedure
  - Risks: Procedure failure, nerve injury, vascular injury, worsening or causing a fracture, ligamentous injury
- Preparation
  - Always check neurovascular status first.
  - Prepare for procedural sedation if required (see p. 49)
  - Provide analgesia
- Procedure: Many reduction methods
  - Allis manoeuvre: Operator stands on bed, assistant pushes anterior iliac, knee and hip flexed at 90 degrees, axial traction
  - Stimson: Patient prone with leg over side of bed, operator pushes on calf
  - Whistler: Both hips and knees 90 degrees, helper holds good ankle, operator stabilises bad ankle, operator's arm under bad knee and their hand grasps the good knee. Operator lifts their arm up and pulls ankle down like a fulcrum

Arterial line insertion

- Indications: Continuous direct BP monitoring, can't use indirect monitoring (e.g. severe burns, morbidly obese, transport), frequent blood sampling or ABGs
- Contraindications
  - Absolute: Infection at site, absent pulse, thromboangiitis obliterans, full-thickness burns over site, inadequate circulation, Raynaud syndrome
  - Relative: Anticoagulation, atherosclerosis, coagulopathy, inadequate collateral flow, partial thickness burns at site, previous operation in area, vascular graft

- Consent: Explain procedure
  - Risks: Haematoma, temporal radial artery occlusion, bleeding, localised infection, sepsis, permanent ischaemic damage, pseudoaneurysm, thrombosis, AV fistula, air embolism, compartment syndrome, carpal tunnel syndrome, paralysis of median nerve, nerve injury, femoral artery dissection, thromboarteritis
- Preparation: Sterile gloves, gauze, drape, antiseptic wash, LA (NO adrenaline), 5 mL syringe, 25 G needle, cannula (many types), suture (with suturing equipment) or skin lock device, dressing, tubing, transducer kit, arm board
- Procedure
  - Choose appropriate vessel. Usually radial, can do brachial (increased risk vascular event) or femoral (higher risk infection, use Seldinger technique and specific kit)
  - Use US to identify vessel for femoral lines and also radial if having difficulty
  - Ensure transducer has been primed and set up prior to starting
  - Position patient prior to scrubbing. Expose area. Tape hand palm up with slight wrist dorsiflexion
  - Aseptic technique
  - Small bleb of LA to skin
  - Insert needle/cannula until flashback and feed line (+/– Seldinger)
  - Remove needle and connect to tubing
  - Zero line, now ready for use
- After care: Regular checks of site for infection and other complications

Lumbar puncture (LP) adult

(See Chapter 18 Paediatrics for child's LP, p. 336)

- Indications
  - Diagnosis: Suspected meningitis/encephalitis, suspected subarachnoid haemorrhage (SAH), suspected central nervous system (CNS) disease (e.g. GBS, MS)
  - Therapeutic: Pseudotumour cerebri
- Contraindications
  - Infected overlying skin, unequal pressure supratentorial to infratentorial (on CT, midline shift, loss of basal and other

cisterns, posterior fossa mass), increased ICP or suspected space-occupying lesion (SOL) (papillo-oedema, focal neurology, abnormal consciousness), coagulopathy

- Perform CT pre-LP in:
  - Suspected meningitis if age > 60, immunocompromised, known CNS lesion, seizure within 1 week, abnormal level of consciousness, focal neuro, papillo-oedema, clinical suspicion of increased ICP
  - All suspected SAH

- Consent: Explain procedure
  - Risks: Failure of procedure (can do x-ray, CT or US guided), false positive, inadequate sample, haematoma, cyst, infection, herniation, nerve root puncture, paraparesis, post LP headache (2–15%)
  - How we will reduce the risks
    - Post-LP headache most common Cx: Use smallest needle size feasible, Sprotte needle with introducer, replace stylet pre-withdraw. Tx: Rest, fluids, analgesia, caffeine, blood patch
- Preparation
  - Document consent, examination including neuro pre-LP, may need procedural sedation
  - Equipment: Sterile drape, sterile gloves and gown, antiseptic solution, LA plus 25 G needle and syringe, spinal needle 22–25 G 12 cm in adult, 6 cm in child, 2 cm in neonate (Sprotte with introducer), manometer, dressing, 3 numbered tubes
  - Position
    - Supine, left lateral, spine fully curved with knees and hips flexed as much as possible, chin to knees. Maintain back perpendicular to bed
    - Sitting up, bent forward over pillow. Often easier; however, can't measure pressure
    - Monitoring for all sedated or seriously unwell
  - Identify anatomical landmarks
    - Posterior iliac crests = L3/4, find corresponding intervertebral space. Can go above or below. Find most open space
    - Spinal cord ends approx. L1/2
    - Mark with marker

- Child or adult with suspected meningitis—Give dexamethasone and antibiotics and delay LP 1–2 hours if:
  - Coma, signs of raised ICP, cardiovascular compromise, respiratory compromise, focal neuro, seizure, coagulopathy, febrile and purpura
- Procedure
  - Aseptic technique. Gown and gloves
  - Skin prep
  - Use LA at chosen site. Wait for effect
  - Insert introducer, bevel up if lateral, bevel to side if upright. Insert towards umbilicus, slightly cephalad
  - Insert needle through introducer
  - Should feel 2 pops (not always)
  - Remove stylet and observe free flow of spinal fluid
  - Attach manometer if measuring pressure. Allow fluid to fill tubing until slows markedly. If ICP is high, don't take further fluid. Stop here
  - Collect 10 drops approx. 0.5 mL in each tube. Use manometer fluid for tube 1
  - Replace stylet
  - Withdraw
  - Apply dressing
- After care
  - Previously advise lay flat for 1 hour. No longer recommended
  - Send sample to lab for cell count and differential, Gram stain, culture, sensitivity, glucose, protein, +/– xanthochromia, viral polymerase chain reaction (PCR)
  - Chase results
  - Give AB if indicated
  - Document findings including cerebrospinal fluid (CSF) appearance

Paracentesis

- Indications: Diagnosis of ascites cause or bacterial peritonitis, symptom control of abdominal pain or respiratory compromise from ascites

- Contraindications: Acute abdomen, INR over 2.0 (give FFP), PLT < 20 (give platelets prior). Pregnancy, distended bladder, abdominal wall cellulitis, distended bowel, intra-abdominal adhesions
  - If no evidence or suggestion of bleeding don't need to check platelets and coags pre-procedure
- Consent: Explain procedure
  - Risks: Fluid leak, bowel perforation, local bleeding, major bleed, infection, pain, other intra-peritoneal injury
- Preparation
  - Place patient in supine position
  - Empty bladder
  - Use ultrasound scan (USS) to avoid adjacent bowel, mark skin
  - Elevate head of bed 30–45 degrees
  - Skin prep: Clean and drape
  - Any LA will be suitable here
  - Aim lower right quadrant lateral to rectus abdominus muscle
  - 22 G needle on 20–50 mL syringe if performing diagnostic paracentesis
  - If therapeutic use: 14–16 G pigtail tip drain with kit
  - Insert needle: Stretch skin and insert obliquely and slowly while aspirating
  - Aspirate intermittently (not continuously) after pop is felt once you are into the peritoneum: Avoiding suction of bowel wall
  - If large amount (> 6 L) to be drained, then replace volume with human albumin solution (no evidence for use if less than this). Once paracentesis complete 100 mL 20% albumin/3 L ascites
  - If therapeutic remove needle rapidly
  - 20 mL into BC bottle + EDTA, biochemistry, urine specimen jar
  - Send for white cell count (WCC), pH, albumin, glucose, LDH, amylase, culture, sensitivities (+/– bilirubin, cytology, triglycerides)

Arthrocentesis

- Indications: Diagnose or exclude septic arthritis, investigation into joint inflammation cause, therapeutic (symptom relief or injection of medications)

- Contraindications: Overlying infection/cellulitis, skin lesions, adjacent osteomyelitis, prosthetic joint (involve ortho first), haemarthrosis, coagulopathy, bacteraemia
- Consent: Explain procedure
  - Risks: Introduce infection, bleeding, structural damage (nerve, vessels, tendons, cartilage), failure of procedure (dry tap)
- Preparation: Sterile gloves and drape, gauze, skin prep, LA, syringes 5 mL and 20 mL, needles 18 G and 25 G, specimen tubes, bandage
- Procedure
  - Analgesia provided if needed
  - Position patient
  - Identify needle insertion site
  - Knee: Patient supine, flex knee 150 degrees (towel under knee), medial or lateral approach, 3–4 mm inferior to patella midpoint
  - Glenohumeral: Sit patient up, arm at side, internal rotation. Medial to humeral head. Just below tip of coracoid
  - Wrist: Neutral position, dorsal approach. Ulnar to radial tubercle and anatomic snuffbox, just ulnar to extensor pollicis longus
  - Ankle: Slight plantar flexion, midway between medial malleolus and tibialis anterior
  - Elbow: Always use lateral approach. Flex 90 degrees, palm down, locate anconeus triangle between radial head, lateral epicondyle of distal humerus and olecranon of ulna. Insert at centre of this triangle
  - Gown and glove
  - Prep and drape, aseptic technique
  - Confirm needle insertion site
  - Administer LA, 25 G needle
  - Use 20 mL syringe and 18 G needle at insertion site perpendicular to skin
  - Aspirate fluid
  - Remove needle and apply bandage
- After care: Send samples to lab (crystals, cell count, cultures, sensitivities). Analgesia as required

Ring block—digital nerve block

- Indications: Any minor surgery or procedure of the digits (e.g. laceration repair, paronychia drainage, trephination, relocation of dislocation)

- Contraindications: Compromised digit circulation, infected injection site, anaesthetic allergy
- Consent: Explain procedure
  - Risks: LA toxicity, allergic reaction, infection, injury to structures (nerve, tendons)
- Preparation: Sterile gloves, drapes, gauze, skin prep, LA (e.g. lidocaine [lignocaine] 1%, syringe 5–10 mL with 25 G needle)
  - Assess neurovascular status prior to block
- Procedure
  - Analgesia if required
  - Position patient. Hand on flat surface palm down
  - Put on gloves
  - Prep skin and drape
  - Insert needle perpendicular to skin, into web space, just distal to metacarpophalangeal joint (MCP) joint. Do not puncture to palmar side
  - Draw back to confirm not in vessel
  - Insert 2 mL of LA, remove needle
  - Massage LA into web space
  - Repeat in other web space of involved digit or lateral side if thumb
  - Note: This is ineffective for big toe which needs a 3- or 4-sided block
  - Perform intended procedure
- After care: Observe for potential LA toxicity, analgesia as required.
- Discharge advice: Wound advice, follow-up, suture out time, safety netting

Biers block

- Indications: Any procedure of arm or leg that requires operating anaesthesia, muscle relaxation and/or bloodless field; e.g. fracture reduction
- Contraindications
  - Absolute: Allergic to anaesthetic agent, uncontrolled hypertension (HT)
  - Relative: Raynaud's, peripheral vascular disease (PVD), sickle cell disease, crushed or already hypoxic extremity,

uncooperative patient (including young children—no absolute age cut off)

- Consent: Explain procedure
  - Risks: LA toxicity (overdosing, malfunction of tourniquet), tourniquet pain, failure of procedure
- Preparation
  - Patient monitored including ECG, BP, sats
  - Equipment: Double tourniquet (test prior to use), IVC in operative hand or foot, IVC in non-operative arm, resus equipment available
  - Ensure adequate staff, preferably 2 doctors and 1 nurse
  - Assess neurovascular status prior to block
- Procedure
  - Place double tourniquet on operative limb
  - Elevate limb for 3–4 minutes to exsanguinate (or wrap in compression bandage)
  - Inflate distal cuff, then proximal cuff, then deflate distal cuff. Proximal cuff should be 250–300 mmHg (100 over sBP) in upper limb or 350–400 in lower limb
  - Remove bandage if applied, lower limb. Confirm absence of pulses
  - Inject 2.5 mg/kg of the LA prilocaine 0.5% IV into operative IVC (can use lidocaine [lignocaine] 0.5%)
  - DON'T EXCEED MAXIMUM DOSE (see Chapter 11 Toxicology, Local anaesthetics, p. 235). DO NOT USE ADRENALINE
  - Check success. Anaesthesia should occur within 5 minutes. Can give normal saline to help circulate anaesthetic
  - Warn patient arm will feel numb or tingle and may appear mottled
  - Remove IVC in operative arm
  - Perform procedure
  - If tourniquet pain, inflate distal cuff, once confirmed successful distal cuff inflation, deflate proximal cuff
  - Leave tourniquet up for 20–60 minutes
  - Release tourniquet
  - Continue to monitor for 15 minutes post
- After care: Watch for anaesthetic toxicity. Analgesia as required, plaster as required

Ankle block

- Indications: Any minor procedure of the foot or ankle; e.g. wound exploration, suturing
- Contraindications: Infected overlying skin. LA allergy
- Consent: Explain procedure
  - Risks: Infection, damage to structures (tendons, nerves)
- Preparation: Sterile gloves, drape, skin prep, LA (e.g. lidocaine [lignocaine] 1%), 5–10 mL syringe, 25 G needle, gauze
  - DON'T EXCEED MAXIMUM LA DOSE (see Chapter 11 Toxicology, Local anaesthetics, p. 235). Use minimum amount required
  - Assess neurovascular status prior to block
- Procedure: Analgesia if required, glove, prep and drape
  - Insert needle, aspirate to confirm not in vessel. Insert 3–5 mL
    - Posterior tibial: Posterior to medial malleolus. Just posterior to posterior tibial artery—anaesthetise sole of foot
    - Saphenous: Between medial malleolus and anterior tibial tendon—anaesthetise arch of foot
    - Deep peroneal: Between anterior tibial tendon and extensor halluces longus—anaesthetise 1st web space
    - Superficial peroneal: Band-like pattern between extensor hallucis longus (EHL) and lateral malleolus—anaesthetise dorsum of foot
    - Sural: Band-like pattern between lateral malleolus and Achilles tendon—anaesthetise lateral foot
- After care: Analgesia as required, observe for LA toxicity
- Discharge advice: Wound advice, follow-up, suture out time, safety netting

Face/dental block

- Indications: Wound exploration, debridement and/or closure, minor dental procedure
- Contraindications: Infected overlying skin, LA allergy, distorted anatomy, uncooperative patient
- Consent: Explain procedure
  - Risks: Infection, bleeding, haematoma, LA allergy or toxicity, failure to anaesthetise, nerve damage, aesthetic result

- Preparation: Sterile gloves, drape, skin prep, LA (e.g. lidocaine [lignocaine] 1%), 5 mL syringe, 25 G or 27 G needle, gauze
  - DON'T EXCEED MAXIMUM LA DOSE (see Chapter 11 Toxicology, Local anaesthetics, p. 235). Use minimum amount required
  - Assess neurovascular status prior to block
- Procedure: Analgesia if required, glove, prep and drape
  - Insert needle, aspirate to confirm not in vessel. Insert 2–3 mL
    - Supraorbital: Supraorbital foramen, 2–3 cm lateral to midline of face inferior edge supraorbital ridge (blocks ipsilateral forehead)
    - Supratrochlear: Supraorbital ridge, 1 cm medial to supraorbital notch (i + ii block the forehead)
    - Infraorbital: Mucobuccal fold, junction of 1st and 2nd maxillary premolar, direct up to infraorbital foramen approx. 2 cm (blocks lower lid, upper cheek, upper lip, canine central and lateral incisors)
    - Inferior alveolar: Mouth wide open, syringe barrel opposite side. Palpate coronoid notch mandible. Insert into corner of gum behind wisdom teeth aiming downwards, hit bone, withdraw 1 mm, aspirate and inject (blocks all teeth ipsilateral mandible and lip)
    - Mental: Junction of mandibular premolar 1 and 2; 1 cm inferior. Hit bone and withdraw (blocks ipsilateral lower lip and chin, not teeth)
- After care: Analgesia as required, observe for LA toxicity
- Discharge advice: Wound advice, follow-up, suture out time, safety netting

Wrist block

- Indications: Minor procedures of hand where local infiltration may be less favourable. For example, simultaneous injury to multiple digits or multiple areas, large abrasions needing thorough irrigation and/or debridement, avoiding distortion of anatomy from local infiltration
- Contraindications: Infected overlying skin. LA allergy. Proximal vascular graft, AV fistula. Prior surgery or injury at wrist may lead to altered anatomy
- Consent: Explain procedure
  - Risks: Infection, damage to structures (tendons, nerves, blood vessels), haematoma

- Preparation: Sterile gloves, drape, skin prep, LA (e.g. lidocaine [lignocaine] 1%), 5–10 mL syringe, 25 G needle, gauze
  - DON'T EXCEED MAXIMUM LA DOSE (see Chapter 11 Toxicology, Local anaesthetics, p. 235). Use minimum amount required
  - Assess neurovascular status prior to block
- Procedure: Analgesia if required, glove, prep and drape
  - Insert needle, aspirate to confirm not in vessel. Insert 3–5 mL
    - Median nerve: 2–3 cm proximal to distal palmar crease. Lateral to palmaris longus, medial to flexor carpi radialis—anaesthetise palmar thumb, palmar and dorsal index, middle and ½ of ring finger
    - Ulnar nerve: 2–3 cm proximal to distal palmar crease. Just medial to flexor carpi ulnaris—anaesthetise palmar and dorsal pinky and ½ of ring finger
    - Radial nerve: Overlying radial styloid, just proximal to anatomical snuff box. Anaesthetise—dorsal lateral hand and thumb
- After care: Analgesia as required, observe for LA toxicity
- Discharge advice: Wound advice, follow-up, suture out time, safety netting

Femoral nerve block

- Indications: Femoral fractures, injuries to patella, wound exploration, abscess drainage
- Contraindications: Infected overlying skin. LA allergy. Open fracture. Anticoagulation is a relative contraindication, high-risk patient for compartment syndrome of thigh
- Consent: Explain procedure
  - Risks: Infection, damage to structures (tendons, nerves, blood vessels), haematoma, bleeding, LA toxicity
- Preparation: US, sterile gloves, drape, skin prep, LA (e.g. ropivacaine 0.75% i.e. 10 mL = 75 mg, use < 3 mg/kg), 20 mL syringe, specific block needle (often has nerve stimulator attachment—not required), gauze, antiseptic swab/wash. Patient on monitoring through procedure
  - DON'T EXCEED MAXIMUM LA DOSE (see Chapter 11 Toxicology, Local anaesthetics, p. 235) 3 mg/kg for ropivacaine. This is not a volume block, unlike fascia iliaca block; use minimum amount to achieve effect
  - Assess neurovascular status prior to block

- Procedure: Analgesia if required, glove, prep and drape
  - Use US to identify nerve/artery/vein bundle
  - Insert needle—usually in plane
  - Ensure can see needle on US
  - Target fascia iliaca overlying the iliopsoas muscle 1 cm from femoral nerve. Push needle beneath fascia iliaca
  - Draw back to confirm not in vessel
  - Insert LA slowly
  - Visualise on US the LA hypoechoic spread around the nerve like a doughnut. Can adjust needle position
  - If at any point can't see spread of LA, cease and suspect endovascular
- After care: Check for effectiveness, observe for LA toxicity. Refer to ortho to manage fracture

Fascia iliaca block

- Indications: Proximal femoral fractures, painful hip
- Contraindications: Infected overlying skin. LA allergy. Open fracture. Anticoagulation is a relative contraindication
- Consent: Explain procedure
  - Risks: Infection, damage to structures (tendons, nerves, blood vessels), haematoma, bleeding, LA toxicity
- Preparation: Sterile gloves, drape, skin prep, LA (e.g. ropivacaine 0.75% 20 mL = 150 mg), 2 × 20 mL syringes, specific block needle (often has nerve stimulator attachment—not required), gauze, antiseptic swab/wash. Patient on monitoring through procedure
  - DON'T EXCEED MAXIMUM LA DOSE (see Chapter 11 Toxicology, Local anaesthetics, p. 235) 2.5 mg/kg for ropivacaine. This is a volume block; therefore, need 30–40 mL of volume. Dilute LA to achieve volume
  - Assess neurovascular status prior to block
- Procedure: Analgesia if required, glove, prep and drape
  - Check landmarks for puncture site: Line between pubic tubercle and anterior superior iliac spine (ASIS), junction of middle and outer third of this line, 2.5 cm inferior to this line, at least 2.5 cm lateral from femoral pulse
  - If using US, ensure lateral to femoral nerve/artery/vein bundle
  - Insert needle until feel 2 pops
  - Can see on US outer layer: Fascia lata and inner layer fascia iliaca, can see injection of LA filling the space

  - Draw back to confirm not in vessel
  - Insert LA slowly with intermit stops to recheck not endovascular
- After care: Check for effectiveness, observe for LA toxicity—prolonged observation not required. Refer to Ortho to manage fracture

Delivering a baby in ED

See Chapter 13 Obstetrics and gynaecology, p. 266

Ultrasound

Note: Ultrasound requires training and practice and is highly user dependent. This is a very simplified guide for jogging your memory under stress. You should not perform US unless you are trained.

FAST (eFAST)

- Used as part of primary survey in trauma patient
- FAST aims to answer a single question: Is there free fluid in the abdomen or not?
- Most useful in haemodynamically unstable trauma patient: If free fluid demonstrated then can go straight for definitive treatment—laparotomy
- eFAST includes lungs: Looking for pneumothorax
- Indications: Blunt/penetrating trauma
- Contraindications: If the scan will delay or get in the way of life-saving procedures
- Probe: Curvilinear probe—frequency 3–5 mHz
- Technique
  - Patient supine
  - Marker probe pointing towards head or towards patient's right
  - Right upper quadrant (RUQ) (Morrison's): Look for liver and kidney, look for solid black between them = fluid/blood
  - Left upper quadrant (LUQ) (splenorenal): Look for spleen and kidney, look for solid black between them = fluid/blood
  - Subxiphoid: Look for apex of heart. Is there effusion, black/fluid around heart?
  - Pelvic (transverse and sagittal): Look at the bladder, check for black/fluid around bladder
  - Lungs: Place probe at highest point on chest to look for pneumothorax (that is the point the air will rise to). Look for

ribs and pleura between 2 ribs. Is it sliding (glittering like ants marching)? Check M mode for the seashore (normal) or stratosphere/barcode (abnormal) signs

- Adjust depth to see everything you need to see but exclude irrelevant deeper images to optimise image
- To improve image: Change focus point to below where you want to look, adjust gain, use appropriate probe, more gel, increased frequency will increase resolution but decrease penetration
- Artifacts: Acoustic shadow (deeper echoes blocked at tissue interface), acoustic enhancement (deeper structure has increased brightness from a more superficial fluid-filled structure), edge shadowing, reverb artifact (repeated reflections between 2 reflective surfaces; e.g. comets), mirror artifact (echo from same surface but delayed—mirror image)

- Can repeat scan to assess evolving issues

Basic ECHO

- Indications
  - Cardiac arrest: Record loop during pulse check and review images once CPR recommenced. Look for cardiac stand still (no movement of heart) to guide further resuscitation attempts
  - PALX view, look for organised cardiac activity among valves and left ventricle (LV)
  - Look for large effusion causing tamponade
  - Look for PE with large RV
  - Look for hypovolaemia with empty LV
- Contraindications: If the scan will delay or get in the way of life-saving procedures
- Probe: Cardiac probe (3–5 mHz, low-frequency phased array), gel
- Technique: 4 main views
  - Parasternal long axis (PLAX): Position marker to right shoulder, transducer at 2nd and 4th intercostal space to left sternum, hunt in small circles for best view
  - Parasternal short axis (PSAX): Start with PLAX view, rotate 90 degrees so that marker is now towards left shoulder, fan probe to get best view
  - Apical 4-chamber view: Move transducer to apex, position marker to left shoulder. Image improved if patient rolls 30 degrees to left

  - Subcostal: Roll transducer below xyphoid process, transverse orientation. Push down. Same as in FAST. Modified 4-chamber view
- Specific findings
  - Pericardial effusion (black/fluid around heart): 1 cm circumferential = large
  - Pericardial tamponade: Effusion + diastolic RV collapse, LV collapse (late sign), IVC dilatation
  - Shock: Hypovolaemic (small LV, hyperdynamic), obstructive (dilated RV in PE, RV collapse in tamponade), distributive (hyperdynamic LV, good size LV), cardiogenic (dilated LV, hypokinetic, wall motion abnormality, IVC dilatation)
  - Dissection: Intimal flap, aortic root dilatation
  - Valve abnormalities: Only trained operators
- Bedside echo in the critically ill patient: RUSH scan (rapid US for shock/hypotension). Five steps—HI FAP
  - Heart: Parasternal long and 2-chamber apical views
  - IVC view
  - FAST scan: Morrison's and splenorenal views including lung slide. Bladder window
  - Aorta views
  - Look for pneumothorax

Aorta

- Aim to answer a single question: Is AAA present or not (> 3 cm)?
- Indications
  - Any presentation where AAA needs to be excluded
  - Unexplained abdominal/back pain older person
  - Syncopal episode older person
  - Renal colic older person
  - Clinical exam indicates AAA
- Contraindications: If the scan will delay or get in the way of life-saving procedures
- Probe: Curvilinear probe—frequency 3–5 mHz
- Technique
  - Orientation by identification of 3 structures
    - Vertebral body: Posterior, large, hypoechoic, dark acoustic shadow

    - IVC, compressible: Thin walled, oval, anterior to spine, on patient's right
    - Aorta: Non-compressible, pulsatile, round, Doppler flow, anterior to spine, on patient's left
  - Measure at 5 sites
    - Proximal (as high as you can go)
    - Mid-aorta
    - Distal aorta (just proximal to bifurcation)
    - Left common iliac
    - Right common iliac
  - Measure from outer wall to outer wall both transverse and longitudinal
  - Improving the image: Gentle pressure to displace bowel gas, bend patient's knees up to relax rectus muscle
- Positive findings: Increased diameter > 3 cm, focal dilation (1.5 × greater than adjacent segment), lack of normal distal tapering, presence of intraluminal thrombus, intra-peritoneal free fluid, pain on probe pressure over aorta

Central lines—general

- Indications: Monitoring, therapeutic (drug delivery), diagnostic (repeat blood tests)
- Contraindications: Relative—coagulopathy, infection over site, uncooperative patient, lack of consent
- Equipment: Lines, cleaning, drapes, LA, USS (and probe cover), sutures, dressing
- Expertise: Person able to do procedure safely +/– helper
- Place: Usually resuscitation bay, need monitoring, ensure rest of department running and safe
- Consent: If able, otherwise make decision in best interest of patient; e.g. if intubated

Central venous catheter (CVC)

- Indications
  - Therapeutic: Delivery irritant drugs like inotropes, replace K quickly, dialysis, temporary pacing, total parenteral nutrition
  - Diagnostic: Taking blood samples
  - Monitoring: CVP, $ScvO_2$, insertion pulmonary art catheter

- Contraindications: Relative depending on clinical situation
  - Infection/burn at chosen site, coagulopathy, uncooperative patient, lack consent, obstructed vein
  - If coagulopathy, respiratory failure, increased ICP: Use femoral site
- Complications
  - Immediate: Arrhythmia, arterial puncture, haematoma, air embolism, pneumothorax, haemothorax
  - Early: Haemopericardium, pneumothorax, catheter block/knot, chylothorax
  - Late: Infection, sepsis, thrombosis, catheter fracture, vessel stenosis, clavicle osteomyelitis (OM)
- Common sites: Internal jugular vein, subclavian vein, femoral vein
- USS guidance: Gold standard
- Pre-procedure check
  - Equipment: Flush all lines with saline
  - Connection ports
  - Drugs: LA
  - Aseptic technique: Gown, mask, gloves, skin prep, drapes
  - USS and probe cover
  - Dressing, suturing
  - Continuous ECG monitoring
  - Consent if able
  - Check patient's coags and platelets
- Procedure
  - Position patient, ensure you and assistant can see ECG trace
  - Check vessel with USS, identify vessel
  - Sterile procedure: Gown up, clean and drape area, sterile probe cover USS
  - Use LA if patient awake
  - Measure, estimate length of insertion needed
  - Ensure all lumens of CVC checked and flushed
  - Under USS guidance insert needle and syringe, pulling back on plunger, enter vessel

  - Remove syringe, ensure blood flow, insert wire, keep eye on cardiac monitor
  - Remove needle. ALWAYS KEEP HOLD OF WIRE
  - Recheck wire inserted into vein with US prior to dilating
  - Dilate vessel using dilator, remove dilator
  - Feed CVC over wire, ensure keep hold of wire, feed to appropriate length
  - Remove wire, show wire to assistant to confirm removal
  - Ensure aspirate and flush all lines
  - Suture in place, transparent dressing
  - CXR: Confirm position, no pneumothorax
  - Should also perform blood gas and transduce to confirm venous
  - Document in patient notes
- Specific sites
- Internal jugular vein
  - Right side better than left
  - Position Trendelenburg, head turned away
  - Needle 1 cm lateral to carotid pulse just above point of triangle formed by 2 heads of sternocleidomastoid (SCM) muscle. Aim parallel to carotid
  - Insertion length: Right 15–17 cm, left 19–21 cm
  - Normal CVP
    - 0–5 in supine breathing patient
    - 0–10 in mechanically ventilated
- Subclavian vein
  - Right better than left
  - Position 15 degrees Trendelenburg, head 30 degrees rotate, towel between shoulder blades
  - Needle middle and medial ⅓ clavicle aim to suprasternal notch
  - Finger over internal jugular
  - Insertion length: Right 14–15 cm, left 18–19 cm
  - Less CVC movement, more patient comfort, lower infection rate, more pneumothorax
  - Difficult to compress artery if accidental puncture

- Femoral vein
    - 1 cm inferior to inguinal ligament, 1.5 cm medial to femoral artery pulse
    - Length not an issue
    - Don't need to confirm on CXR
    - Don't need to watch cardiac monitor when wire inserted
    - Easier to perform, fewer major complications
    - No specific contraindications
    - Higher infection and thrombus rate

CHAPTER 3

Cardiology

Approach to chest pain

- Assessment
  - Differential diagnosis to consider
    - The big immediately life-threatening diagnosis to always consider and exclude to appropriate certainty: AMI/acute coronary syndrome (ACS), PE, aortic dissection
    - Potentially serious conditions to consider: Pneumonia, pneumothorax, pericarditis, angina
    - Other conditions to consider: Oesophageal or gastric pathology, abdominal pathology causing referred pain, chest wall pain
  - History
    - Pain history (onset, duration, character, radiation, aggravating and relieving factors), PHx (including risk factors, HT, cholesterol, diabetes, vascular disease, inflammatory conditions, family history [FHx]), medications, smoking, drug use (especially cocaine), allergies, systems review (consider conditions that may exacerbate ischaemia such as bleeding)
  - Examination
    - Observations, haemodynamics, appearance, murmurs, lung pathology, heart failure, BP difference between limbs, abdominal exam, DVT
- Investigations
  - ECG
  - Bloods: EUC, FBC, troponin, coags if on thinners, +/– D-dimer (for PE or dissection)
  - Imaging: CXR. Consider computed tomographic pulmonary angiography (CTPA) or computed tomography angiography (CTA) if indicated for PE, dissection
- Example strategy for assessment and management of chest pain—in sequential order

  Within 10 minutes do the following

  - ECG
    - If ST elevation myocardial infarction (STEMI)/STEMI equivalent on ECG, transfer immediately to cath lab if able

  - o If no cath lab, thrombolyse unless contraindicated (see STEMI management)
  - o Other significant concerns about ECG or patient: Discuss immediately with cardiology
- ▪ Attach monitoring for ECG and BP
- ▪ Aspirin 300 mg if considering ischaemia and no contraindications
- ▪ If saturations below 93% give supplemental O_2
- ▪ Try to relieve pain. Pain increases cardiac demand and worsens ischaemia
  - o Glyceryl trinitrate (GTN) 300–600 micrograms (up to 1800 micrograms) SL, watch BP
  - o Morphine 2.5–5 mg IV q5min to relieve pain
  - o IVC, order investigation (Ix): CXR, bloods with troponin + other Ix case-specific to patient

Based on the results of your work up

- ▪ Risk stratify (see below for details) and do one of the following:
  - o Definitive treatment of ACS (cath lab, thrombolytics)
  - o Admission for monitoring and/or further investigations
  - o Need Ix/management (Mx) of significant non-cardiac cause of chest pain; e.g. PE
  - o Discharge with serious and life-threatening causes of chest pain excluded. Consider what follow-up is needed

- HEART score: 0–3 = low risk, > 3 = high risk (Table 3.1)
- Other risk-stratifying tools (MDCalc), pulmonary embolism rule-out criteria (PERC), Wells etc.

Table 3.1 HEART score

	2	1	0
History	Highly suspicious	Moderately suspicious	Slightly suspicious
ECG	Significant changes	Non-specific changes	Normal
Age	≥ 65	45–65	< 45
Risk factors	≥ 3	1–2	0
Troponin	≥ 3 × normal	1–3 × normal	0

- Accelerated chest pain assessment protocol: Heart Foundation 2016
  - High risk: *admit all* +/– urgent coronary intervention
    - Ongoing or repetitive chest pain despite management
    - Elevated trop
    - Sustained ventricular tachycardia (VT)
    - Syncope
    - Persistent or dynamic ST changes or new T inversion > 2 contiguous leads
    - Transient ST elevation > 2 contiguous leads
    - Haemodynamic compromise (low BP, cool peripheries, sweating, new mitral regurgitation (MR), Killip > 1)
    - Known left ventricular systolic dysfunction (ejection fraction < 40%)
    - Prior myocardial infarction (MI), percutaneous coronary intervention (PCI) or bypass in last 6 months
  - Intermediate risk: Admit +/– coronary intervention
    - No to high-risk features
    - Initial ECG repeated with serial troponin
    - Patient either developed further symptoms or symptoms unrelieved, had new ECG changes or elevated serial troponin
  - Low risk: Discharge home
    - No to high- and intermediate-risk features
    - Check the following: Age < 40, normal ECG, normal serial troponin, no ongoing symptoms, atypical symptoms for angina
      - If yes to all of the above can be discharged home with no further tests needed
      - If no to any of the above will need further follow-up and investigations

STEMI management

- Aspirin 300 mg PO
- Heparin 5000 units IV/100 U/kg max. 7000 OR enoxaparin
  - Heparin preferred in severe renal impairment

- Try to relieve pain. Pain increases cardiac demand and worsens ischaemia
  - GTN 300–600 micrograms (up to 1800 micrograms) SL, watch BP, avoid in RV infarction or severe aortic or mitral stenosis, careful in inferior infarction
  - Morphine 2.5–5 mg IV q5min to relieve pain
- Oxygen if saturations below 93% or in shock
- Clopidogrel 300–600 mg or ticagrelor 180 mg, PO (don't use in intracerebral haemorrhage [ICH], liver disease)
- Indications for urgent intervention with PCI or thrombolysis
  - ECG: Persistent ST elevation ≥ 1 mm in 2 limb leads

    OR
  - ≥ 2 mm in 2 chest leads or new left bundle branch block (LBBB)

    AND
  - History consistent with AMI
- PCI if:
  - < 1 hour of symptoms and can perform PCI within 60 minutes

    OR
  - 1–3 hours of symptoms and can perform PCI within 90 minutes

    OR
  - 3–12 hours of symptoms and can perform PCI within 2 hours

    OR
  - Symptoms over 12 hours and haemodynamically unstable
  - Different cardiologists might consider PCI under other circumstances. Talk to your cardiologist if you feel PCI may benefit patient; e.g. patient with very convincing history and exam without ECG matching STEMI criteria
- Thrombolysis
  - If can't meet the time criteria above and chest pain > 30 minutes and < 12 hours
    - Reteplase 10 units IV bolus, repeat in 30 minutes

      OR
    - Alteplase accelerated infusion 15 mg over 1–2 minutes then 0.75 mg/kg (max. 50 mg) over 30 minutes then 0.5 mg/kg (max. 35 mg) over 60 minutes (note: at > 67 kg max. dose is reached; total max. dose = 100 mg)

      OR
    - Tenecteplase (weight-based dosing)

- Contraindications (these vary between texts)
    - Absolute: New neuro symptoms, suspected aortic dissection, any ICH, intracranial neoplasm, intracranial vascular malformation, significant trauma within 2 weeks, ischaemic stroke within 3 months
    - Relative contraindications: Bleeding diathesis, active bleeding, gastrointestinal (GI) bleed in the last month, non-compressible puncture, anticoagulant use, active PVD, refractory HT, pregnancy, advanced liver disease, infective endocarditis, recent neurosurgery
- Complications: Arrhythmia, failure, cerebrovascular accident (CVA), bleeding, hypotension, allergy, cardiac rupture, bone pain

Non-STEMI

- Aspirin, clopidogrel/ticagrelor
- Enoxaparin or heparin
    - Studies show enoxaparin is better: 1 mg/kg BD subcutaneously (SC)
- Morphine, GTN
- PCI within 48 hours
- Should be started on a beta-blocker

Pericarditis

- Causes: Viral, idiopathic, bacterial, myocarditis, autoimmune, serum sickness, cancer, radiation, cardiac surgery, AMI, uraemia, Dressler's syndrome, tuberculosis (TB)
- Assessment
    - History: Pleuritic chest pain, positional pain (usually decreased leaning forward), pain that radiates to left trapezius and scapula. Background of recent virus, connective tissue disease, recent AMI
    - Examination: Pericardial rub (increased sitting forward and with inspiration)
    - **Tamponade**: Hypotension, muffled heart sounds, jugular vein distension. Tachycardia, pulsus paradoxus, increased JVP on inspiration, hepatosplenomegaly, ascites, peripheral oedema
- ECG
    - Normal (uraemic pericarditis usually ECG normal)
    - Phase I (hours to days): Concave ST ↑, PR ↓ and QT ↓

    - Phase II (transient): Normal ST, PR ↓
    - Phase III (days to weeks): T inversion, SR tachycardia, electrical alternans
    - Phase IV (up to 4 months): Normal
    - **Tamponade**: Electrical alternans, low voltage
- Other investigations
    - CXR: Normal, pleural effusion, globular heart, pericardial fat pad (= effusion), calcification if chronic
    - Bloods: Troponin (exclude other causes of chest pain or associated myocarditis), WCC, CRP (↑ CRP = patient more likely to get recurrence), erythrocyte sedimentation rate (ESR)
    - Echo: Fluid (effusion) seen as black around cardiac echo
        - **Tamponade**: Effusion + diastolic RV collapse, LV collapse (late sign), IVC dilatation

- Treatment
    - **May need urgent relief of tamponade**: See Pericardiocentesis, p. 45
    - Analgesia
    - Paracetamol
    - Colchicine 0.5 mg daily (BD if > 70 kg) PO
    - Aspirin 600 mg 4-hourly PO

      OR
    - Ibuprofen 400 mg TDS PO

      OR
    - Indometacin 25–50 mg TDS PO
    - If connective tissue disease: Use prednisone 50 mg/day PO, taper if required
    - If uraemia: Need dialysis, steroids
    - If bacterial: Antibiotics, aspirate, ICU

Aortic dissection

See Chapter 8 Coagulation, anticoagulation and vascular, p. 183

Syncope

- Causes
    - HEAD: Hypoxia, Epilepsy, Anxiety, Dysfunction of the brainstem

  - HEART: Heart attack, Emboli, Aortic obstruction, Rhythm disturbance, Tachycardia
  - VESSELS: Vasovagal or volume depletion, Ectopic, Situation, Subclavian steal, Low systemic vascular resistance (SVR), Sensitive carotid sinus
- Assessment based on identifying potential causes and high-risk features and cardiac vs non-cardiac
- High-risk criteria
  - Age > 55
  - PHx: Congestive cardiac failure (CCF), coronary artery disease, pacemaker, abnormal echo
  - Onset sitting, no prodrome
  - FHx sudden death
  - Abnormal ECG
  - Significant trauma from syncope
  - Exertional
- San Francisco Syncope Rule: If any of the following, there is a 12% risk of serious outcome within 7 days
  - **C**CF prior
  - **H**aematocrit < 30
  - **E**CG changes
  - **S**OB
  - **s**BP < 90
- If any high-risk features or positive CHESS findings
  - Need to investigate further
- Investigations
  - All patients: ECG, postural BP, EUC, FBC, troponin
  - Consider CXR, CTB, other more specific bloods
  - Other investigations directed at potential causes to be excluded after Hx and Ex

Heart failure—acute pulmonary oedema

- Causes
  - Cardiac
    - Arrhythmia, AMI, anaemia, acute valvular dysfunction
    - PE, poor compliance with medications, perforated septum
    - Hypertensive crisis

    - Drugs and diet; e.g. EtOH, excess H_2O, opiates
    - Iatrogenic
    - Non-cardiac
        - Airway obstruction, asthma, aspiration, drowning, lung re-expansion
        - Eclampsia, DIC
        - Sepsis
        - Pancreatitis
        - ICH
        - High altitude
- Assessment
    - History: Of precipitating event or PHx of specific cause
    - Examination
        - ↑ RR, ↑ PR, ↓ CR, ↑ or normal BP (↓ BP has poor prognosis)
        - Agitated, sitting up, use of accessory muscles
        - Ashen or pale, sweaty, cool
        - Widespread crepitations or wheeze, frothy sputum
        - Elevated JVP, murmur

  Note: APO is fluid misplaced; patient may be vascularly fluid overloaded, hypovolaemic or euvolaemic
- Investigations
    - CXR: Cardiomegaly, upper lobe diversion, basilar/hilar infiltrate, Kerley B lines, pleural effusion
    - US: Homogenous comet tails (B lines) > 3 per field
    - Bloods: Hb, electrolytes, trop, lipase
        - Brain natriuretic peptide (BNP) > 500 / proBNP > 450 = APO likely
- Management
    - Sit upright, O_2 15 L NRB titrate to sats > 92%, monitor ECG/BP/sats/PR
    - Decrease preload with nitrates: Must monitor BP
        - GTN 5–10 microgram/min IV (50 mg GTN in 500 mL 5% glucose), double every 5 minutes as per response and BP
        - Can use topical, sublingual while getting access
        - CAUTION in severe AS and inferior/RV AMI
        - DON'T USE with sildenafil, other PDE5 inhibitors or hypertrophic obstructive cardiomyopathy (HOCM)

- Non-invasive ventilation with:
    - CPAP 5–10 cm H_2O or
    - BIPAP: 10 cm IPAP / 4–8 cm expiratory positive airway pressure (EPAP)
- Other drugs
    - Furosemide: Consider once fluid has been shifted with above treatments and have reassessed to see if patient is fluid overloaded, hypovolaemic or euvolaemic. Don't use high doses; start with 20 mg IV (or if patient already on frusemide then give their usual PO dose but give as IV; max. 80 mg)
    - Aspirin if suspected AMI
    - Morphine: No study shows benefit
- Not responding, consider dobutamine 2.5–10 microgram/kg/min IV (beware ↓ BP) or milrinone
- PCI if Hx/ECG changes suggest AMI
- May need intubation if ↓ level of consciousness, ↑ pCO_2, ↓ pO_2
- If hypotensive/shock: Further strategies which may be considered
    - Consider gentle fluid bolus
    - Inotropes: Adrenaline 0.05 microgram/kg/min or 1 microgram/min start rate, dobutamine (as above)
    - Intubation
    - Invasive monitoring
    - Intra-aortic balloon pump
    - PCI if suspecting AMI
- Identify and treat precipitating factors
- Correct electrolytes, calcium, magnesium, phosphate (CMP)
- If patient in rapid AF consider adding
    - $MgSO_4$ 10 mmol IV over, e.g. 1 hour
    - Digoxin (if not already taking) traditionally 250–500 microgram PO/IV load but new guidelines suggest no need to load; use 62.5–125 microgram (as per age/creatinine [Cr])

Arrhythmias

(For a detailed ECG guide see Chapter 19, p. 362)

- **All arrhythmias**: *investigate* and *treat* precipitates:
    - Dehydration
    - Electrolytes, CMP

  - Stimulants
  - Infection
  - AMI
- Monitor, ECG, IVC, bloods (CMP, FBC, EUC)

Atrial flutter

- Usually 2 : 1 AV block
- Regular with rate 150: flutter waves II, V_1, narrow QRS
- Treat as AF. Often need less electricity with DCCV; e.g. 50 J

Atrial fibrillation

- Irregularly irregular
  - If haemodynamically unstable
    - Immediate DC cardioversion (see Cardioversion, p. 46)
    - If AF duration > 48 hours need enoxaparin 1 mg/kg SC BD or heparin 5000 U IV bolus, 1000 U/hr, as per APPT
  - Treat the cause
    - Often no other treatments needed if the cause is identified and treated
    - Cardiac examples: Ischemic heart disease (IHD), pericarditis, HT, pre-excitation, myxoma, postoperative
    - Non-cardiac examples: Electrolytes, sepsis, PE, intoxication, chronic obstructive pulmonary disease (COPD), thyroid, drugs
  - Rhythm control (not always necessary)
    - If symptoms < 48 hours can cardiovert with DCCV or drugs
    - Symptoms > 48 hours transoesophageal echocardiogram (TOE) first and anticoagulate before cardioversion
    - DC shock: Sedate (see Procedural sedation, p. 49); start 100 Joules or 50 Joules in flutter. See cardioversion in procedures
    - Drugs for rhythm control
      - Flecainide (must be structurally normal heart) 2 mg/kg PO, max. 150 mg
      - Amiodarone 200 mg TDS PO for 1 week then wean
    - Maintenance of SR with amiodarone; flecainide (50–100 mg BD PO); sotalol (40–160 mg BD PO, monitor for ↑ QT)
  - Rate control options
    - $MgSO_4$ 10 mmol IV over 1 hour
    - Digoxin 62.5–250 microgram PO/IV daily (as per age/Cr)

- Atenolol 25–100 mg PO
- Metoprolol 25–100 mg PO or 5–10 mg IV
- In young, active patients, structurally normal hearts, can use:
  - Diltiazem CR 180–300 mg PO

    OR
  - Verapamil SR 160–480 mg PO

    OR
  - Verapamil 1 mg/min IV to max. 15 mg as per BP

- Anticoagulants
  - Consider in all patients
    - Do not use if AF < 48 hours and CHA2DS-VASc score 0
    - Consider use if AF > 48 hours or CHA2DS-VASc score > 0
    - Weigh up use of anticoagulant versus bleeding risks
    - Warfarin, DOAC, enoxaparin, heparin
  - CHA2DS-VASc:
    - CCF—1 point
    - HT—1 point
    - Age 65–74—1 point
    - Diabetes—1 point
    - Stroke or transient ischemic attack (TIA) prior—2 points
    - Vascular disease—1 point
    - Age ≥ 75—1 point (in addition to the point given above for age 65–74; i.e. a patient that is 75 will now have 2 points for age)
    - Sex female—1 point

Supraventricular tachycardia (SVT)

- Narrow QRS; rapid rate
- If QRS > 0.14 sec consider VT!
- If any doubt treat as VT
- DCCV if unstable
- Place patient head down and give reassurance (a good explanation and calm attitude while filling up those neck veins can revert patients)

- Vagal manoeuvres
  - Valsalva: Perform with patient head down or place patient head down immediately postprocedure
  - Babies and infants: Wrap child, dunk face in ice cold water
- Drugs
  - Adenosine 6 mg IV as a push via large cubital fossa cannula then flush. If no response increase dose to 12 mg. If still no response increase to 18 mg
  - Verapamil (can make hypotensive) 1 mg/min up to 15 mg (can pre-treat with 5 mL Ca gluconate 10%)
    - NEVER give if Wolff-Parkinson-White syndrome (WPW) and in AF, VT, heart disease, beta-blockers
- Long term consider electrophysiology studies (EPS), ablation, prophylaxis (e.g. atenolol, flecainide)

Ventricular tachycardia (VT)

- More likely to be VT if: Axis deviation, previous MI, active angina, age > 35, absent RS complex in any praecordial lead. Praecordial QRS concordance
- Regular, wide QRS, rate 120–220
- *If in doubt treat as VT*
  - Conscious, stable VT (rate usually > 140, can be 110–140, 5% < 110 msec), can try:
    - Amiodarone 5 mg/kg IV (up to 300 mg) over 10–20 minutes then 15 mg/kg (up to 900 mg) over 24 hours
    - Sotalol 1–2 mg/kg IV over 20–30 min
  - If unstable, LOC, drugs fail progress to DCCV
  - Pulseless VT as per ALS algorithm
  - Investigate for and treat cause
  - Long-term treatment: ICD, EPS, amiodarone, sotalol, atenolol, metoprolol

Torsades (polymorphic VT)

- Investigate for and treat cause
  - Examples: Low Mg, low Ca, antiarrhythmic medications, TCA overdose, poisoning, drug interactions
- URGENT K^+ level. Maintain K^+ 5–5.5 with potassium chloride (KCl)
- If brady: Atropine 0.5–1.5 mg IV q15min

- Treatments
  - $MgSO_4$ 2 g IV over 10–15 min +/– IV infusion
  - Isoprenaline 20 microgram IV repeated then can run infusion
  - Lidocaine (lignocaine) 75–100 mg IV over 2 min then can run infusion
  - Overdrive transvenous pacing rate 90–100
  - DON'T use amiodarone, flecainide or sotalol
- If haemodynamic collapse treat as VF in ALS algorithm with lidocaine (lignocaine) instead of amiodarone

Acute bradyarrhythmias

- Sinus brady
  - Treat only if symptomatic
- Sick sinus syndrome
- Atrioventricular junctional rhythm
  - Treat if hypotensive
- Slow idioventricular rhythm
  - Start with atropine, pacing if fails
  - Don't use antiarrhythmic
- AV block
  - 1° no treatment
  - 2° may require pacing
  - 3°/complete
    - Treatment required (see below but atropine likely won't work)
- Management of bradyarrhythmias: Stepwise approach
  - Identify and treat causes; e.g. AMI, meds (beta-blockers)
  - Atropine 0.6–1.2 mg IV (repeat q15min)
  - Isoprenaline 20 microgram IV repeat then IV infusion 1 microgram/min
  - Adrenaline infusion 1 microgram/min
  - Transcutaneous pacing
  - Temporary pacing wire transvenous

Hypertensive emergencies (rare)

- Causes: Malignant hypertension, hypertensive encephalopathy, pulmonary oedema, thoracic aortic dissection, catastrophic intracranial event, pre-eclampsia/eclampsia, autonomic dysreflexia, clonidine/beta-blocker withdrawal

- Treatment: ↓ BP by ≤ 25% in first 2 hours. Check end-organ function
- IV treatments
  - Metoprolol 1–5 mg repeat (max. 15 mg)
  - Esmolol 500 microgram/kg bolus then 50 microgram/kg/min
  - Hydralazine 5–10 mg q20min
  - Clonidine 150–300 microgram q10min
  - GTN (DON'T use with Viagra) 1–10 microgram/min titrate to BP (50 mg GTN in 500 mL glucose)
  - Sodium nitroprusside 0.3 microgram/kg/min for 10 minutes then ↑↓ by 0.3 microgram/kg/min every 10 minutes (max. 10 microgram/kg/min)
- PO treatments
  - Increase dose of patient's current anti-HT medication
  - Amlodipine 5–10 mg
  - Prazosin 2–5 mg
  - Captopril 6.25–50 mg or other angiotensin-converting enzyme (ACE) inhibitor
  - Metoprolol or other beta-blocker

Permanent implanted pacemakers

- Indications: Brady/tachyarrhythmias, heart failure
- Can have a pacing or defib function or both
- Usually a code which tells you what that pacemaker is doing
- Code is 5 letters. First 3 are the most important
- Can interpret this using PaSeR acronym
  - P: Chamber paced (O = none, A = atrium, V = ventricle, D = dual)
  - S: Chamber sensed (as above)
  - R: Response to sensing native cardiac activity (O = none, T = trigger pacing activity, I = inhibit, D = dual)
  - Fourth letter in code refers to programmability and the fifth letter refers to special functions; e.g. defib
- DDD most common first 3 letters

- Magnet mode: Applying a magnet will usually revert pacemaker back to a default asynchronous mode—it will deliver a constant paced rhythm regardless of native rhythm
- ECG: See pacing spikes, often not in all leads
  - Atrial: Before each p, usually p normal morphology
  - Ventricle: Spike before each QRS, causes a bundle branch block (BBB) morphology
  - ST and T waves should be discordant
- Complications of pacemakers
  - Early: Pneumothorax, pericarditis, haematoma
  - Latter: Lead dislodgement, skin erosion
  - Failure to sense: Poor lead position, low battery. Can lead to ROT (R on T phenomenon) and VF
  - Failure to pace: No spikes. Battery low, over-sensing, lead break
  - Failure to capture: Battery low, MI, drugs, metabolic, low amplitude, cardiac rupture
  - Runaway pacemaker: Rare, rate > 200
- Management of complications
  - Magnet
  - Praecordial thump
  - Isoprenaline infusion 1 microgram/min titrated
  - Adrenaline infusion 0.05 microgram/kg/min or start at 1 microgram/min
  - Temporary pacing: External, venous, oesophageal
- Pacemaker technician

Bacterial endocarditis

- Risk factors
  - Predisposing abnormal valve; e.g. rheumatic heart disease, prosthetic valve
  - Intravenous drug user (IVDU) consider tricuspid valve disease
  - Poor dentition
  - Immunocompromised: HIV, diabetic, dialysis
- Signs and symptoms: Wide spectrum of presentations
  - History

    - o Recent surgery or dental treatment, malaise, risk factors, fevers, anaemia, haematuria (glomerulonephritis), symptoms of organ infarction
  - Examination
    - o Fever, petechiae, rash, new murmur, heart failure
    - o Embolic complications: Abnormal neurology, hepatosplenomegaly, Janeway lesions (non-tender, haemorrhagic, fingers and toes), splinter haemorrhages
    - o Immune phenomenon: Osler nodes (tender nodes fingers and toes), Roth spots (retinal haemorrhages)
- Investigations
  - Elevated CRP
  - EUC (look at renal function), FBC, LFT
  - Urine (look for glomerulonephritis)
  - 3 × blood cultures from different sites
  - Echo, CXR
  - ECG
- Diagnosis: Based on Duke Criteria. Probably won't be officially Dx in ED
- Management (check local guidelines)
  - Empiric treatment: Benzylpenicillin 1.8 g IV 4-hourly + flucloxacillin 2 g 4-hourly + gentamicin 3–5 mg/kg daily
  - If prosthetic valve or hospital acquired or penicillin allergy use vancomycin 1.5 g BD + gentamicin
  - Change antibiotic as per organism
  - Treat complications: Resuscitation, support
  - Consult: Infectious diseases specialist, cardiology, cardiothoracic surgeons

CHAPTER 4

Respiratory

Asthma

(See Chapter 16 Paediatrics for asthma guide for children, pp. 326–329)

- Risk factors for severe/fatal asthma
  - Previous ICU/tubed/non-invasive ventilation (NIV), poor lung function, sudden attack, known brittle asthma
  - Asthma admission in the last year, multiple ED visits in the last year
  - 3+ asthma medications, frequent short-acting beta agonist (SABA; e.g. salbutamol) use, poor compliance, current oral steroid use, oral theophylline use
  - Depression/social issues, no GP, drug abuse, comorbidities including psychiatric, smoker, advanced age
- Evaluate severity: Monitor/vitals/sats. Note: Wheeze is a poor indicator of severity (Table 4.1)
  - Normal peak flow > 480 (160 cm tall) > 620 (180 cm tall); varies with age and gender
- Treatment
  - Mild
    - SABA/salbutamol
    - 100 microgram inhaler with spacer 12 puffs or 5 mg nebuliser = one dose
    - Repeat as needed. Treat as moderate if no effect or if needing repeat dose within 1–2 hours
    - If = or > 3 hours between SABA can discharge home
  - Moderate
    - SABA as above ×3 doses 20 minutes apart. Repeat as needed
    - Ipratropium bromide 20 microgram Inhaler with spacer ×8 or 500 microgram neb, max. 3 doses
    - O_2 to keep sats > 94%
    - Prednisone PO 50 mg in adult
    - Consider $MgSO_4$ IVI (dose below)
    - Consider discharge home if improves and > 3 hour between SABA

Table 4.1 Evaluating severity of asthma presentation

Feature	Mild	Moderate	Severe	Extremis
Level of consciousness	Alert	Alert	Drowsy	Coma
Exhaustion	No	No	Yes	↓ RR
Talks in	Normal sentences	Phrases/some difficulty talking	Single words	Unable
Pulse (normal 60–100)	< 100	100–120	> 120	> 140 or ↓
PEF (% predicted)	> 75%	50–75%	< 50%/unable	Unable
Sats RA	> 95%	92–95%	< 92%	–
Central cyanosis	No	Possible	Likely	Yes
ABG	–	–	$PaCO_2$ > 40	↓ PaO_2 ↑ $PaCO_2$

- Severe
  - Salbutamol 5 mg nebuliser with high-flow O_2 continuous, monitor/check K^+ and glucose. Watch lactate
  - Ipratropium bromide 500 microgram nebuliser up to 3 doses
  - Hydrocortisone 200 mg IV or dexamethasone 8 mg IV
  - IV $MgSO_4$ 2 g or 10 mmol (10 mmol = 2.5 g) over 20 minutes
  - Nebulised $MgSO_4$ potentially beneficial
- Extremis: Other things to try
  - Salbutamol infusion: 5 mg/5 mL ampoule
    - Dilute with 95 mL normal saline to 100 mL total
    - Commence at 10 microgram/min (12 mL/hr)
    - ↑ to 20 microgram/min if req (max. 42 microgram/min = 50 mL/hr)
  - IV adrenaline infusion
  - Start at 0.05 microgram/kg/min (1 microgram/min in an adult)
  - NIV: 3–5 cm CPAP or BIPAP 7–15 cm/3–5 cm H_2O. Keep pressures < 15 cm

  - Aminophylline 5 mg/kg (max. 500 mg) load over no more than 25 mg/min. (Not too rapid. Keep monitored) Then 0.5 mg/kg/hr IVI
  - Ketamine (may also be required to enable NIV), heliox
  - External compression on expiration (long expiration time)
- Things are getting worse!
  - Intubation:
    - AVOID IF POSSIBLE! Only intubate if cardiac and/or respiratory compromise and other treatments failing, RR↓↓, altered CNS/agitated, ↑↑ pCO_2, ↓↓ pO_2, exhaustion: despite maximal treatment
    - Agents preferred for RSI = ketamine and rocuronium
  - Ventilation: Humidified, hand bag until stable
    - FiO_2 100% and wean to keep sats > 95%
    - RR 6–8, I:E = 1:4
    - Permissive hypercapnia
    - Tidal volume 4–6 mL/kg, minimal PEEP 0–5 cmH_2O
    - Target plateau pressure to < 30 cmH_2O, allow peak inspiratory pressure up to 40 cmH_2O
  - If ↓↓ BP briefly stop ventilation to ↑ venous return, PEEP 0–5
  - Once intubated: sedation, analgesia, paralysis (avoid prolonged paralysis), monitor electrolytes
- Deteriorations: Always think DOPE
  - Displaced ETT, Obstructed ETT (e.g. mucus), Pneumothorax, Equipment failure
  - Is the issue breath stacking? Could this be anaphylaxis?
- Arrest or PEA
  - Trial apnoea, external chest compressions, volume challenge, adrenaline
  - Look for and treat: Tension, acidosis, high/low K, low oxygen, ETT complications, cardiac ischaemia

- Investigations
  - Bloods: Usually not needed. Take if placing IVC
    - EUC, FBC, CRP—look for signs of infection, electrolyte disturbance
    - VBG—to check pH, CO_2, electrolytes and lactate (secondary to SABA use)
    - Arterial blood gas (ABG)—usually unnecessary

- CXR: Usually not needed for mild and moderate asthma unless not responding to treatment. Indicated for severe/life-threatening. Look for infection, pneumothorax

- Disposition
  - ICU—severe or life-threatening
  - Admit—moderate
  - Discharge—mild or appropriately treated moderate
    - Not needing SABA more than 3-hourly
    - Review triggers, review maintenance medications, compliance
    - Provide Action plan
    - Provide Weaning management plan
    - Education if needed
    - Follow-up

Chronic obstructive pulmonary disease (COPD)—acute exacerbation

- Signs and symptoms
  - ↑ SOB, ↑ RR, cough, sputum, +/– fever, ↓ exercise tolerance
- Complications
  - Arrhythmia, pneumothorax, PE, pulmonary HT, cardiac failure, infection, bullae, GI bleed, stress ulcer
  - Steroid SE
  - Hypoxic, hypercapnia
- Management
  - SABA
    - Salbutamol 100 microgram 6–12 puffs inhaler with spacer or 2.5–5 mg neb as needed (PRN)

    AND/OR
  - Ipratropium bromide 20 microgram 4–8 puffs inhaler with spacer or 250–500 microgram neb maximum 3–4 doses in a day
  - Steroids
    - PO prednisone 25–50 mg daily

      OR
    - IV Hydrocortisone if severe 100 mg IV 6-hourly
    - Only need to taper if course > 5/7 (some books say 5, others say 14)

- Oxygen: To keep sats ~90, start 2 L nasal prongs or 28% venturi (beware ↑ pCO_2 but oxygenation always comes first)
- Antibiotics if potential infection
  - Amoxicillin 500 mg TDS PO or doxycycline 100 mg BD
  - Consider IV if severe
- NIV: Consider if pH < 7.35 and/or RR > 30
  - Contraindications: Pre-arrest, decreased level of consciousness, massive secretions/vomit, patient can't protect own airway, untreated pneumothorax, base of skull fracture, maxillofacial operation, marked haemodynamic instability, airway obstruction, patient refusal
  - NIV can be considered under the above contraindications as a bridge to ETT or other situations; e.g. where NIV is ceiling of care
- Intubation if all else fails and if deemed appropriate
- Respiratory consult and/or admission

Cough

- Differential diagnosis
  - Smoking
  - Asthma
  - Infection (upper respiratory tract infection [URTI], pneumonia, TB, pertussis)
  - Rhinitis
  - Gastro-oesophageal reflux disease (GORD)
  - Aspiration
  - Drugs (ACE inhibitors, beta-blockers)
  - Cancer
  - Bronchiectasis
  - Heart failure
  - Psychogenic
  - Interstitial lung disease

Pleural effusion

- Presentation
  - Symptomatic: SOB, cough, pain
  - Preexisting: e.g. patient with malignancy
  - New finding on CXR: Need to consider potential causes

- Investigations
  - CXR, ECG, bloods: EUC, FBC, LFT, CRP, +/– coags (if considering drainage, on anticoagulation)
  - + other Ix specific to potential causes
- Diagnosis
  - Sample fluid
  - Lights criteria: Fluid is exudate if:
    - Pleural fluid protein/serum protein > 0.5
    - Pleural LDH/serum LDH > 0.6
    - Pleural LDH > ⅔ upper normal limit serum LDH
  - Transudate
    - Heart failure, cirrhosis, nephrotic syndromes, ascites, dialysis, PE
  - Exudate
    - Infection, cancer, autoimmune, Dressler's syndrome, PE
  - Cytology (for suspected malignancy), pH, culture
- Drain if:
  - Large, severely symptomatic, purulent, loculated bacteria present, pH < 7.2, LDH > 1000 U/L, fever/sepsis
- Drainage: See Intercostal catheter insertion, p. 50
  - Use 8–10th rib space mid scapular, posterior puncture
  - Patient position: Leaning over pillow
  - US guidance
- Antibiotics
  - Amoxicillin + clavulanate if well
  - If sick IV piperacillin and tazobactam
  - Change as per cultures

Haemoptysis

- Massive = any volume which is life-threatening due to blood loss or airway obstruction
- Causes
  - TB
  - Cancer
  - Bronchiectasis

- Others
  - Other infections
  - Medications: Anticoagulants, amiodarone, chemo, propylthiouracil (PTU)
  - Coagulopathy, trauma
  - PE/infarct, AV malform, ruptured aneurysm, vasculitis (systemic lupus erythematosus [SLE], Goodpasture's syndrome, Wegener's granulomatosis)

- Management: Resuscitation
  - Airway: May need intubation, double-lumen ETT—get expert help
  - Breathing
    - Oxygen
    - Traditionally, nurse bleeding-side down to decrease aspiration risk
  - Circulation
    - Large-bore IVC (send cross-match, FBC, coags, VBG)
    - Volume resuscitation
    - Massive transfusion protocol initiated if needed
    - Coagulant reversal; e.g. warfarin
- Consults and imaging
  - Discuss with cardiothoracic surgeons urgently
  - URGENT CT, bronchoscopy
  - Embolisation

Pneumonia

- Presentation
  - Obvious signs: Cough, SOB, chest pain, sputum, fever
  - Beware less obvious presentations: Fever of unknown origin, abdominal pain, back pain, headache (can present like meningitis without any lung signs)
- Investigations
  - CXR (can be normal initially)
  - Bloods: FBC, EUC, LFT, CRP, VBG
  - Cultures: Sputum, blood cultures
  - +/– urine antigens for pneumococcal and *Legionella*, or specific atypical serology; e.g. mycoplasma

- Assess severity: Lots of different scoring systems
  - SMARTCOP: sBP, Multilobar, Albumin low, RR high, Tachycardia, Confusion, Oxygen low, pH low
- Management: Always base antibiotic choice on most up-to-date local guidelines. These change frequently. The suggestions below will likely have changed by the time this book is printed!
  - Mild: Consider discharge
    - Amoxicillin 1 g TDS 5/7 (30 mg/kg in child max. 1 g)
    - And if suspecting atypical add doxycycline 100 mg BD 5/7
    - If allergic: Clarithromycin 250 mg BD
  - Moderate: Admit
    - IV benzylpenicillin 1.2 g QID (60 mg/kg in child max. 1.2 g)
    - If allergic: Ceftriaxone 1 g daily or moxifloxacin in severe allergy 400 mg PO daily

      AND
    - Doxycycline 100 mg BD PO (or clarithromycin PO)
    - If from tropical region or significant comorbidities: Use ceftriaxone 2 g IV and gentamicin 5 mg/kg IV (adjusted for renal function)
  - Severe
    - IV ceftriaxone 2 g (moxifloxacin if allergic) daily

      AND
    - Azithromycin 500 mg IV daily
    - If suspecting staph: Add flucloxacillin or vancomycin if suspecting methicillin-resistant *Staphylococcus aureus* (MRSA)
    - If from tropics: Meropenem 1 g IV 8-hourly and azithromycin 500 mg IV daily
  - Aspiration pneumonia
    - Minor: Often no treatment required
    - Benzylpenicillin 1.2 g QID IV and metronidazole 500 mg BD IV

Pneumothorax

- Causes
  - Primary: Blebs, bullae, smoker, tall and thin stature, Marfan's syndrome
  - Secondary: Trauma, airway disease, infection, cancer, IVDU, Valsalva

- Investigations
  - CXR: Absent peripheral lung markings, deep sulcus, subcutaneous emphysema, increased diaphragm definition
  - US: Absent pleural slide, absent comets, stratosphere on M-mode instead of seashore
- Assessing severity
  - Is there tension: High peak pressures, chest pain, respiratory distress, increased PR, decreased air entry, (less reliable or late signs are decreased sats, decreased BP, elevated JVP, tracheal deviation)
  - British Thoracic Society guidelines
    - Visible rim on posteroanterior CXR < 2 cm size = small, ≥ 2 cm size = large
- Management options: See Chapter 2, pp. 50–52
  - No absolute correct answer. Base management on individual patient and joint and informed decision-making
  - Observation
    - Can consider in: Small primary, large primary and when patient refuses intervention, very small secondary (but must always admit)
    - Repeat CXR at 1 and 3–5 days
  - Aspiration
    - Considered in: Large primary, iatrogenic, small secondary and age < 50
    - Repeat CXR post aspiration to confirm success
  - Pigtail
    - Considered in: Large primary, symptomatic, secondary, failed conservative treatments
- Recommendations
  - No diving ever: Unless definitive management (i.e. with a cardiothoracic surgeon)
  - No flying for at least 2 weeks following full resolution of pneumothorax

Acute respiratory distress syndrome (ARDS)

- Causes
  - Top 3 causes: Sepsis, respiratory infections, gastric aspiration

- Other examples: Trauma (pulmonary and non-pulmonary), blood transfusion, drowning, airway obstruction, toxic gas, overdose, altitude, neurogenic, rapid lung re-expansion, organ failure

- Diagnosis
  - Diffuse lung injury, non-cardiac, high permeability pulmonary oedema
  - Berlin definition
    - < 1 week of clinical insult/new or worsening symptoms
    - CXR opacities not explained by other pathology
    - Oedema non-cardiac, not explained by overload or CCF
- Assessing severity
  - Based on Berlin criteria
  - Calculate PaO_2/FiO_2 on a PEEP of 5 cm H_2O
    - 200–300 = mild mortality 27%
    - 100–200 = moderate mortality 32%
    - < 100 = severe mortality 45%
- Management
  - Oxygenation
  - Ventilation: Protective lung strategy
    - Low tidal volume 6 mL/kg
    - Permissive hypercapnia (keep pH > 7.2)
    - Can ventilate prone (once in ICU!)
    - High PEEP, recruitment manoeuvres. Set pressure alarm to plateau pressure not peak pressure
  - Fluids: Use caution, restrict if possible. Use CVP to guide
  - Support: Aim euglycaemic, provide nutrition
  - No steroids

Pulmonary embolism (PE)

- Presentation
  - Obvious: Chest pain, SOB, cough, haemoptysis, cyanosis, signs of deep vein thrombosis (DVT), increased RR
  - Less obvious/beware: Fever, tachycardia, syncope, sweats, arrhythmia (e.g. AF), collapse, arrest

- Diagnosis and scoring systems
  - Wells score to assess high or low risk: Simple and most validated
    - Worth 3 marks each: DVT symptoms/signs, PE at least as likely as alternative diagnosis
    - Worth 1.5 marks each: PR > 100, immobility/operation last 4 weeks, prior PE/DVT
    - Worth 1 mark each: Cancer Hx, haemoptysis
    - Score ≥ 5 = PE likely, 0–4 = unlikely
  - PERC rules: Patient must be low risk to use this tool; PE very unlikely if answers yes to the following
    - Age < 50
    - PR < 100
    - Sats > 95%
    - No unilateral leg swell
    - No haemoptysis
    - No recent trauma, surgery
    - No PE/DVT patient history
    - No hormone use
- Investigations
  - CXR: Rule out other causes
  - ECG: Rule out other causes, look for strain
    - May see: Normal ECG, sinus tachycardia, RBBB, RAD, S1Q3T3, AF, T inversions
    - T inversions V1–4 and inferior are highly specific 99%
  - D-dimer: High sensitivity. Useful in low-risk patients. Doesn't exclude PE in high-risk patients
    - Positive result if > 0.5 mg/L
    - Age adjusted for patients > 50 years,
      - In general, positive D-dimer is > 0.5 mg/L
      - In patients > 50 years, positive age-adjusted D-dimer is > age × 0.01 mg/L
    - Pregnancy adjustments by trimester have also been suggested
  - Troponin and BNP: Used to identify patients at high risk of poor outcomes
  - Ventilation/perfusion (V/Q) scan: Less risk to breast tissue therefore good in pregnant and lactating women, not useful if prior lung disease or abnormal CXR; often get equivocal result

    - CTPA: Can see clot burden; good for alternative diagnosis, contrast and radiation risk
- Risk stratify and risk-based management
    - High/massive = haemodynamically unstable
        - Shock, low BP, +/– RV dysfunction markers
        - Heparin, thrombolysis, embolectomy
    - Intermediate
        - No shock, haemodynamically stable but evidence of RV dysfunction
        - Admit, low-molecular-weight heparin (LMWH), monitor
        - In some cases embolectomy and thrombolysis might be considered
        - Thrombolysis if patient crashes
    - Low
        - Normal BP, no haemodynamic compromise, no RV dysfunction
        - LMWH/NOAC (new oral anticoagulants) and early discharge
- General management
    - Support
        - ABC, careful IV fluids, may need inotropes
    - Heparin
        - Enoxaparin 1 mg/kg BD or 1.5 mg/kg daily (adjust for creatinine clearance)
        - Unfractionated heparin 80 units/kg bolus IV then infusion 18 units/kg/hr, adjust as per APTT
    - Warfarin or NOAC—longer term
    - Thrombolysis
        - Use thrombolytics in arrest or high-risk patients with compromise
        - In arrest: r-TPA (alteplase) 50 mg IV bolus, then further 50 mg after 15 minutes if no ROSC with ongoing CPR—CPR should continue for 45–60 minutes post thrombolysis
        - Protocols vary
        - Non-arrest: Alteplase 10 mg over 2 minutes then 90 mg over 2 hours
        - **Stop heparin while giving the thrombolytic**

CHAPTER 5

Gastroenterology and surgery

Treating nausea and vomiting

- Acute vertigo
  - Prochlorperazine 12.5 mg IM or 5–10 mg PO or 25 mg PR
  - Promethazine 25–50 mg PO or 10–25 mg IM/slow IV
- Pregnancy related
  - Investigate causes (infection especially pyelonephritis, metabolic cause, molar/multiple pregnancies)
  - Pyridoxine vitamin B6 12.5 mg PO mane (in the morning) and midi (at midday), 25 mg nocte
  - Doxylamine succinate (Category A) 25 mg PO nocte
  - Metoclopramide (Category A) 10 mg PO/IV/IM TDS
  - Prochlorperazine (Category C) 5 mg PO (see doses above)
  - Promethazine (Category C) 25 mg PO TDS
  - Ondansetron (Category B1) 4–8 mg PO/IV daily
- Other causes of nausea and vomiting; suggested order of treatment
  - IV fluids; e.g. normal saline
    - Can improve symptoms without medications
  - Metoclopramide OR prochlorperazine (doses above)
  - + Ondansetron (doses above)
  - + Dexamethasone 4–8 mg PO, IV
  - Consider droperidol 0.625 mg IV
  - Consider promethazine
  - Cyclical vomiting related to cannabis use: relieve with hot shower
  - If needing to use more than 2 medications:
    - Consider sinister causes
    - Have patient on monitor (beware ↑ QT from medications)
    - Check electrolytes (especially K, Mg), VBG (metabolic alkalosis) and ECG (check QT) first

Foreign body GI

- Assessment
  - History of the present illness (HPI)
    - What was ingested? Is it causing symptoms; e.g. abdominal pain, vomiting, difficulty swallowing?
    - Adults: Often food bolus
    - Children: Could it have been a high-risk object such as button battery, magnet (need 2 magnets or 1 magnet + something metal to cause significant issues), object made of lead (e.g. fishing sinker), very large object (e.g. > 6 cm), other concerning or unknown object
  - PHx
    - Adults: Consider underlying cause; e.g. GORD, stricture, cancer
    - Children: Consider those at increased risk; e.g. with prior GI abnormalities, strictures
  - Initial investigations
    - Adults: Usually IVC, +/– bloods, +/– CXR, +/– lateral airways x-ray
    - Children: May not need any investigations if good history in an asymptomatic child without any concerning past history and the object ingested is not a high-risk object. If any concern, order plain x-ray (should see most metal objects)
- X-ray assessment
  - Is the foreign body in the airway or oesophagus?
    - On CXR a coin in the oesophagus will be circular on the AP and a thin line on the lateral
    - On CXR a coin in the trachea will be a thin line on the AP and circular on the lateral
  - Is it a button battery? Look for double shadow ring
  - Where is the object in the GI tract? Is it in the oropharynx, oesophagus, stomach, intestine?
- Management: Adults
  - URGENT if patient can't swallow saliva needs endoscopy ASAP
  - Removal of foreign body
    - Some studies suggest medical therapy should not be attempted as these delay endoscopy and usually not successful.

        - May need CT to localise site
        - Basic rule of thumb: Above sternal notch consult ENT, below sternal notch consult gastro
    - Dissolution (if food bolus)
        - Only if normal x-ray, normal airway reflexes, soft object, no perforation, non-complete obstruction
        - 25–50 mL carbonated drink, soft food
        - Beware aspiration
    - GTN 600–1200 microgram SL (little evidence to support)
    - Glucagon: Has minimal evidence and significant risk of vomiting
- Management: Children
    - URGENT ENT consult: If object is lodged in the oropharynx, difficulty breathing
    - URGENT GASTRO consult: Objects lodged in oesophagus, button battery that has not passed to stomach, magnet(s) (if there is one, assume there are more), very large object in the stomach, can't swallow saliva
    - Note: If a button battery has passed the oesophagus 90% will pass asymptomatically (still need consult and follow-up)
    - Any other symptoms (e.g. can't tolerate food/fluids, abdominal pain, vomiting, fevers): Consult gastro team
    - If asymptomatic child, no high-risk past history, no high risk of ingestion. Can discharge home with instructions for follow-up and when to return

Peptic ulcer disease (PUD) and epigastric pain

- Risk factors for PUD
    - Smoker, FHx, alcohol, stress, medications (NSAIDs, steroids), Zollinger-Ellison syndrome
- Complications of PUD: Causes of ED presentations
    - Epigastric pain, reflux
    - Penetration: Can cause pancreatitis
    - Perforation: Present with acute abdomen, severe pain, sepsis
    - Bleeding: See upper GI bleed
    - Gastric outlet obstruction
    - Cancer

- Assessment and investigations
  - Exclude sinister causes of chest pain like AMI
  - Exclude acute abdomen
  - Consider other causes of abdomen pain; e.g. pancreatitis
  - Bloods: EUC, FBC, LFT, lipase, VBG (↑ lactate—perforation, hypokalaemia and metabolic alkalosis—gastric outlet obstruction)
  - CXR: Look for perforation (e.g. subcutaneous emphysema, subdiaphragmatic gas)
  - May need CT; if suspect perforation, look for alternative diagnosis
- Management
  - Ulcer
    - *Helicobacter pylori* eradication
    - H_2 antagonist
    - Proton pump inhibitor
    - Other: Sucralfate, bismuth
  - Complications
    - Gastroenterologist consult
    - Endoscopy
    - Urgent operation

Upper GI bleeding

- Causes
  - PUD, oesophagitis, varices, Mallory-Weiss tear
  - Erosions (secondary to EtOH, NSAID, smoking, stress)
  - Cancer, angiodysplasia, aortoenteric fistula
- Presentation
  - May be obvious, haematemesis
  - May be vomiting without reported haematemesis, generally unwell, symptoms of anaemia or blood loss, syncope, melaena
  - Beware an isolated increase in urea
- Investigations
  - FBC, EUC, LFT, coags, G&H
  - EUC: Elevated K, elevated Ur, Ur:Cr > 200 (specific, not sensitive)

  - ECG, erect CXR
  - Consider:
    - Faecal occult blood
    - NGT for diagnostic purposes
    - Gastroscopy, angiography (only useful if bleed > 0.5 mL/min)
- General management
  - Proton pump inhibitor infusion (see below)
  - Transfusion of packed red cells if significant anaemia; e.g. Hb < 7 g/dL (or higher if history of IHD or vascular disease)
  - Discussion with gastroenterology +/– haematology
  - Cease +/– reverse anticoagulants depending on reasons for use
  - Endoscopy semi-urgent, angiography or surgery in selected cases
- Management in severe bleeding
  - Resuscitation
    - ABC, team approach
    - Large-bore IVC ×2
    - Cross-match blood
    - Initiate massive transfusion protocol if needed
    - Fluid resuscitation for shock with blood products
    - Permissive hypotension
    - Guide blood products to end points, consult haematology
    - FFP if INR > 1.5, platelets if < 50×10^9/L
    - Consider tranexamic acid (1 g IV over 10 minutes then 1 g IV over 8 hours)
    - Reverse anticoagulants
  - Broad-spectrum antibiotics: Ceftriaxone IV 1 g if suspect varices
  - Proton pump inhibitors
    - Pantoprazole 80 mg IV bolus then:
      - 8 mg/hr IVI (80 mg in 100 mL normal saline or 5% dexamethasone) infusion

        OR
      - Pantoprazole 80 mg IV BD
  - Urgent consult with gastroenterology and urgent endoscopy

- Potential discharge with early outpatient follow-up
  - Glasgow-Blatchford score
    - Must answer yes to all of the following:
      - No Hx of liver or heart disease, no syncope, no melena, sBP > 110, PR < 100, Ur < 6.5, Hb > 120–130
  - Not everyone uses this; check what your hospital does. Make sure that if you're sending someone home you have discussed with a gastroenterologist, have follow-up arranged and are happy your patient will comply

Bleeding oesophageal varices

- General
  - Enlarged portosystemic vein, result of portal hypertension
  - 20–40% mortality
  - Presentation usually more severe. Large haematemesis. Shock
  - Usually history of varices or causes such as EtOH or chronic liver disease
- Management
  - Resuscitation as per severe upper GI bleed
  - Octreotide 50–100 microgram IV bolus then 25–50 microgram/hr IVI
  - Broad-spectrum antibiotics: Ceftriaxone 1 g IV
  - URGENT endoscopy
  - If no scope or OT available and patient unstable/ongoing massive haemorrhage:
    - Tamponade with Minnesota tube
    - Requires patient to be intubated first
    - Insert tube into stomach, inflate balloon (to volume on packet), x-ray to confirm, traction

Ascites and spontaneous bacterial peritonitis (SBP)

- Chronic cirrhosis, ↑ portal vein pressure, ↓ Alb, ↑ Na retention
  - Exudate
    - High protein > 25 g/L
    - Low serum-ascites albumin gradient (SAAG) < 11
    - Causes: Infection, nephrotic syndrome, cancer, pancreatitis

    - Transudate
        - Low protein < 25 g/L, high SAAG > 11
        - Causes: Cirrhotic ascites, heart failure, portal HT
- Investigations
    - EUC, FBC, LFT, check coags
    - Diagnostic tap: See Paracentesis, p. 57
- General management
    - Consult gastroenterology
    - Spironolactone 50–100 mg starting dose mane PO
    - Frusemide 40 mg + PO mane
    - Restrict fluids
    - Therapeutic tap: See procedures paracentesis
- Spontaneous bacterial peritonitis
    - At risk: Cirrhosis, ascites, nephrotic syndrome, peritoneal dialysis, secondary SBP from pancreatitis or from perforate viscous
    - Symptoms and signs
        - Fever, abdominal pain, nausea, vomiting, diarrhoea
        - Ascites, tender abdomen without peritonism, encephalopathy, confusion, cloudy ascitic fluid, renal failure
    - Diagnose with ascitic tap
        - WCC > 250/mm^3 especially if neutrophils
        - Runyon's criteria: 2 or more—protein > 10 g/L, glucose < 2.8 mmol/L, LDH > upper serum normal
        - Other markers: ↑ amylase, ↑ bilirubin, ↑ alkaline phosphatase (ALP), ↑ CEA, polymicrobes
    - Management
        - Ceftriaxone 2 g IV daily
        - + Ceftazidime intra-abdominally in peritoneal dialysis patient
        - IV albumin 2–5 mL/kg 20% up to 100 mL BD

Acute hepatic encephalopathy

- Causes
    - Drugs: Antibiotics (e.g. amoxicillin, ciprofloxacin, azithromycin), antiseizure (e.g. phenytoin, valproate), antifungal (e.g.

ketoconazole), chemo agents, NSAIDs (e.g. diclofenac), paracetamol, propylthiouracil (PTU), duloxetine, salicylates, illicit, herbal (e.g. some Chinese herbal remedies), mushroom etc.

- EtOH
- Viruses: Hepatitis A virus (HAV), hepatitis B virus (HBV), hepatitis C virus (HCV), cytomegalovirus (CMV), Epstein–Barr virus (EBV), herpes simplex virus (HSV)
- Sepsis
- Others: HELLP, metabolic, autoimmune ischaemic necrosis, vascular

- Presentation
  - Symptoms: Irritable, lethargic, confusion, coma, jaundice, ↓ BSL
  - Signs: Organomegaly, asterixis, increased reflexes
  - Precipitants: Renal impairment, GI bleed, infection, toxins, drugs, increased protein intake, low K, progressive deterioration
  - Grading: 1 = drowsy, 2 = confused, 3 = stupor alternating agitation, 4 = coma
- Investigation
  - Bloods: FBC, EUC, CMP, LFT, coags, VBG, BSL, paracetamol level, culture, hepatitis serology, CMV, EBV, ANA, ammonia
  - Usually: ↑ ammonia, ↓ Mg, ↓ K, ↓ Na, ↓↓ BSL
    - ↓ phosphate = good prognosis
- Management
  - Resuscitation: A, B, C. Fluids. May need intubation, monitor ICP, ICU
  - Treat the cause/precipitants/complications
    - Bleeding (vitamin K, platelets, FFP, packed cells)
    - Infection (antibiotics)
    - ↓ BSL (IV glucose and monitor)
    - Hepatorenal syndrome (albumin IV)
    - Cerebral oedema (hyperventilate, mannitol 0.3–0.4 g/kg)
    - Antidotes; e.g. N-acetylcysteine (NAC) in paracetamol OD
    - Correct electrolytes

- Encephalopathy
  - Lactulose 30 mL 1–2-hourly then daily (consider NGT if altered GCS)
  - Empirical IVAB ceftriaxone 1 g daily, metronidazole 500 mg BD
  - + Ampicillin 1 g QID if already on AB
- Consider transplant: King's College Criteria
  - pH < 7.3 or INR > 6.5 + Cr > 300 + grade 3 or 4 encephalopathy

Inflammatory bowel disease

- Reasons for ED presentations
  - New diagnosis
    - Abdominal pain and cramping
    - Stools: Diarrhoea, mucus, irregular, nocturnal diarrhoea or diarrhoea that wakes (not usual with simple gastroenteritis), bloody, constipation, tenesmus, incontinence
    - Systemic: Fever, weight loss, fatigue
  - Complications
    - Bowel obstruction, perforation, cancer
    - Extra-abdominal complications: Arthritis, DVT/PE, uveitis, pyoderma, rash
    - More likely with Crohn's disease: Perianal disease (fistula, abscess, fissure)
    - More likely with ulcerative colitis: Toxic megacolon, haemorrhage, fluid/electrolyte abnormalities, severe diarrhoea
    - Toxic megacolon: see p. 122
- Investigations
  - FBC, EUC, CMP, B12, folate, iron, ESR/CRP, stool culture
  - Imaging as needed: X-ray abdomen, erect chest, CT abdomen/pelvis
- Management: Consult gastroenterology and surgery if needed
  - General in acute flare ups
    - Prednisone 25–50 mg daily, topical/rectal steroids
    - Sulfasalazine 500 mg BD

- Fulminant ulcerative colitis (> 10 stools per day + systemic features)
    - o IV piperacillin/tazobactam/broad-spectrum AB, IV steroids, NGT
- Toxic megacolon: For management, see p. 122
- Management of other complications

Thiamine deficiency

- To prevent Wernicke's encephalopathy
- Any patient with suspected EtOH excess
- Thiamine 300 mg IV for 3/7
- Up to 500 mg IV TDS if already has confusion

LFTs

- Bilirubin: ↑ in jaundice
- Liver disease causes ↓ vitamin K leading to ↑ PT time
- Transaminases: Intracellular enzymes; ↑ in hepatocyte injury. AST non-specific (also in other cells), alanine aminotransferase (ALT) more specific
    - AST/ALT > 2 = alcoholic; ratio < 1 = viral hepatitis
    - May be in the thousands with severe injury or near normal if end-stage chronic injury
- ALP ↑ = biliary obstruction
    - > 4 × ↑ = cholestasis
    - Also ↑ in bone production, children, EtOH, pregnancy etc.
- Gamma-glutamyl transferase (GGT) ↑ = cholestasis, EtOH, medications, AMI etc.
- Synthetic liver function: Albumin, bilirubin, prothrombin time and glucose
- Patterns
    - Alcohol abuse: AST 2× > ALT, ↑ GGT
    - Ischaemic/toxic injury: AST = ALT > 10× normal, bilirubin < 5× normal
    - Ischaemia: ↑ AST = ALT, ↑ LDH, ALT/LDH < 1, bilirubin normal
    - Viral acute hepatitis, hepatocellular: ↑ ALT > AST, ↑ bilirubin 5–10× normal, ALP normal or ↑, ↑ LDH
    - Cholestasis: ↑ ALP, ↑ GGT, ↑ bilirubin, normal or ↑ ALT

General surgery

Acute abdomen

- Acutely unwell + abdominal signs and symptoms
- Pain location and potential causes to consider
  - Epigastric: AMI, peptic ulcer, acute cholecystitis, perforated oesophagus
  - RUQ: Acute cholecystitis, duodenal ulcer, hepatitis, congestive hepatomegaly, pyelonephritis, right-sided pneumonia
  - LUQ: Ruptured spleen, gastric ulcer, aortic aneurysm, perforated colon, pyelonephritis, left-sided pneumonia, splenic artery aneurysm
  - Central: Intestinal obstruction, acute pancreatitis, early appendicitis, mesenteric thrombosis, AAA, diverticulitis
  - Left or right lower quadrant (LQ): Appendicitis, renal/ureteric stone, incarcerated hernia, Crohn's disease
  - RLQ: mesenteric adenitis, Meckel's diverticulum, perforated caecum, psoas abscess, appendicitis
  - LLQ: Sigmoid diverticulitis, ulcerative colitis
  - *In females* consider ectopic pregnancy +/– rupture, cyst accident, ovarian torsion, pelvic inflammatory disease (PID), salpingitis, tubo-ovarian abscess
- Examination
  - As a minimum: Cardio exam, respiratory exam and abdominal exam
  - Always look for hernias
  - Always check genitals, testicles, perineum
  - Is the patient writhing around? Consider renal stones, ischaemic pain
  - Is the patient still with legs drawn up? Consider peritonitis
  - Signs to look for: Murphy's, Cullen's/Grey Turner's (especially patient on thinners; indicate retroperitoneal bleeding), cough test (cough worsens pain = peritonitis), hop/bump test (jumping or hopping or bumping the bed causes pain = peritonitis)
    - Appendicitis signs: Iliopsoas (external rotation of right hip causes pain), obturator sign (internal rotation of flexed right hip causes pain), Rovsing's sign, heel drop sign (examiner drops or bangs heels causing pain)
- Investigations
  - Bloods: FBC, EUC, LFT, lipase/amylase, +/– lactate +/– CRP. *In females always check* ***βhCG***

  - Urine
  - Erect CXR, ECG, +/– CT abdomen, +/– US abdomen/pelvis
- General management
  - IVC, IV fluids, NBM, analgesia
  - If severe/shock: A, B, C, fluid resuscitation etc.
  - Consider imaging required
  - Consults: Surgery, gynaecology, gastroenterology etc.
  - Urgent surgical consult if peritonitis (shock, lying still, tender with cough, rebound, rigidity)

Pancreatitis

- Causes
  - EtOH, gallstones
  - Other: Post endoscopic retrograde cholangiopancreatography (ERCP), idiopathic, trauma, cancer, hereditary, drugs, mumps and other virus, peptic ulcer penetrating, autoimmune, hypothermia, hypotension, hypercalcaemia, hyperlipidaemia
- Presentation
  - Abdominal pain, epigastric or upper abdomen, often radiates to back, vomiting, better sitting forward
  - May be febrile, ↑ HR, jaundice, shock, nausea, vomiting
- Investigations
  - Bloods: FBC, EUC, CMP, LFT, VBG, BSL
  - Amylase ↑↑, lipase ↑↑
  - Imaging: CXR to exclude alternative diagnosis
    - CT if severe
    - US looking for stones and duct dilation
- Prediction tools for severe acute pancreatitis (SAP)
  - SIRS, APACHE II
  - Ranson (score takes 48 hours): ≥ 4 = ↑ mortality
    - Presentation: Age > 55, WCC > 16, BSL > 10 mmol/L, LDH > 350, AST > 250
    - 48 hours: HCT ↓ ≥ 10%, urea rise > 1.79 mmol/L, Ca < 2 mmol/L, pO_2 < 60 mmHg, base deficit ↑ > 4, fluid sequestration > 6000 mL
- Management: Consult surgery
  - Severe
    - Resuscitation; ABC, +/– intubation
    - Fluid resuscitation, strict fluid balance, IDC, NGT

- o Invasive monitoring, ICU
- o Sedation
- ▪ IVC, NBM, +/– NGT
- ▪ Analgesia, antiemetics
- ▪ Nutrition
- ▪ Treat cause; e.g. ERCP
- ▪ Antibiotics only if proven infection, septic, necrotising; e.g. IV piperacillin/tazobactam 4.5 g 8-hourly (check local guidelines)
- ▪ Necrotising pancreatitis: Operate/debride

Gall bladder/ducts

Biliary colic

- Risk factors: Overweight, female, FHx, increased age, haemolysis, rapid weight loss (e.g. post bariatric operation)
- Symptoms: Severe constant RUQ or epigastric pain, vomit at end of attacks, precipitated by rich food, decreased pain leaning forward
- Examination: Afebrile, RUQ tender no peritonism, negative Murphy's sign
- Investigations: LFT—transient raised ALP and GGT, US
    - ▪ Exclusion tests: Urine, lipase, FBC, βhCG, ECG, CXR, +/– abdominal x-ray or CT
- Management
    - ▪ Analgesia
    - ▪ Discharge if pain free, no fever, non-tender, tolerating diet, no obstruction
    - ▪ Abdominal US can be managed by LMO
    - ▪ Surgical follow-up: Cholecystectomy (not urgent)

Acute cholecystitis

- Causes: Stone (risk factors as above), acalculous (elderly, diabetic, already unwell patient [e.g. sepsis, inpatient])
- Symptoms: Severe RUQ pain, patient usually unwell
- Examination: ↑ HR, tender RUQ, Murphy's sign positive, febrile
- Investigations: US (thick gallbladder wall, stones, gas in wall, sonographic Murphy's sign, dilated CBD), elevated WCC, CT (less sensitive, may be good if need to exclude other diagnosis)

- Management
  - IVC, NBM, IV fluids
  - Analgesia: Fentanyl, morphine (can cause sphincter of Oddi dysfunction)
  - IVAB ampicillin 1 g IV QID + gentamicin 3–5 mg/kg (adjusted)
  - Surgical consult

Ascending cholangitis

- Risk factors: Stent or instrumentation, stones, obstructions
- Signs and symptoms: Fever, rigor, pain, +/– jaundice, ↑ HR, ↓ BP, +/– shock, +/– altered level of consciousness. Can rapidly become very unwell
- Investigations: ↑ neutrophils, ↑ bilirubin, ↑ AST and ALT, ↑ ALP, blood cultures. Can have renal failure, pancreatitis, abnormal coags
- Imaging: US, +/– CT, CXR for diagnosis exclusions
- Management: Urgent surgical consult, resuscitation and support, IVAB ampicillin and gentamicin as above, add metronidazole 500 mg BD IV if recent instrumentation. Urgent relief obstruction (e.g. ERCP)

Diverticular disease

Terminology

- Diverticula: Herniation mucosa through muscle
  - Large bowel. Most sigmoid and descending colon
  - Right-sided disease more common in those of Asian descent, young people
- Diverticulosis: Uncomplicated diverticula. Most asymptomatic
  - Can get colicky abdominal pain, irregular bowel habit
  - General advice: High fibre, keep stool soft

Diverticulitis—inflamed diverticulum

- Mild
  - Mild abdominal pain + tender (usual LLQ)
  - No peritonism, no systemic symptoms
    - Can discharge home
    - PO AB: amoxicillin + clavulanate forte 1 tab BD 5–10/7 OR cephalexin 500 mg QID + metronidazole 400 mg BD for 5–10/7

  - If 1st episode colonoscopy in 6/52 to confirm
  - If symptoms do not improve CT abdomen
- Severe or complicated
  - Systemic features, peritonism, failed output treatment
  - Admission
    - Bowel rest, IV fluids, IVAB
    - Ampicillin 2 g QID and
    - Metronidazole 500 mg BD
    - + (as per renal function) gentamicin 4–6 mg/kg daily
  - CT abdomen + surgical review
  - Surgery usually if: Peritonitis + perforation, abscess and can't percutaneously drain, obstruction, recurrent episodes, fistula

Lower GI bleed

- Causes
  - Diverticular bleed: 50%
    - Can be massive especially if on NSAIDs, antiplatelets. Abrupt onset. 80% settle
  - Angiodysplasia, cancer, ischaemic colitis, infection, inflammatory bowel disease (IBD)
  - In younger patients: Peutz-Jeghers syndrome, Henoch-Schönlein purpura (HSP), Meckel's diverticulum
- Differentiating site
  - Upper GI bleed: Haematemesis, tarry black offensive stool
  - Haemorrhoid: Fresh blood, on wiping/in toilet bowl around stool
  - Lower intestine: Bright blood
  - Higher up in intestine: Mixed with stool
- Investigations
  - FBC: WCC increased with infection, increased platelets indicates acute bleeding, if decreased platelets this may be the cause or contributing to bleeding
  - EUC: Increased Ur/Cr ratio and increased K = upper GI bleed
  - LFT, G&H, coags
  - ECG, CXR

- Management
  - Large-bore IVC ×2, G&H, cross-match blood, NBM
  - Resuscitation, fluids and early use of blood if needed
  - Reverse anticoagulants (consider risks versus benefit)
  - Consider massive transfusion protocol if needed
  - Consult surgeon +/– radiology
  - If bleeding was significant but has ceased or eased: Will need scope, CT angiogram unlikely to be helpful
  - Ongoing severe bleeding, localise bleeding site with CT angiogram +/– embolisation. CT with embolisation is often the better choice even in unstable patients as it is potentially diagnostic and curative
  - May require surgery

Appendicitis

- Presentation
  - Typical: Generalised abdominal pain then localising to right iliac fossa (RIF). Nausea, vomiting. Can have fever. Anorexia
  - Atypical: Any location of abdominal pain or no pain obvious, generally unwell. Diarrhoea and vomiting mistaken as gastroenteritis. Febrile illness
  - Beware: Can get appendicitis at any age. Elderly and young children often delayed or incorrect diagnosis. Children < 1 year of age with appendicitis almost always have delayed diagnosis. Elderly patients often perforate. Not uncommon in pregnancy and often pain in later pregnancy is RUQ or flank
- Examination
  - Typical: Tender RIF with rebound pain. Tender at McBurney's point. Peritonism localised (rebound and percussion tenderness, pain with cough or hop) or generalised in perforation. Rectal tenderness
  - Signs: Rovsing (pain RIF when pressing on LIF), psoas (flex right hip causes pain), obturator (internal rotation right hip causes pain)
  - Atypical: Pain can be generalised especially early in illness. May not have tenderness especially where appendix is not in typical location. Children can present as ileus, rupture, small bowel obstruction (SBO). The younger the child, the more likely the diagnosis is initially missed
  - Look for signs of complications: Perforation, abscess, shock, sepsis, SBO

- Investigations
  - Bloods: Don't change the yield! Often an argument with surgical team. Normal bloods don't exclude anything! CRP, WCC, neutrophilia, left shift, does make diagnosis more likely
  - Positive urine does not exclude appendicitis! Patients with appendicitis: 15% will have bacteria, 30% will have elevated RBC or WBC
  - US: Very good if appendix visualised but no use if appendix can't be found
  - CT abdomen: Good for diagnosis and excluding alternative diagnosis. Newer approaches—don't need contrast. Use low-dose radiation
  - MRI especially in children
  - Alvarado score
    - 2 points each: Tender RIF, WCC > 10,000
    - 1 point each: Anorexia, nausea/vomit, migratory pain, rebound pain, temp > 37.3°C, neutrophils > 75% and/or left shift
    - Score 1–4, appendicitis unlikely; score > 6, straight to OT
- Management
  - IVC, IV fluids, NBM
  - Analgesia
  - IV antibiotics if systemic symptoms or concerns of perforation
    - Ampicillin 1 g QID, metronidazole 500 mg BD, +/– gentamicin (dose adjusted)
  - Alternative to operation: IV antibiotics with ceftriaxone 1 g daily and metronidazole 500 mg BD for 24 hours then change to PO for 10 days
    - Effective in approximately 60%
    - Consider if no evidence of perforation, compliant patient with good access to return to hospital if needed, and/or patient refusing surgery

Mediastinitis

- Causes
  - Direct: Trauma, cancer, post cardiac operation, post endoscopy, oesophageal rupture, Boerhaave's syndrome (oesophageal rupture from sudden increased pressure; e.g. severe vomiting)
    - Infection: Pulmonary, rib osteomyelitis, TB, lymph node

  - Extension (descending necrotising mediastinitis): Teeth, pharyngeal, sinus infections
- Presentation
  - Symptoms: URTI, fever, pain retrosternal/interscapular
  - Signs: Sepsis, trismus, stridor, Hamman's sign (crunch with heartbeat), neck crepitus/swelling
- Investigations
  - Bloods: ↑ WCC/CRP/ESR, ↓ Na, abnormal BSL, ↓ protein
  - Culture, swabs
  - CXR: Suspect if subcutaneous emphysema, left pleural effusion, pneumoperitoneum
  - CT neck and chest
- Management
  - Depends on cause: If well and post endoscopy, for example, often managed conservatively with observation only
  - Resuscitation
    - Airway: Preferably awake fibreoptic intubation before CT. If have to do crashing airway GET HELP
    - Fluids
  - IV antibiotics
    - Piperacillin/tazobactam 4.5 g

      OR
    - Ceftriaxone 2 g (50 mg/kg), metronidazole 500 mg (7.5 mg/kg) and gentamicin (6 mg/kg adjusted)
    - +/– vancomycin 15 mg/kg max. 1.5 g
  - Urgent surgical/ENT consult

Oesophageal perforation/rupture

- Causes
  - Iatrogenic: ETT, endoscopy, operation etc.
  - Trauma: Blunt (e.g. motor vehicle crash [MVC] on a full stomach), penetrating, caustic ingestion
  - Barrett's syndrome, foreign body, infection, tumour, aneurysm
  - Boerhaave's syndrome: Sudden increase in intra-oesophageal pressure; e.g. vomit, birth, strain and cough. Often EtOH background

- Presentation
  - Symptoms: Severe, sudden (in Boerhaave's syndrome), diffuse pain, SOB, cyanosis, haematemesis
  - Signs: Subcutaneous emphysema, peritonism, rigid abdomen, shock, Hamman crunch (crunch with heartbeat—pneumomediastinum)
  - Can be initially subtle, delayed onset; e.g. post trauma—slow development of pain and peritonism as contents leak
- Investigations
  - Bloods: EUC, FBC, G&H, LFT (if EtOH background)
  - CXR: Most abnormal in some way. Left pleural effusion, pneumothorax, pneumomediastinum
  - CT chest for diagnosis and localisation of perforation to guide surgery
  - Don't scope
- Management
  - Resuscitation as required
  - IV antibiotics
    - Ampicillin 1 g, metronidazole 500 mg and gentamicin (5 mg/kg adjusted)
  - Urgent surgical consult or meet them in OT

Ischaemic gut/small bowel ischaemia

- Causes
  - Thrombosis, embolism, atherosclerosis, vasculitis, decreased perfusion; e.g. shock, hypovolaemia
- Presentation
  - History: Ask about vascular risk factors, other vascular disease—IHD/PVD/atherosclerosis, AF, valvular heart disease
  - Symptoms: Abdominal pain usually severe, nausea, vomiting, diarrhoea, can have PR blood
  - Signs: Pain and illness $\gg$ clinical signs or no abdominal signs, peritonism, shock, hypovolaemia, AF, lack of bowel sounds
  - Chronic ischaemia—'gut claudication': Severe, colicky, post prandial pain (usually LLQ), diarrhoea, PR blood
  - Abdominal pain + AF: Beware ischaemic gut!!

- Investigations
  - Bloods: FBC, EUC, LFT, VBG, lipase, +/– coags, G&H
  - ↑ Hb, ↑ WCC, metabolic acidosis, ↑ lactate
  - Normal bloods don't exclude. You don't have to have high lactate!
  - Abdominal x-ray (AXR): Gasless abdomen, thumb print, gas in wall
  - CT angiogram
  - MRI very good but usually not available
- Management
  - Resuscitation as needed
  - IVC, IV fluids, NBM
  - Analgesia, antiemetics as needed
  - IVAB (ampicillin 1 g, gentamicin 3–5 mg/kg adjusted, metronidazole 500 mg)
  - Urgent surgery (remove dead bowel)

Venous thrombosis

- Ask about history of thromboembolic disease, hypercoagulability
- Treat with heparin

Bowel obstruction

- Signs and symptoms: Anorexia, nausea and vomiting, colicky abdominal pain, distension, constipation (may be absolute; i.e. no faeces/flatus), tinkling bowel sound, bowel sounds can be increased
- Causes
  - Small bowel: Adhesion, hernia, Crohn's disease, intussusception, tumour, foreign body, gallstone ileus, radiation, bezoars, abscess
  - Large bowel: Tumour, volvulus, diverticular, stricture
- Investigations
  - Bloods (EUC, FBC, LFT, lipase), erect CXR (exclude perforation), urinalysis (UA), ECG, lactate/VBG (consider ischaemia)
  - Erect and supine AXR
    - Small bowel obstruction (no gas in large bowel, central gas, diameter > 3.0 cm, > 5 fluid levels)
    - Large bowel (gas proximal to block, > 6 cm diameter)

- Note:
  - Small bowel = valvulae conniventes cross lumen, ladder
  - Large bowel = haustra don't cross whole lumen width
- CT abdomen now usually investigation of choice

- Management
  - IV fluids, NBM, NGT, correct electrolytes
  - Surgery
    - URGENT if strangulation (↑↑ pain, ↑ WCC, fever, peritonism)
    - URGENT if large bowel + gross dilation + tender over caecum
- Specific causes
  - Sigmoid volvulus: Bowel twists on mesentery, severe-rapid strangulation
    - Cause: Usually severe chronic constipation
    - Usually elderly and debilitated
    - AXR: Inverted U-shaped loop of bowel, no haustra, absent rectal gas, coffee bean sign
    - Manage with rectal tube decompression, sigmoidoscopy or operation if fails
  - Caecal volvulus
    - Risk factors: Previous abdominal operation, pregnancy, congenital
    - Usually young people
    - AXR: Single gas-filled caecum with air fluid level can be anywhere in abdomen. 1 or 2 haustra. Caecal valve makes distended caecum kidney shaped. Marked distension of small bowel
    - Manage with surgical reduction +/– resection
    - Perforation common, high mortality
  - Stomach volvulus: Gastro-oesophageal obstruction
    - Vomiting/retching, regurgitate saliva, can't pass NG
    - Risk factors: Pyloric stenosis, congenital bands
    - AXR: Gastric dilatation, double fluid level on x-ray
    - Management: Resuscitation, laparotomy

Toxic megacolon

- Causes: IBD, ischaemic gut, pseudomembranous colitis, infection, inflammation
- Assessment
  - Fever, tachycardia, anaemia, shock, abdominal pain, dehydration
  - WCC elevate, abnormal electrolytes
- AXR: Dilated without obstruction > 5.5 cm, caecum > 9 cm, haustra loss, lead pipe colon
- Management: Resuscitation, fluids, may need inotropes, IV piperacillin/tazobactam 4.5 g, NGT and NBM, may need surgery

CHAPTER 6

Orthopaedics and rheumatology

Lower back pain

- Pain below costal margin, above inferior gluteal folds +/– sciatica (sharp/burning radiating down lateral/post leg[s])
- Sciatica usually = herniated lumbar disc or canal stenosis in elderly
- Red flags
    - Trauma
    - Weight ↓
    - Past history of cancer or osteoporosis
    - Fever, infection
    - IVDU
    - Steroid use
    - > 50 years old
    - Severe, night-time pain
    - ↑ pain lying down or at rest OR no ↑ pain with movement
    - Cauda equina syndrome (urine retention/incontinence, bilat neuro signs and symptoms, saddle anaesthesia)
- Examinations (Table 6.1)
    - Posture, spinal tenderness, ROM, abdominal examination, pelvic examination, hip irritability, bedside AAA USS
    - Straight leg raise (elevate straight leg with ankle dorsiflexed; pain radiates down leg = positive sign for nerve root involvement)
    - Signs of nerve root involvement (Table 6.1)
- Management
    - If red flags:
        - Imaging: Plain x-ray/CT/MRI (choice depends on Hx)
        - If neuro/nerve involvement discuss with spinal team
        - Cauda equina = URGENT imaging and spinal team consult
    - No red flags or neuro
        - Explain and reassure; advice: Stay active, avoid bed rest, exercise/physio, heat packs, limit opioid use, imaging if symptoms persist beyond 6 weeks

Table 6.1 Signs of nerve root involvement

Nerve root	Muscle power ↓	Sensation ↓	Reflex ↓/absent
L3/L4	Quadriceps	Anterior/lateral thigh	Knee
L5	Dorsiflex ankle big toe	Dorsum foot	
S1	Plantar flex ankle	Lateral foot	Ankle
Cauda equina	Progressive foot/leg bilat	Saddle	↓ anal tone, distend bladder

    - Increased risk of chronic pain if: Stress, psychiatric PHx, depression, workplace factors
  - Analgesia options
    - Paracetamol, NSAIDs preferred
    - Oxycodone 5–10 mg QID PO but limit opioid use especially on discharge
    - Tramadol (many side effects and drug interactions)

Upper limb

Rotator cuff disease

- Tears, nerve impingement, calcific tendonitis, bursitis, tendinopathy, etc.
- Shoulder +/– lateral arm pain, night pain, can't sleep, pain on resisted shoulder abduction
  - Severe and rapid usually = calcific
  - Impingement = pain on resistance with patient's hand on contralateral shoulder
- X-ray to exclude fracture
- Consider US or MRI to assess ligaments and bursa
- Management
  - Analgesia (paracetamol, NSAID, oxycodone, tramadol, morphine; minimise opioid use)
  - Physiotherapy
  - Some may inject depot steroids with US especially if calcific and night pain
  - Surgery

Adhesive capsulitis (frozen shoulder)

- Usually 50–60 years old, female > male
- Initial slow development, severe disabling shoulder pain: Intermediate stiff phase
- ↓ motion: Recovery phase
- Usually self-limiting over 2–3 years
- Treat symptomatically: Analgesia, short course of steroids

Lateral and medial epicondylitis (tennis, golfers' elbow)

- Pain/tender epicondyle, pain with resisted movements, night pain, stiffness
- Management: Analgesia, NSAIDs PO and topical, injected steroids, acupuncture, surgery

Lower limb

Hip and groin pain

- Red flags
  - Swelling, erythema, ↓↓ ROM, systemic features with no trauma (infection, inflammation)
  - Rapid swelling post trauma (haemarthrosis)
  - Pain +/– abnormal sensation +/– changed reflexes + ↓ power (radiculopathy)
  - Persistent, localised, no change with movement (bone disease)
  - Diffuse, no other signs (somatic referred)
  - Steroid use, EtOH abuse (atraumatic avascular necrosis)
  - Trauma, fracture head/neck femur (traumatic avascular necrosis)
- Most common cause: Arthritis
- Fracture neck of femur (NOF): Can't weight bear (can if impacted subcapital) externally rotated + short leg
- Investigate with x-rays hip/pelvis, other imaging (e.g. CT), bloods—FBC, ESR, CRP, UA
- Management: Depends on cause—analgesia including fascia iliaca block; if concerned about septic joint/infection consult ortho prior to antibiotics
  - Consult ortho

Knee pain

- General treatment with rest, ice, compression and elevation (RICE), NSAIDs

- Red flags as with hip pain
- Atraumatic: Monoarthritis causes, acute atraumatic haemarthrosis (consider if on warfarin), infection (aspirate joint [see arthrocentesis, p. 58] and test—microscopy, culture and sensitivity [MCS])
- Traumatic—x-ray if any of the following (Ottawa knee rules): Age ≥ 55, isolated patella tenderness, fibular head tenderness, unable to flex 90 degrees, unable to bear weight immediately and in ED.

Meniscal tear

- Rotatory movement on semi-flexed knee. Medial joint line tender, effusion, ↓ flex, McMurray test (flex knee, extension and rotation—positive result if clunk/click felt), Apley's grind test. Orthopaedic review URGENT if true 'locked' knee otherwise 1/52

Collateral ligament tear

- Valgus (medial collateral) or varus (lateral collateral) force to knee. Local tenderness, swelling, pain with valgus/varus stress with knee 20-degree flex
- Treatment: Brace, physio
- Complete tear/unstable needs surgery

Anterior cruciate injury

- Marked valgus stress or injury post landing from a jump
- Rapid effusion, haemarthrosis
- Lachman test most sensitive (knee flex 15–20 degrees, stabilise femur, draw tibia forward, excess translation and lack of firm end point = positive compared with other side). Other tests: Pivot shift, anterior draw (least sensitive)
- Investigations: X-ray, MRI. (Note: 70% of haemarthroses due to ACL injury; Segond fracture (#) on x-ray suggest ACL injury)
- Management: Physio, analgesia +/– reconstruction

Posterior cruciate injury

- Rarely isolated. Associated with hip injury/dislocation, femur and tibia fractures
- Godfrey's sign (both legs, hips, knees at 90 degrees; look for knee sag/lag), posterior draw test

Knee pain and swelling

Bakers cyst

- Herniation of chronic knee effusion between 2 heads of gastrocnemius
  - Posterior knee joint mass +/– tenderness
  - Multiple causes: Must look for underlying pathology

Bursitis

- See p. 127 for details
- Semimembranosus bursitis and prepatellar bursitis
  - Consider gout and infection

Lower leg

- Red flags as before
  - **Ruptured Baker's cyst**: Causes acute calf pain. Look for effusion, exclude DVT
  - **Compartment syndrome**: See Compartment syndrome, p. 139

Ankle

- Red flags
- Usually trauma associated
- X-ray as per Ottawa = malleolar pain + bony tenderness tibia/fibula or can't weight bear
- Treat non-fracture with RICE, analgesia +/– physio

Ruptured Achilles tendon

- Usually male > 40 years old
- Acute pain in lower leg usually post rapid acceleration; e.g. squash, sprint. May hear snap
- Other associations/causes: Rheumatoid arthritis (RA), CRF, SLE, steroids, AB/fluoroquinolones (ciprofloxacin)
- Tear may be partial
- Can't weight bear, can't stand on toes
- Rapid swelling at site of rupture
- Examination: Palpable defect/discontinuity of tendon and weak or no plantar flex with resistance. Thompson test (with patient prone, squeezing calf should cause plantar flex if Achilles intact)
- Investigate with US, x-ray if need to exclude fracture
- Management: Controversial—discuss with local ortho, equinus cast, consider DVT prophylaxis

Ruptured quadriceps tendon

- Divot in thigh proximal to patella
- Unable to straight leg raise. Needs operation

Bursitis

- Fluctuant, warm swelling
- Mild pain. Exclude infective bursitis
- Aspirate with US to differentiate septic verses aseptic

- DON'T aspirate the joint!!
- Management usually conservative
- **Semimembranosus bursitis**: medial side popliteal fossa. Look for knee joint pathology
- **Prepatellar bursitis**: Anterior to patella post trauma acute/chronic

Fractures

- Always look for:
  - Lipohaemarthrosis (knee x-ray)
  - Avulsion fracture
  - Fat pads (e.g. sail sign)
  - Joint above and below in significant injury
  - Effusions
- Describing a fracture
  - Open/closed
  - Side (left/right)
  - Site (bone; prox, mid, distal)
  - Fracture line (transverse, oblique, spiral)
  - Comminuted (> 2 fragments), impacted, intraarticular (involves articular surface)
  - Deformity, displaced (anterior [ant], lateral [lat] etc.)
  - Angulation (direction of tilt of the distal fragment)
  - Rotation
- Is distal limb neurovascularly intact?
- Salter-Harris classification in children where fracture involves the physis (growth plate). To remember use S-A-L-T-eR (Table 6.2)
- ALWAYS consider admission for: Calcaneal fracture, supracondylar humerus, femoral
- ALWAYS discuss: Comminuted, intraarticular, open, deformed, associated dislocations, pain out of proportion, abnormal neurovascular exam
- Neurovascular assessment
  - Pulses, capillary refill, warmth: Compare with opposite side
    - Axillary nerve: Lateral sensation shoulder
    - Musculocutaneous nerve: Extensor forearm
  - Other nerves for assessment depending on fracture site (Fig. 6.1)
- Specific fractures and general management (Table 6.3)

Table 6.2 Salter-Harris classification

Salter-Harris 1 (S = straight across): Separation through physeal plate (x-ray may be normal)	
Salter-Harris 2 (A = above): # through some of the physis then extends through metaphysis (above the physis)	
Salter-Harris 3 (L = lower/below): # through some of the physis then extends though epiphysis (below the physis) and into joint	
Salter-Harris 4 (T = through): # through the metaphysis, physis and epiphysis	
Salter-Harris 5 (eR = rammed): crush injury. Direct damage to part or all of physis. May be no displacement—may miss it!	

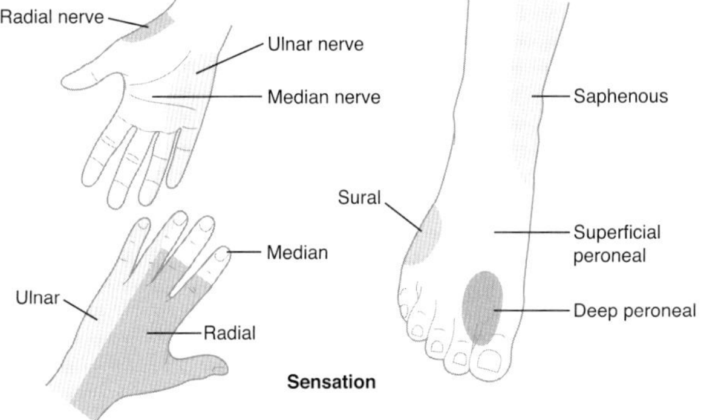

Figure 6.1 Other nerves for assessment depending on fracture site

Table 6.3 General management for specific fractures
NOTE: Practice will vary with different institutions and specialists

Fracture	Definition, classification and complications	Management
Jones	Transverse#base of 5th metatarsal Cx: Non-union	• Discuss with ortho • May need operation
Clavicle	A = middle ⅓ (most) B = outer ⅓ (classed 1–5) C = inner ⅓ Cx: Non-union, chronic pain, dissatisfaction of patient	• Comminuted, skin tented or significantly displaced: Need ortho • High variability in management
Surgical neck of humerus	Minimally displaced • 2 parts • 3 parts • 4 parts	• Majority non-operative management • Involvement of greater tuberosity, lesser tuberosity and articular surface, or multiple parts: Discuss with ortho
Mid-shaft humerus	Oblique, spiral or transverse Cx: Radial nerve palsy, neuropraxia, entrapment	• Operation if angulated, nerve palsy, multi-trauma, open#, pathologcal#, floating elbow
Supracondylar humerus	On a normal x-ray, radial shaft line should intersect capitellum, anterior humeral line should intersect with capitellum Gartland classification I = undisplaced (look for fat pad/sail sign) II = displaced, posterior intact (look at anterior humeral line) III = disrupted anterior and posterior Cx: Nerve injury (ulnar, radial and medial), brachial artery injury	• Admit all II and III • Need operation. True emergency if significant displacement or compromised
Epicondylar	Medial (50% associated with dislocation) Lateral (very prone to moving)	• Ortho review

Table 6.3 General management for specific fractures *NOTE: Practice will vary with different institutions and specialists—cont'd*

Fracture	Definition, classification and complications	Management
Radial head	Mason classification 1 = no/minimum displacement, no mechanical block to rotation 2 = displaced > 2 mm, suspecting block to rotation, angulation 3 = comminuted, block to motion 4 = + elbow dislocation	• Type 1 immobilisation • All others likely to need operation; consult ortho
Olecranon	Mayo classification 1 = not displaced 2 = displaced and ulnohumeral joint stable 3 = displaced and unstable ulnohumeral joint	• Type 1 immobilisation • All others likely operation needed, consult ortho
Radius/ulnar shaft fractures	OTA classification A = simple ulnar A1, radius A2, both A3 B = wedge ulnar B1, radius B2, both B3 C = complex fracture 'Nightstick' = isolated midshaft ulnar	• Isolated, non-displaced, non-angulated, distal ulnar#usually no operation needed • All other ulnar#and all radial shaft usually need operation
Monteggia	#proximal ulnar, dislocated head of radius	• Open reduction internal fixation (ORIF)
Galeazzi	#mid-radius, dislocated ulnar/ radius distally	• ORIF
Essex-Lopresti	#radial head, dislocated ulnar/ radius distally	• ORIF
Colles	#distal radius, transverse dorsal angulation/displaced hand Cx: Stiffness, median nerve compression, malunion, delayed union, compartment syndrome, extensor pollicis longus (EPL) rupture, complex regional pain syndrome	• ORIF if: tilt > 20 degrees, displaced > 1 cm, radius shortened > 5 mm, comminuted, intraarticular
Smith's	Reverse Colles' fracture, volar displacement	• Consult ortho

Continued

Table 6.3 General management for specific fractures
NOTE: Practice will vary with different institutions and specialists—cont'd

Fracture	Definition, classification and complications	Management
Barton's	Either a Colles' or a Smith's#; where the radius fracture extends intraarticularly	• Consult ortho
Hutchinson/ Chauffeur	Radial styloid#extends to radiocarpal joint. Associated with carpal dislocations	• Consult ortho
Scaphoid fracture	Need specific views Cx: Avascular necrosis, non-union, missed Dx	• Consult ortho • Thumb spica cast
Bennett's	Thumb fracture, extends to joint, dislocated carpo-metacarpal joint	• Consult ortho
Roland's	Comminuted#base of 1st metacarpal	• Consult ortho
Skier's thumb	#proximal phalanx ulnar collateral	• May need operation
Neck of femur	Intracapsular: 1 = incomplete, 2 = complete, 3 = displaced, 4 = fragments Extracapsular: 1 = non-displaced, 2–5 = displaced with 2, 3, 4 parts Cx: Operation related, medical (UTI, LRTI), avascular necrosis, non-union	• Ortho review • 1 and 2: Screws • 3 and 4: Hemiarthroplasty
Greater trochanter	1 = No intertrochanteric#, not displaced 2 = > 1 cm displaced	• Conservative • ORIF
Femoral shaft	1 = not comminuted, 2 = comminuted 3 = severe 4 = all contact lost Cx: Bleeding into tissue, fat embolism, compartment syndrome, delayed/non/mal union, limb shortening	• Ortho review • Usually nails • Manage blood loss
Supracondylar	A = extraarticular B = unicondylar C = bicondylar	• Ortho and operation

Table 6.3 General management for specific fractures
NOTE: Practice will vary with different institutions and specialists—cont'd

Fracture	Definition, classification and complications	Management
Tibial plateau (oblique and tunnel x-ray views)	1 = wedge#, lateral plateau 2 = type 1 + depression 3 = pure depression, no# 4 = medial plateau# 5 = wedge#medial and lateral 6—tibial shaft and plateau Cx early: Popliteal artery injury, compartment syndrome, tibial nerve injury, DVT Late: Osteoarthritis (OA), malunion, stiff knee, deformity Associated ligament injuries: Medial plateau—posterior cruciate ligament (PCL) and lateral collateral ligament (LCL); lateral plateau—anterior cruciate ligament (ACL) and medial collateral ligament (MCL)	• 1: Conservative • 2: Review, consider operation • 3: Conservative • 4: Operation (worst prognosis) • 5: Operation • 6: Operation
Segond (need tunnel x-ray)	Small avulsion# proximal lateral tibia = capsular ligament tear and ACL tear. Most tear meniscus	• Operation
Patella (skyline view)	Undisplaced, comminuted Displaced	• Zimmer • ORIF
Tibial shaft	A = simple (spiral, oblique, transverse) B = wedge (spiral, bend, fragments) C = complex (spiral, segment, irregular) Toddler's = spiral Cx: Peroneal nerve injury, vascular compromise, compartment syndrome, infection, non-union	• Ortho review for possible operation • Can't cast if shortened or tibia #and fibula okay
Fibula	Rare in isolation. Look for tibia#	• Conservative

Continued

Table 6.3 General management for specific fractures
NOTE: Practice will vary with different institutions and specialists—cont'd

Fracture	Definition, classification and complications	Management

Ankle	Weber A = fibula#below level of syndesmosis
	B = #at level of syndesmosis
	C = #above syndesmosis
	Alternative classification:
	• Unimalleolar (medial or lateral)
	• Bimalleolar (medial and lateral)
	• Trimalleolar (medial, lateral and posterior tibia)
		• A: Usually conservative
		• B & C: Consult ortho
		• Unimalleolar: Consult ortho
		• Bimalleolar: Operation
		• Trimalleolar: Always operate

Maisonneuve	Proximal fibula#with ruptured intraosseous membrane	• Consult ortho
Dupuytren's#	Maisonneuve + disrupted syndesmosis	• Consult ortho
Wagstaffe-Le Fort	Avulsion#distal fibula	• Consult ortho
Tillaux-Caput	Avulsion#tibia	• Consult ortho
Talar neck	1 = non-displaced 2 = displaced + sublux/ dislocated subtalar (ankle normal) 3 = displaced (dislocated subtalar and ankle) Cx: Avascular necrosis. 10% of type 1, 30% type 2, 90% type 3	• All usually need operation
Calcaneal (look at Böhler's angle)	A = anterior B = middle C = posterior Cx: Swelling, neurovascular (high risk of other injury and fractures [e.g. pelvis, spine, limb], Lover's triad = forearm#, lumbar compression#and calcaneal#)	• Deferred operation, admit and elevate all
Lisfranc (see also Dislocations, p. 135)	Horizontal: All 5 metatarsals move in same direction Partial: 1 or 2 displaced Divergent: 1st metatarsal moves medially, others move laterally Cx: High risk pain and disability	• Ortho review for all

Dislocations

- Shoulder: X-ray pre-reduction if > 40 years old, suspected fracture, trauma, 1st episode. Otherwise can consider reducing first. For x-ray changes see Table 6.4
  - Anterior dislocation (95%)
    - Examination: Arm abducted, held by patient, loss of shoulder roundness. Inferior to acromion feels empty. Head may be palpable subcoracoid. Assess neurovascular
    - Associated injuries: Rotator cuff, greater tuberosity #, artery compromise, Bankart (avulsion anterior glenoid), Hill–Sachs (compression # head)
    - Complications: Brachial plexus injury, axillary nerve injury
  - Posterior dislocations
    - Injury mechanism: Electricity, seizure, anterior blow
    - Examination: Internal rotation and adduction, fullness posterior shoulder
    - Associated injuries: Reverse Bankart (# posterior glenoid), reverse Hill–Sachs (anterior, medial compression #)
    - Complications: Acute re-dislocation, osteonecrosis
  - Inferior dislocations: Luxation erecta
    - Examination: Severe pain, arm abducted, hand stuck overhead, head inferior to glenoid (can look like anterior but shaft will be parallel to scapula)
    - Complications: High # rate, 80% rotator cuff injury, 60% nerve injury especially axillary
    - Management: Urgent reduction, will need deep sedation

Table 6.4 X-ray changes with shoulder dislocations

Dislocation type	AP x-ray	Oblique armpit x-ray	Y view x-ray
Anterior dislocation	Humerus head moved DOWN (subcoracoid, subclavicular or subglenoid)	Golf ball off tee, moved down and in	Humerus medial to Y
Pseudosubluxation	Haemarthroses		
Post dislocation	Light bulb, wide glenohumeral space	Golf ball off tee, moved up and out	Humerus lateral to Y

- When to reduce in ED
    - Simple anterior dislocation
    - Use procedural sedation if required and safe to do so
    - Usually do not relocate posterior dislocations (should discuss with ortho first, usually harder to reduce), inferior dislocations need urgent reduction in OT
    - Usually do not relocate dislocated shoulder if suspected fracture surgical neck
    - NEVER REDUCE A CHRONIC DISLOCATION. Dislocation for > 4 weeks has significant risk of vascular injury on reduction
    - Always assess nerves pre and post reduction (median, axillary, radial, ulnar)
- Methods of reduction: Shoulder reduction (see procedures, p. 53)

- Hip
    - Posterior (80–90%)
        - Mechanisms: Prosthetic, major trauma
        - Examination: Leg shortened, adducted, internally rotate
        - X-ray: Femur superior and lateral (pushed up and out)
        - Reduction: Can usually reduce prosthetic in ED
        - Complications: Acetabular #, sciatic nerve injury, arthritis
    - Methods of reduction: Posterior dislocation (see procedures, p. 54)
    - Central dislocation
        - # through acetabulum
        - Need general anaesthetic and operation
    - Anterior dislocation
        - Mechanisms: Usually MVC
        - Examination: External rotation, abduction, flexion
        - X-ray: Femoral head inferior and medial (down and in)
        - Consult ortho
- Knee
    - URGENT consult!
    - Often spontaneously reduce pre-hospital
    - Must suspect this injury as there is a high rate of complications
    - Cx: Popliteal artery and vein, compartment syndrome, ligament injury and peroneal nerve injury

   - If reduction is delayed > 8 hours: Significant risk of needing amputation
   - Management: URGENT
      - Assess for vascular injury: Will need angiography
      - Reduce with longitudinal traction. Usually easy to reduce
- Patella
   - Usually lateral
   - Examination: Knee flexed, internally rotated. Patella apprehension sign
   - Management: Reduce with medial pressure and knee extension
   - Cast or Zimmer splint unless injury is recurrent
- Ankle
   - URGENT
   - Relocate quickly before there is neurovascular compromise
   - Most dislocations posterior
   - Grasp toes, traction on foot
   - Continue traction post reduction while applying backslab
   - Need operation
- Lisfranc injuries
   - Mechanisms: High-velocity MVC, fall off horse with foot caught in stirrup
   - Involve 2nd metatarsal joint
   - Examination: May be normal. Midfoot pain, swelling, passive movement supine or prone causes pain
   - X-ray: Gap between 1st and 2nd metatarsal bases
   - Suspect if x-ray not following normal patterns of alignment
      - Medial edge of base of 2nd metatarsal aligns with medial 2nd cuneiform
      - Lateral edge of 3rd metatarsal aligns with lateral edge lateral cuneiform
      - Oblique: 2nd and 3rd metatarsal spaces continuous with space between lateral and medial cuneiform. Medial 4th metatarsal aligns with medial cuboid
      - Metatarsal should never be more distal than tarsals
   - Associated fractures: Base of 2nd metatarsal, 3rd metatarsal, 1st/2nd cuneiform, navicular

- Classified
  - Horizontal: All 5 metatarsals move in same direction
  - Partial: 1 or 2 displaced
  - Divergent: 1st metatarsal moves medially, others move laterally
- Complications: Arthritis, disability, non-union

- Radiocarpal dislocations
  - Lunate dislocation
    - Mechanism: Fallen onto an outstretched hand (FOOSH), MVC, usually young adult
    - X-ray: AP—disrupted Gilula lines, lunate overlaps, looks like a piece of pie. Terry-Thomas sign—increased distance between the scaphoid and the lunate. Lateral—lunate has appearance of crescent moon or spilled teacup
    - Urgent reduction
  - Perilunate dislocation
    - Mechanism: High energy, young adult
    - X-ray: AP—disrupted Gilula lines, lunate overlaps capitate. Lateral—radius and lunate remain in line. Lunate does not intersect capitate
    - 60% associated with scaphoid fracture
- Sternoclavicular (SC) and acromioclavicular (AC) dislocations
  - Sternoclavicular joint dislocation
    - Mechanisms: MVC, sport, direct blow, FOOSH
    - Anterior: Can't abduct shoulder, head turned to injury. On x-ray clavicular head looks magnified. Usually need operation
    - Posterior: Anterior chest tender and swollen, may have cough/SOB/dysphagia/dysphonia. Complications include vascular compromise, tracheo-oesophageal fistula, nerve injury. Need CT and general anaesthetic reduction
  - AC joint dislocation
    - Mechanisms: Fall on shoulder
    - Clinically deformed
    - X-ray: AC joint > 6 mm or > 2–3 mm different to other side

Hand injuries

- Jersey finger
  - Flexor digitorum profundus rupture
  - Mechanisms: Object pulled from grasp
  - Examination: Can't flex distal interphalangeal (DIP) joint, can flex at proximal interphalangeal (PIP) joint
  - Management: Needs operation
- Central slip rupture
  - Mechanism: Associated with PIP dislocation
  - Examination: Tender PIP, +/– Boutonnière deformity
  - Management: Reduce and splint
- Mallet finger
  - Mechanism: Sudden flexion, rupture of extensor tendon
  - Examination: Can't extend distal phalanx
  - Management: Operation if penetrating or # otherwise splint
- Digit amputation
  - History: Injury mechanism, ischaemia time, occupation, handedness, comorbidities (e.g. smoker, diabetes)
  - Investigations/management
    - Wrap parts in saline-soaked gauze, place in bag, put sealed bag in very cold water (around 4°C)
    - X-ray all parts
    - ADT (may need tetanus immune globulin [Tet Ig]), antibiotics (e.g. cefazolin 1 g TDS IV)
    - OT indications: Thumb or index finger, multiple fingers, child, distal phalanx
    - Relative contraindications to operation: Other severe injury taking priority, chronic disease, age > 50 years, crush, contaminated, delayed cooling, very proximal injuries

Compartment syndrome

- Causes
  - Fractures: Usually closed, tibia, humerus, radius/ulnar, supracondylar
  - Soft tissue injury: Crush, snake bite, exertion, immobilisation, constrictive plaster/bandage, infection, seizure, burn, tourniquet, extravasation

  - Increased risk: Coagulopathy, young male, anabolic steroid use, muscular individual
- Examination
  - Pain: With passive stretch, pain not improved with immobilisation, pain out of proportion
  - Pallor
  - Perishingly cold
  - Pulseless (late sign)
  - Paralysis
  - Paraesthesia (on 2-point discrimination)
  - Tense, swollen compartment
  - For anterior leg: Weak toe extension, back pain with passive toe flexion, decreased sensation 1st toe space
  - For posterior leg: Weak toe flexion, pain with passive toe extension, decreased sensation sole
- Diagnosis
  - Measure the pressure: Stryker device or angiocath and arterial line
    - Stryker: 3 mL saline in syringe, connect to chamber and then to needle. Remove air from chamber by injecting the saline (leave no air in chamber), put in Stryker device, close drawer, zero device (holding at angle you will insert in patient). Insert into compartment, inject small amount of saline (< 0.5 mL) and see pressure rise
    - Anterior compartment lower limb: 1 cm lateral to anterior border of tibia, at the junction of the proximal and middle thirds of the lower leg. Depth 1–3 cm. Confirm location—plantarflex foot should increase pressure
    - Posterior compartment lower limb: Just medial to medial border of tibia at the junction of the proximal and middle thirds of the lower leg. Depth 2–4 cm. Confirm location—toe extension should increase pressure
    - Others: Forearm dorsal and volar, lateral leg, superficial thigh
  - Diagnosis: Pressure > 30 mmHg (normal 0–10) or delta pressure < 30 mmHg
    - Delta pressure = diastolic BP – compartment pressure
- Management
  - URGENT ORTHO REVIEW
  - Treat cause if able; e.g. remove plaster, reduce fracture

  - Elevate limb
  - Fasciotomy
- Complications
  - Gangrene, ischaemic contracture, loss of function, rhabdomyolysis, renal failure, amputation

Fat embolism syndrome

- Fat embolism syndrome = multi-organ dysfunction. Rare
- Causes
  - Long bone fractures, CPR, severe burns, liver injury, bone marrow transplant, liposuction, pancreatitis, total parenteral nutrition
- Clinical picture
  - ARDS-like: Hypoxia, increased RR, haemoptysis
  - Petechial rash: Usually anterior chest, axillae
  - Neurological: Confusion, altered GCS. Often transient
  - Cardiovascular: Hypotension, tachycardia
  - Other: DIC, anaemia, renal compromise, hepatic compromise
  - Investigations
  - Bloods: ↓ platelets, ↓ Hb, DIC, elevated ESR, elevated alveolar–arterial (A–a) gradient
  - Fat seen in urine, blood, sputum
  - CXR: ARDS-like, bilateral opacities
  - Other imaging: CT, MRI, TOE; may show changes
- Management
  - Prevent with early fixation of fractures
  - Supportive, ICU

Crush injuries

- Causes
  - Trauma: Limb #, compression, electrocution, burns, long lie, immobilisation
  - External compression: Plaster, military antishock trousers (MAST) suit
- Complications: Rhabdomyolysis, compartment syndrome, fluid loss, ulcerations

Rhabdomyolysis

- Skeletal muscular injury causing intracellular contents released (myoglobin, CK, LDH, K^+ etc.)
- Causes
    - Direct muscle injury: Crush, electrical, ischaemia, post ischaemia, compartment syndrome
    - Drugs of abuse: EtOH, amphetamines, cocaine, opiates, caffeine, withdrawal
    - Medications: Benzodiazepines, steroids, lithium, narcotics, tricyclic antidepressants, statins, theophylline
    - Excessive muscle activity: Sport, seizure, psychosis, dystonia
    - Genetic and immune: Glycolysis disorder, polymyositis
    - Infection: Sepsis, necrotising fasciitis, toxic shock, clostridium, group A *Streptococcus* (GAS), salmonella, Legionnaire's disease, *Streptococcus pneumoniae*, *Staphylococcus aureus*. Viral: CMV, EBV, HIV, hepatitis
    - Toxins; e.g. snake envenomation
    - Thermal and endocrine: Neuroleptic malignant syndrome, malignant hyperthermia, serotonin syndrome, environmental, thyroid storm, ↓↑ Ca, ↓ K^+, ↓↑ phosphate
    - Others: Acute respiratory failure (ARF), ↑ uric acid, DIC, peripheral neuropathy
- Signs and symptoms: Myalgia, stiff, weak, low fever, dark urine, nausea and vomiting, ↑ HR, abdominal pain, mental change, tender swollen muscle, red muscles
    - Can be asymptomatic
- Investigations
    - CK > 1000, usually > 10,000 (rises at 2–12 hours, peaks at 24–72 hours post injury)
    - ↑ myoglobin/myoglobinuria (note: Dipstick will show positive blood, no RBC on analysis)
    - EUC: Renal impairment, ↑ K, ↑ phosphate, ↑ uric acid, ↓ Ca
    - ↓ albumin, coagulants (can indicate DIC), ↑ LDH
    - Imaging/MRI to localise
- Management
    - Treat the cause
    - Fluid resuscitation, IDC to monitor fluid balance
    - If anuric: Haemodialysis, replace losses, restore euvolaemia

- If oliguric: Aim for high urine output (e.g. > 2 mL/kg/hr), IV fluids, consider mannitol, CVP monitoring, avoid overload, alkalinise urine (e.g. HCO_3^- 50 mmol/hr titrated to urine pH), aim urine pH > 7, may need dialysis
- If decreasing urine output and euvolaemic consider dopamine
- Monitor electrolytes, urine pH and calcium
- Treat ↑ K^+
- Avoid suxamethonium

Gout

- **Acute**
  - 1st attack usually 1 joint, acute, often big toe
  - History/exam: Joint is very painful, red, swollen; pain usually onset over hours, maximum 6–12 hours. No systemic symptoms
  - Risk factors: Male, familial, chemotherapy, psoriasis, renal transplant, EtOH, diuretics, renal disease
  - Investigations: X-ray/US, urate level (< 0.45 mmol/L makes gout highly unlikely in untreated patients), FBC (↑ WCC without toxic changes), LFT, CRP/ESR (slight ↑), joint aspirate (see procedures for arthrocentesis, p. 58; fluid is cloudy, yellow, WBC 2000–50,000, polymorphonuclear/PMN cells > 50%, needle shaped negative birefringent crystals)
  - If age < 30 always investigate cause
  - Always consider and exclude septic arthritis
- Management
  - NSAIDs; e.g. indomethacin 50 mg PO TDS for 3–5/7 then 25 mg TDS until resolved
  - Colchicine 0.5 mg TDS PO on the first day then daily or BD until symptoms resolve
  - Consider prednisone PO (e.g. 25 mg daily for 3/7) unless contraindicated or intraarticular steroids
  - LMO follow-up: Address lifestyle, diet
  - Prophylaxis: Allopurinol 50 mg daily ↑ by 50 mg each week to 300 mg daily
- **Chronic gout**
  - Recurring attacks eventually fail to completely resolve: Crippling destructive arthritis, gouty tophi (elbows, knees, peripheral joints)
  - Can use steroids if other treatment fails
  - Note: MUST use allopurinol **with** NSAID or colchicine cover

- **Pseudogout** (calcium pyrophosphate deposition disease)
  - Presents like gout—knee most common joint, can be polyarthropathy
  - Investigate with joint aspirate (rhomboid-positive birefringent crystals), bloods, x-ray (calcific intraarticular cartilage)
  - Treat with indomethacin or colchicine + paracetamol
    - Can use steroids if resistant

Septic arthritis

- Risk factors: RA, IVDU, diabetes mellitus, prosthesis, immune suppression, age > 80, superficial infection
- Presentation: Post trauma or spontaneous monoarticular arthritis, joint swelling, red, pain, fever, systemically unwell. Usually gradual onset
- Investigations
  - Bloods: Cultures, EUC, FBC (WCC > 11), CRP, ESR > 30
  - Joint aspirate (see arthrocentesis, p. 53): Fluid is cloudy, yellow, WCC > 50,000, PMN cells > 50–80%, no crystals. Await culture. Get ortho opinion prior to performing if hardware in joint
  - Imaging: X-ray
  - Diagnosis: Kocher criteria—non-weight bear, WCC > 12, ESR > 40, fever > 38.5
- IVAB (usually *Staphylococcus aureus*): Often ortho want to do washout and take samples in OT prior to antibiotics
  - Empiric = flucloxacillin 2 g (50 mg/kg) IV QID if septic and can't wait for OT
  - Add ceftriaxone 2 g daily IV if suspect Gram-negative or gonococcal
  - Adjust to cultures
  - Add gentamicin in IVDU, children
- Surgical review, drainage URGENT

Osteomyelitis

- Risk factors: IVDU (sternoclavicular, vertebral), diabetes mellitus, alcoholics, chronic steroids, neonate, sickle cell anaemia, open fractures, chronic ulcers, elderly, urine/bladder procedures, gonorrhoea

- Investigations
  - X-ray; progression: Soft tissue swelling—periosteal new bone formation—focal bone radiolucency—joint effusion
  - ↑ WBC, cultures ↑ ESR/CRP
  - MRI (if spinal) +/or CT +/or bone scan
- Child versus adult (Table 6.5)

Polyarthritis

Table 6.6 compares the more common types of polyarthritis and their typical features.

Giant cell arteritis

See Facial pain, p. 161.

Table 6.5 Osteomyelitis in children versus adults

Child	Adult
Usually long bone—hip, knee	Usually axial
Usually haematogenous spread	Usually direct spread
Usually no underlying cause	Usually underlying disease
Most—*S. aureus*	Most—*S. aureus*
Other—GAS, Hib, *Enterobacter*	Others—GAS, Hib, *Enterobacter*, gonorrhoea, *E. coli*, salmonella (sickle cell anaemia)
Symptoms: • Infant—Failure to thrive, swelling can be hidden • Child—increased pain over hours, fever, look unwell, not using limb, pain with hip rotation	Symptoms: Local pain, tenderness, increased with movement
Management: • Flucloxacillin 50 mg/kg (max. 2 g) IV QID • If < 5 years old add ceftriaxone 50 mg/kg IV daily (or cefotaxime)	Management: • Flucloxacillin 2 g QID IV • If suspect MRSA add vancomycin 1 g BD IV, if suspect Gram-negative add cefotaxime or ceftriaxone 2 g daily IV

Table 6.6 Features of the more common types of polyarthritis

Osteoarthritis	Rheumatoid arthritis	Ankylosing spondylitis	Reiter's syndrome
Universal age > 70 years; associated with obesity; genetics	Female > male, age 40–50 years, genetics	Age 15–40 years; genetics; associated with Reiter's syndrome, IBD, *Yersinia*	Associated with urethritis/cervicitis or dysentery (chlamydia, salmonella, *Yersinia*, mycoplasma, genetics) within 1 month
Gradual onset. Pain with exercise. Morning stiffness improves < 30 min	Insidious. Morning stiffness +++ longer duration. Symmetrical. C1/C2 sublux, popliteal cyst. Extraarticular—heart, lungs, vessels, ocular, nodules	Mild constant symptoms, sacroiliac (SI) joint always involved, +/– hips and shoulders. Pain back/butt/chest. Extraarticular features—heart, ocular, pulmonary fibrosis	Onset days to weeks, recurrence common. Asymmetrical. Extraarticular—ocular, aortic root dilatation, mucocutaneous ulcer, rash
Ex: Joint enlarged, ↓ ROM, crepitus, nodes Bouchard (PIP) and Heberden's (DIP)	Ex: MCP, wrist, knee warm/tender/swell, deformity (Boutonnière, swan neck)	Ex: Tender SI joint, decreased chest expansion	Ex: Asymmetric arthritis usually lower limbs, sausage-shaped fingers, conjunctivitis or iritis, genital ulceration
X-ray: Narrow irregular joint space, ↑ subchondral bone, pseudocyst, osteophyte	X-ray: Narrow joint space, erosion, subchondral destruction. Blood: Rh Fc, ↓ Alb, CRP, ↓ Hb, LFT abnormal	X-ray: SI blurred, bamboo spine (only see abnormal x-ray after years). Blood: Rh factor negative, ESR ↑	X-ray: Erosion, narrow joint, syndesmophytes, spurs. Blood: Rh factor negative, ESR ↑, WCC ↑
Mx: Analgesia, weight loss, exercise	Mx: Support, disease-modifying antirheumatic drugs (DMARDs), operation	Mx: Analgesia, NSAIDs, physio	Mx: NSAIDS, steroids

CHAPTER 7

Neurology

Headache

- Concerning headache patterns (Table 7.1)
- History and examination
  - History
    - Onset, pattern, location, associated symptoms, trauma, medications, toxins, PHx, FHx
  - Examination
    - Vitals, palpate (sinus, temporomandibular joint and temporal artery), check dentition, eye exam, ear exam, fundoscopy, full neuro exam, meningism, Kernig's sign, and usual cardio, respiratory and abdominal exam
  - **Red flags**
    - Onset: Sudden or exertional. Onset after the age of 50
    - Associated symptoms: Neurology, papillo-oedema, mental state change, seizure, systemic symptoms, fever, vision change, pain with cough/straining, pain positional
    - Associated conditions: Pregnancy (including postpartum), SLE, Behçet's disease, cancer, sarcoid, vasculitis
    - PHx: No previous headache history (i.e. new headache), pain significantly different from previous headaches, recent trauma
    - Medications: Anticoagulants/antiplatelets, recent antibiotic use, immune suppressants, drugs (e.g. cocaine), toxicology

Specific headaches

Tension

- Recurrent, bilateral, heavy/band-like around head +/– photophobia. Nausea and vomiting rare. Secondary to contraction masseter or neck muscles. Females ≫ males

Migraine

- Recurrent, throbbing, often unilateral, severe, associated photophobia, nausea and vomiting, limits activity
  - Features
    - POUNDing: Pulsating, Onset gradual 4–72 hours, Unilateral, Nausea, Disabling

- o Aura: Focal neurology; usually visual; can have unilateral weakness, sensory and speech change and mimic stroke. Last 5–60 minutes. Can occur without headache. Most migraines don't have aura

Table 7.1 Headache patterns and possible causes

Headache patterns	Possible causes
Sudden onset; associated confusion, drowsy, vomit, stroke-like neurology	SAH, ICH, vertebral artery dissection, cerebral venous thrombosis
Recent onset; Confusion, drowsy, fever	Meningitis, encephalitis, abscess, severe hypertension
Recent onset; young, obese	Idiopathic intracranial hypertension (AKA BIH [benign intracranial hypertension])
Recent onset; patient > 50	Tumour, giant cell arteritis, subdural, herpes, medications, cervicogenic, sinusitis
Recent onset with cough, exertion or sex	SAH, tumour
Post head injury especially if LOC	ICH
Associated with: • pregnancy • HT • vision loss	 • preeclampsia • malignant hypertension, phaeochromocytoma • glaucoma

Cluster

- Male ≫ female. Age 30–50 years. Centred around orbit, autonomic symptoms (ptosis, tearing, red eyes, stuffy nose), seasonal
  - Lasts 15–180 minutes. Multiple attacks each day for weeks or months

Abnormal CSF pressure

- Intracranial hypotension; e.g. post LP. Headache resolves with lying down
- Benign/idiopathic intracranial hypertension: Pain with cough, bending or valsalva. Due to raised ICP. Examine for papillo-oedema. Associated with obesity. Management: Refer to neurologist

- Neoplasm
- Head trauma
- Postconcussion syndrome—associated symptoms: Dizziness, tinnitus, blurred vision, depression, memory loss, insomnia. May last months
- Hydrocephalus
  - Adult: Increased ICP symptoms, altered level of consciousness, incontinence, symptoms of cause
  - Child: Abnormal feeding, high pitched cry, seizure, large head, thin scalp, tense fontanelle, sclera visible above iris = setting-sun sign

Cerebral venous thrombosis

- Pattern: Slow-onset headache, ↑ severity over days (can be sudden), seizure, stroke symptoms may be present, can have fever
- Associated/previous history: Recent sinusitis, facial cellulitis, malignancy, pregnancy, postpartum, coagulopathy, oral contraceptive pill (OCP) or trauma
- Headache, fever, eye (chemosis, proptosis, oedema, papillo-oedema), cranial nerve (CN) palsies (III, IV, VI), neurological signs
- Magnetic resonance venography (MRV) more sensitive than CT with contrast
- Treat with anticoagulation

Other significant causes of headaches

- Vascular disorders: Hypertensive encephalopathy, dissection (e.g. carotid artery), temporal arteritis, post encephalopathy, cavernous sinus thrombosis
- Infection: Meningitis, encephalitis, sinus infection
- Medication overuse/rebound: Paracetamol, opioids
- Trigeminal neuralgia: Usually > 50 years old, sudden brief face spasms often triggers (e.g. brushing, shaving)
- Shingles: Unilateral
- Eye pathology: Glaucoma, iritis, optic neuritis, giant cell arteritis (GCA)
- Temporomandibular joint (TMJ) dysfunction

Investigation

- Aim in ED is to exclude serious cause
- Bloods FBC, CRP/ESR, EUC, LFT

- Consider CT head if:
  - Limited neck flexion, neck pain/stiffness, vomiting
  - Thunderclap/peak pain within 1 hour/1st or most severe headache/different headache, ↑ age (some studies suggest > 40) history of cancer, any neurology, ↓/change in level of consciousness, symptoms associated with ↑ ICP (e.g. pain on cough)
  - Onset during exertion, BP > 160/100
  - Other red flags (e.g. immunosuppressed with fever)
- Other imaging: Contrast CT (if consider space-occupying lesion, vascular cause), MRI (especially venous thrombosis, children, space-occupying lesion)
- LP if suspect meningitis (don't usually need CT first) or suspect SAH (post CT), although some new guidelines suggest LP not needed

Management

Tension

- PO aspirin 600–900 mg QID, ibuprofen 400 mg TDS (exclude bleed before aspirin/NSAID), paracetamol 1 g QID

Migraine

- Aspirin, ibuprofen, paracetamol (see Tension above)
  - IV fluids
  - Metoclopramide 10–20 mg IV, PO

    OR
  - Prochlorperazine 5–10 mg PO or 12.5 mg IV

    OR
  - Domperidone 20 mg PO
  - If fails can use: sumatriptan 50–100 mg PO
  - Severe/persistent attack use:
    - IV fluids + chlorpromazine 0.1 mg/kg (12.5 mg) IV over 30 minutes (can repeat ×3)

      OR
    - Droperidol 1.25–2.5 mg IM
    - Must monitor, ECG prior; can prolong QT
    - DON'T use if heart disease or abnormal K^+, Mg
    - CAUTION if has already had prochlorperazine
- Prevent recurrence of migraine with 10 mg IV dexamethasone

Cluster

- 100% oxygen, sumatriptan

Abnormal CSF pressure

- Consult neurosurgeons

Cerebral venous thrombosis

- Treat with anticoagulation
- May need mannitol

CNS infections

- **Note: Meningococcal sepsis**—not the same as meningococcal meningitis. Can have both
  - Pain: Neck, back, arms, legs (early sign)
  - Relatives concerned: Never ignore
  - Rash: Petechial, purpura (late sign)

Bacterial meningitis

- Often symptoms are ↓↓ in infants and elderly
- History: Fever, headache, stiff neck, prodromal URTI, photophobia, change in mental state, seizure
- Risk factors: Trauma, immunocompromised, unimmunised, Age < 5 years particularly neonates, living conditions (dorms, day care etc.)
- *Beware* of partial treatment with PO antibiotics. Signs and symptoms will be less and can be missed. Always ask about antibiotic use
- Examine: Vitals, meningisms—head jolt (lateral head rotation), resist passive neck flex, Brudzinski's sign (hip/knee flex in response to passive neck flex), Kernig's sign (patient lying flat—flex hip to 90 degrees then extend knee; if pain/resistance sign is positive), rash, extracranial infection focus (otitis media, sinusitis, pneumonia, urinary tract infection [UTI]), fundi, evolving neurology
- Investigations: DON'T DELAY ANTIBIOTICS FOR INVESTIGATIONS
  - Bloods: EUC, FBC, CRP, procalcitonin, cultures
  - CT before LP if suspect ↑ ICP (CT may be normal with ↑ ICP)
  - LP without CT if: < 60 years, not immune compromised, no CNS disease, no seizures, level of consciousness normal, no focal neurology or papillo-oedema, cognitive function normal

    - CXR: Often pneumococcal meningitis patients have pneumonia
- Treatment
    - Treat with empiric antibiotics aimed at *Neisseria meningitidis*, *Streptococcus pneumoniae*, *Haemophilus influenzae* type b (Hib)
        - Ceftriaxone (BD) or cefotaxime (QID) 50 mg/kg max. 2 g IV
        - If immunosuppressed or suspect listeriosis add benzylpenicillin 60 mg/kg max. 2.4 g 4-hourly IV
        - If suspect pneumococcal add vancomycin 12.5 mg/kg max. 500 mg QID IV
        - In a baby under 3 months of age use cefotaxime, benzylpenicillin, +/– vancomycin, +/– aciclovir
    - Treat with dexamethasone before or with 1st dose antibiotics 0.15 mg/kg (max. 10 mg) IV 6-hourly for 4/7
    - Support: ABC, analgesia, monitor, fluid resuscitation, treat seizures, correct electrolytes. Cerebral oedema (head elevate, hyperventilate $PaCO_2$ 25–30, mannitol)
    - Chemoprophylaxis for contacts if *N. meningitidis* or Hib, get Public Health input

Viral meningitis

- CSF PCR: Consider testing for enterovirus, CMV, HSV, adenovirus, mumps, HIV
- Can have same signs and symptoms as bacterial usually less severe
- Usually treat with empiric AB until LP results

Lumbar puncture

- See procedures, p. 55
- Check Table 7.2 for interpretation of LP results and CSF characteristics
- If traumatic LP basic rule is to allow 1 WBC for every 1000 RBC

Viral encephalitis

- Viral infection of brain parenchyma usually coexists with viral meningitis
    - Signs and symptoms: New psychiatric symptoms, confusion, seizure, movement disorder, fever, meningism, headache, abnormal behaviour, decreased/altered level of consciousness
        - HSV involves limbic system leading to psychiatric symptoms, ↓ memory, aphasia. Arbovirus involves basal ganglia lead to Parkinsonism

Table 7.2 Lumbar puncture result interpretation for adults

Parameter	Normal CSF	Bacterial infection	Viral infection	Neoplasm	Partially treated bacterial infection
Mononuclear cells	< 5	< 50	10–100	10–100	Varying
Polymorphs	Nil	> 200–300	Nil		Varying
Glucose	2.5–3.5 mmol/L	↓, CSF:serum ratio < 0.4	↑/normal	↓	↓/normal
Protein	0.2–0.4 g/L	↑ 0.5–2.0	↓/normal	↑	↑/normal
Gram stain	–	+ve in 80%	–ve		Can be –ve
Culture	–ve	+ve	–ve		Can be –ve Perform PCR
Appearance	Clear	Turbid	Clear		
Pressure	5–20 cmH_2O	↑	normal		

- Investigations: Bloods, imaging (CT, MRI), LP (CSF looks like viral meningitis), electroencephalogram (EEG) (almost always abnormal), CMV, EBV, PCR for HSV, viruses in CSF, NMDA receptor antibodies
- Management
  - Empiric: Only HSV proven to respond. Aciclovir 10 mg/kg TDS for 14–21/7. (May give IVAB if initially suspecting bacterial meningitis)
  - Support: ABC, behaviour control, hydration, seizure management
  - Steroids if suspect anti-NMDA receptor encephalitis: Usually young, most female, commonly have teratoma, viral-like prodrome, psychiatric symptoms, autonomic dysfunction, dyskinesia

Brain abscess

- Predisposing factors: Paranasal sinus focus, otic source/middle ear, penetrating injury, neurosurgery, systemic hypoxemia (e.g. heart disease), immunosuppressed (e.g. HIV)
- Signs and symptoms: Non-specific, usually don't look acutely unwell; fever, headache, focal neurology, poor balance, ICP ↑, vomiting, confused, signs of origin (e.g. acute otitis media [AOM])
- Investigations: CT with contrast—ring of enhancement around low density centre + white matter oedema. MRI
- Management: IVAB and neurosurgery
  - Benzylpenicillin 2.4 g 4-hourly + metronidazole 500 mg TDS + ceftriaxone 2 g BD
  - If post neurosurgery use vancomycin + piperacillin/tazobactam 4.5 g QID

Epidural abscess

- Back pain red flags: Immunocompromised (HIV, diabetes mellitus [DM], steroid use, chemotherapy etc.), fever, systemic symptoms, IVDU, spine surgery/procedure (including epidural, LP, cortisone injection), bowel or bladder change, decreased saddle sensation, decreased PR tone
- Not all patients have back pain!
- Signs and symptoms: Evolution of signs and symptoms
  - Pain, fever, local tenderness
  - Radicular pain, increased reflex, nuchal rigidity
  - Bladder and bowel change, neurology
  - Paralysis

- Investigations: Blood cultures, ESR/CRP elevated, MRI better than CT, x-ray useless
- Management: Urgent spine surgeon review
  - Start IV antibiotics if neuro deficit present, sepsis or delay to OT
  - Vancomycin 25 mg/kg stat IV and ceftazidime 2 g and gentamicin
  - Operation versus IVAB alone versus CT-guided drainage

Movement disorders

Drug induced

- Usually caused by dopamine blockers; e.g. metoclopramide
- Can be acute, tardive or on withdrawal
  - Acute dystonia (e.g. oculogyric crisis), acute akathisia, drug-induced Parkinson's disease
    - Stop offending drug
    - Benztropine 1–2 mg PO/IM/IV
  - Tardive dyskinesia and dystonia
    - Side effect of long-term antipsychotics
    - Attempt slow taper of drug; if severe can use tetrabenazine 12.5 mg PO/day ↑ to eventually 25 mg TDS max. May need levodopa, antidepressant, dopamine agonist pergolide, change antipsychotic to clozapine, anticholinergic etc.

Multiple sclerosis

- Females > males. Typically, 20–50 years old
- Symptoms
  - Common symptoms: Numbness, tingling, limb(s) weakness, incoordination, dizziness, vision ↓/blurred, urgency, constipation, sexual problems, anxiety/depression, fatigue, heat sensitive
  - Less common: Leg spasticity, pain, tremor, dysarthria, mood disorder, incontinence, cognitive change, neuralgias, paraesthesia on neck flex, psychiatric symptoms, face twitch, seizure, dysphasia, hemiplegia, headache
- Investigations
  - Look for potential inter-current illness: Infection etc.
  - LP: Target cells, IgG oligoclonal bands
  - Only MRI/image in ED if in doubt as to cause

- Acute treatment
  - Consider and treat: Infections, fever, ↑ environmental temperature, depression (these all can produce pseudorelapses)
- Mild relapse: Rest, reassurance
- Moderate: Some disability or unpleasant symptoms or worsening symptoms
  - Prednisone 75 mg PO/day for 4/7 then 50 mg 4/7 25 mg 4/7 (treat as outpatient)
- Severe; e.g. optic neuritis with vision loss, paraplegia, brainstem symptoms
  - Admit, methylprednisolone 1 g IV over 1 hour then daily for 3/7 (slow infusion if arrhythmia/cardiac risk factors)
  - Must do full bloods pre-treatment
  - Acute side effects: Anaphylaxis, arrhythmia, psychiatric symptoms, GI, sleep disturbance.
  - Chronic side effects: Osteoporosis, myopathy, aseptic necrosis femoral
  - Note: Steroids don't alter extent of final recovery; therefore, if in doubt, observation doesn't harm
- Long-term management
  - Immunosuppressants, immunomodulators (e.g. interferon)
  - Symptom control: Spasticity (baclofen), tremor (clonazepam), bladder (oxybutynin) and paroxysmal symptoms (e.g. trigeminal neuralgia) (carbamazepine)

Parkinson's disease

- Usually treating patients with other presentations and already diagnosed Parkinson's disease. Not usually diagnosed from ED
- Consider complications/secondary conditions
  - Delirium (from meds or infection)
  - Infections; e.g. aspiration pneumonia, UTI
  - Falls
  - Neuroleptic-like malignant syndrome (can get from med withdrawal)
- Very important to chart Parkinson's medications early; missing a dose can cause serious outcomes. Keep the same dose, medication, brand, preparation and times where possible
- If can't give patient their correct meds discuss with the specialist neurologist

- If can't give oral medications (e.g. strict NBM), can use patches (most hospitals now stock). Get help to calculate dose (neurologist/ pharmacist)
- Medications patients may be taking:
  - Levodopa combination with dopa decarboxylase inhibitors
  - Anticholinergics
  - Bromocriptine
  - Amantadine
  - Others: Rotigotine
- AVOID antipsychotic medications such as haloperidol and chlorpromazine. If sedation required, consider benzodiazepines

Neuromuscular disorders

Myasthenia gravis

- Autoantibodies against acetylcholine receptor
- Young adults, muscle fatigue, extraocular, bulbar, neck, limb girdle, voice weakens with counting, myasthenia snarl, ptosis, diplopia
- Symptoms ↑ by: Pregnancy, ↑ K^+, emotion, infection, climate, exercise, medications (gentamicin, opiates, beta-blockers, calcium channel blockers, tetracycline)
- 75% of myasthenia gravis (MG) patients have thymic hyperplasia, 10% have thymoma
- Investigations: Tensilon test (10 mg edrophonium versus normal saline placebo), anti acetylcholine receptor antibody (AchR), neurophysical, CT thymus
- Management
  - Treat if urgent; e.g. breathing, swallowing affected. **Call for help**
  - Otherwise await diagnosis (may need plasmapheresis)
  - Pyridostigmine 60 mg PO (↑ up to 6×/day)
  - Immunosuppression
  - Thymectomy
  - Note: Lots of drugs make MG worse! Steroids, barbiturates, phenytoin, quinines, Hartmann's, aminoglycosides, sulfonamides, tetracycline, lithium, haloperidol, chlorpromazine, colchicine, quinidine, procainamide, beta-blockers, lidocaine (lignocaine), morphine, levothyroxine, diuretics, **all neuromuscular blockers including sux (suxamethonium chloride)**!

- Myasthenia crisis
  - Diagnosis: (Not usually done in ED, seek expert advice) Differentiate MG crisis from cholinergic crisis (from excess cholinergic medications): IV edrophonium
    - If this causes fasciculation, ↓ respiration, cholinergic symptoms then diagnosis is cholinergic crisis
    - If weakness improves diagnosis is MG crisis
    - NOTE: Edrophonium can lead to bradycardia, paralysis, AV block, AF, arrest (treat with atropine; have resus equipment ready)
  - Assessment
    - MG crisis and cholinergic crisis can present with respiratory distress
    - Can develop sudden apnoea
    - Look for respiratory failure: Pulse oximetry, ABG, spirometry
    - Once airway/ventilation addressed can look for causes of crisis; e.g. infection, inadequate treatment or over medication
- Management
  - Treatment for MG crisis and cholinergic crisis same
  - ABC; may need intubation (get expert help—patients often sux resistant, rocuronium preferred, use propofol in small doses, not ketamine)
  - MG crisis: Neostigmine 0.5–2 mg SC/IM or 15 mg PO
  - Can use pyridostigmine PO, IVI
  - steroids
  - IVIg
  - Plasma exchange
  - **AVOID** neuromuscular blockers, aminoglycosides, benzodiazepines, calcium channel blockers, beta-blockers

Guillain-Barré (AIDP)

- Rapid, progressive, weakness and sensory change begins peripherally then usually ascending, with reflex loss (deep tendon), pain with passive movement
- Symmetric usually sensation normal on examination
- Rare symptoms: Facial weakness, ophthalmoplegia, autonomic instability and respiratory failure. Several rarer variants exist; e.g. Miller-Fisher syndrome (paralysis begins in head/eyes not legs)

- Often preceding viral illness; ⅔ occur post *Campylobacter* infection
- Autonomic dysfunction: Poor prognosis
- Investigations
  - LP (post CTB): ↑↑ protein, normal glucose, normal cell counts
  - Respiratory function test (do spirometry in ED to help determine disposition)
- Management
  - Admit, observe, if FVC < 20 mL/kg admit to ICU, if < 15 mL/kg intubate—check spirometry 4-hourly
  - DON'T use sux—associated with sudden death!
  - Plasma exchange
  - IV immunoglobulin 0.4 g/kg IV/day 5/7 or 1 g/kg IV/day for 2/7
  - Plasmapheresis
  - DVT prophylaxis
  - Treat neuropathic pain
- Differential diagnosis: Tick bite paralysis, spinal cord compression, acute intermittent porphyria (weakness, psychosis, abdominal pain, +/– seizure; usually precipitated by medications), Lyme disease—if travel Hx indicates (look for a tick, CSF Lyme antibodies)

Metabolic paralysis

- Hypokalaemic periodic paralysis
  - Increased in Asians, male > female
  - Precipitants: Carbohydrates, alcohol, stress, insulin, exercise followed by rest, humidity
  - Flaccid paralysis, lasts minutes to days
  - Potassium decreased during attack (< 2.9)
  - Managed with potassium
- Others: Normokalaemic periodic paralysis, hyperkalaemic periodic paralysis, thyrotoxic periodic paralysis

Botulism

- Food-borne ingestion of enterotoxin. Poorly stored food
- Descending symmetric paralysis
- 95% are < 6 months old: Constipation, floppy baby, death

- Investigations: Check stool/serum/vomit/suspected food for bacteria and toxin. CSF is normal
- Management: Respiratory support, antitoxin. Lavage and charcoal considered

Tetanus

- Tetanus-prone wounds
  - Puncture, penetrating, crush fracture, compound fracture, foreign body, burns, contamination, pyogenic, ischaemic. Note: ⅔ cases post trivial wounds
- Signs and symptoms: Stiff neck, stiff jaw, trismus, seizure, opisthotonos, respiratory muscle spasms and autonomic instability. Note: Consciousness is normal
- Diagnosis is clinical
- Complications: Pneumonia, rhabdomyolysis, respiratory failure, clotting
- Management: Support, sedate, ventilate, paralyse, neutralise toxin—tetanus immunoglobulin (IG), remove source (debride), penicillin + metronidazole
- Prevention (these often change—check most up-to-date guideline)
  - Vaccinate at 2, 4, 6 and 18 months, 5 years then every 10 years
  - If patient sustains wound and is immunised
    - Last dose within 5 years: No treatment
    - Last dose 5–10 years with minor wound: No Tx
    - Last dose 5–10 years with infection-prone wound: Give tetanus toxoid vaccine
    - Last dose > 10 years: Give tetanus toxoid vaccine
  - If patient sustains wound and was never immunised or unsure
    - Give all patients tetanus toxoid vaccine
    - If infection-prone wound also give tetanus IG

Diphtheria

- Toxin of *Corynebacterium diphtheriae*
- Signs and symptoms: Fever, very unwell patient, pharyngitis (grey membrane on pharynx, easily bleeds), myocarditis, cranial nerve palsy, motor paralysis, nephritis
- Investigations: Serum antibodies, Schick test, culture pseudomembrane
- Management: Support, antitoxin available, isolation, penicillin, reportable

Facial pain—differential diagnosis

- Trigeminal neuralgia
  - Sudden, severe, brief, paroxysmal, unilateral face in CN V maxillary or mandibular branches distribution; consider MS in young person; treat with carbamazepine 50–100 mg PO BD increasing dose gradually to 200 mg BD
- Glossopharyngeal neuralgia
  - As above but in CN IX distribution; treat same; exclude malignancy/structural cause, may need operation
- Facial migraine
- Temporomandibular pain syndrome (from abnormal temporomandibular joint movement)
  - Joint crepitus on palpation, treat with dental splint, NSAIDs
- Tooth pain
- Glaucoma
- Angina
- Sinusitis
  - Tender over maxillary (cheek or teeth) frontal (supraorbital) sinuses
- Barotrauma
- Postherpetic neuralgia
  - Burning, ache, stabbing pain; allodynia
  - Occurs/persists 4–6/52 post crusting of herpetic vesicles
  - Usually elderly
  - Treatment: Paracetamol, ice massage, TENS, lidocaine (lignocaine) gel. May need tricyclic antidepressant (TCA)
  - Amitriptyline 10–25 mg PO nocte, gradually increases dose to 100 mg
  - Gabapentin 300 mg daily, gradually increase dose
  - Pregabalin 75 mg nocte, gradually increase dose

Giant cell arteritis

- Rare < 50 years old, often have features of polymyalgia rheumatica
- Clinical features
  - Severe headache (temporal, occipital), visual changes, jaw claudication, symptoms of TIA, cough, sore throat, voice hoarse,

arm claudication, thoracic aortic aneurysm, fever, swelling/ tender temporal artery

- Investigations: ↑ ESR (almost always > 50, usually > 100), ↑ CRP, FBC, ↑ LFT, normal or low Hb, temporal artery US, biopsy
- Treatment
  - Prednisone 40–60 mg/day

    OR
  - Methyl prednisolone 1 g IV if vision loss
  - Urgent review from rheumatologist, ophthalmologist, and/or neurologist depending on your hospital

Seizures

(For paeds see p. 345)

- Types
  - Generalised (both hemispheres): Absence, myoclonic, tonic-clonic, tonic, atonic
  - Partial (one hemisphere): Simple (no altered level of consciousness), complex (↓ level of consciousness), secondary generalised
  - Non-convulsive status
- Causes
  - BATH TIME
    - **B**rain lesion
    - **A**lcohol/drug withdrawal
    - **T**rauma
    - **H**ereditary
    - **T**oxins
    - **I**nfections
    - **M**etabolic
    - **E**pilepsy
- Assessment and investigations
  - History: Ask about the following
    - Pre-event: Precipitants, preceding symptoms, systems review
    - The event: Incontinence, tongue biting, cyanosis, trauma sustained, situation (e.g. were they in a bath)
    - Post event: Post ictal, recovery time

  - Investigations to diagnose seizure
    - Blood gas soon post seizure most will have lactic acidosis
    - Serum lactate ↑ resolves 15 minutes to 1 hour
    - Blood prolactin level ↑ 15 minutes to 1 hour
    - Elevated WCC, low bicarbonate and phosphate
    - EEG
  - Investigations for precipitants and alternative diagnosis
    - BSL, inflammatory markers, pregnancy test, antiepileptic medication levels
    - ECG: Especially if first seizure—arrhythmias often present with 'seizure'
  - Identify and treat complications
    - Respiratory (hypoxic, hypercapnic), cardiac (hypotension, arrhythmia), metabolic (electrolyte imbalance, temperature, rhabdomyolysis, DIC), trauma (fracture, dislocation—perform imaging), circumstance (burns, drowning)
  - DON'T EVER FORGET GLUCOSE
- Differential diagnosis
  - Syncope, pseudoseizure, hyperventilation, migraine, movement disorder, narcolepsy, arrhythmia
  - AEIOU TIPS (differential for decreased level of consciousness)
    - **A**cidosis/alcohol
    - **E**pilepsy
    - **I**nfection
    - **O**verdose
    - **U**raemia
    - **T**rauma
    - **I**nsulin
    - **P**sychiatric
    - **S**troke
- Management
  - During seizure: Maintain airway and vitals; patient on side
  - Usually self-terminate
  - 1st line: Benzodiazepines
    - Midazolam 5 mg (0.1 mg/kg) IM/IV/IO, 10 mg (0.3 mg/kg) buccal/intranasal

- o Diazepam 10 mg (0.3 mg/kg) IV/IO—***beware extravasation***—10–20 mg (0.5 mg/kg) PR
- o If prophylaxis from further seizures required, follow immediately with:
  - – Levetiracetam 20–40 mg/kg

    OR
  - – Phenytoin 20 mg/kg (monitor heart: causes ↓ heart, ↓ BP, brady max. 50 mg/min). Don't dilute with glucose

    OR
  - – Phenobarbitone 20 mg/kg, max. rate 1 mg/kg/minute (max. 60 mg/minute). Monitor

- ■ 2nd line: More benzos (doses above)
- ■ 3rd line: Levetiracetam 20 mg/kg and/or phenytoin 20 mg/kg (10 mg/kg in children), whichever one you have not given yet
- ■ 3rd line/refractory
  - o Midazolam infusion 1–5 microgram/kg/min
  - o Valproate
  - o Phenobarbitone 20 mg/kg IV
  - o Intubation and IV infusions midazolam, propofol and/or barbiturate
  - o Propofol IV/IO 2.5 mg/kg stat (for intubation) then 1–3 mg/kg/hr
  - o Thiopentone IV/IO 2–5 mg/kg slowly stat (for intubation) then 1–4 mg/kg/hr
  - o Continuous EEG
- ■ Avoid phenytoin in toxicity or alcohol withdrawal
- ■ Pyridoxine 100 mg slow IV if < 6 months with refractory seizure

- • Managing patients with previous seizures
  - ■ Look for precipitate: Low therapeutic levels of medications, other medications/infections etc. that ↓ seizure threshold, poor compliance
  - ■ Consider changes in regular medications, may need loading, consult neurologist
  - ■ Admit/neurology consult if: Focal neuro, persistent change in mental state, new intracranial lesion, change in seizure pattern, poor control, pregnant
  - ■ CT head if: Focal neuro, change in pattern, change in mental state, head trauma, HIV/immunosuppressants, alcoholism, coagulopathic/on thinners

- Managing a first ever seizure
  - Look for precipitants: Trauma, ICH, drugs and toxins, EtOH/drug withdrawal, structural (mass, vascular [e.g. aneurysm], congenital), infection (HIV, meningitis etc.), metabolic (↓↑ BSL/Na, uraemia, ↓ Ca, ↓ Mg), eclampsia, hypertension encephalopathy, anoxic ischaemic injury (e.g. cardiac arrest, hypoxemia)
  - Usually all get CT head/imaging
  - If all bloods (FBC, EUC, CMP, LFT) and CT normal and examination normal and patient young, consider discharge and outpatient MRI and neurology follow-up
- If discharge must advise: Can't drive, can't work with hazardous tools, caution with heights, avoid swimming and baths

Cerebrovascular accident (CVA)/transient ischaemic attack (TIA)

Risks and causes

- Risk factors: AF, hypertension, smoking, diabetes mellitus, ↑ cholesterol, cardiovascular disease, age
- Causes of TIA: Atherosclerosis, cardiac emboli, inflammatory artery diseases, dissection, hypotension, hyperviscosity, subclavian steal, sympathomimetics
- CVA/TIA leads to ↑ risk AMI!

Signs and symptoms—general overview

- Fig. 7.1 shows the vessels of the circle of Willis. The 3 main vessels (anterior, middle and posterior cerebral arteries) are shaded with different patterns to correspond to Fig. 7.2 showing roughly what part of the brain they supply and therefore what symptoms the patient will have when occluded
- **Upper motor neuron (UMN) lesion**: Weakness, spasticity/↑ tone/clonus, ↑ reflexes, ↑ plantar
- **Lower motor neuron (LMN) lesion**: Weakness, wasting, ↓ tone, ↓ reflexes, normal plantar, fasciculations
- **Anterior cerebral artery stroke**: Leg > arm contralateral hemiparalysis, confusion, behaviour change, mild contralateral hemiasthesia, can develop anarthria
- **Middle cerebral artery stroke**: Contralateral hemiparesis (arm > leg upper limb, trunk lower face)
  - Contralateral hemianaesthesia (body and face)
  - Dominant hemisphere (usually left) causing aphasia

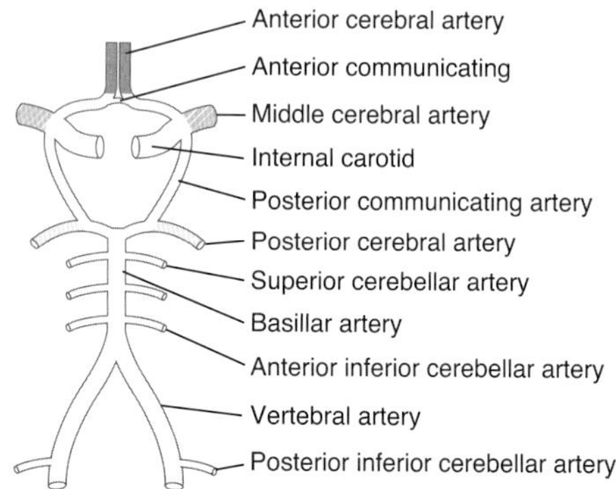

Figure 7.1 Circle of Willis

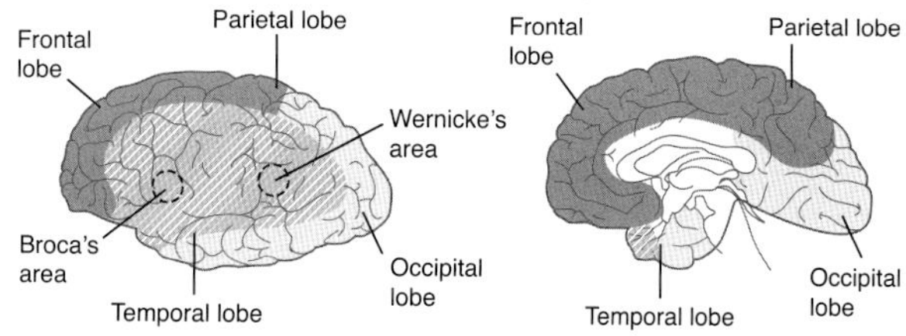

Figure 7.2 Vascular supply to brain

- Non-dominant (usually right) causing neglect, dysarthric, gaze to infarct side, homonymous hemianopia

- **Posterior cerebral artery stroke**: Contralateral hemianopia with macular sparing, memory problems, patient may be unaware hemianaesthesia, usually minimal hemiplegia, hemiballismus
- **PICA**
  - Ipsilateral: Horner's syndrome (miosis, ptosis, anhidrosis) pharyngeal and laryngeal paralysis, sensory loss face, cerebellar signs (dysarthria, ataxia, nystagmus, vertigo)
  - Contralateral: Sensory loss limbs/trunk

- **Vertebrobasilar syndrome**: Posterior circulation supplies brain stem, cerebellum, visual cortex. Stroke causes: Ipsilateral CN deficits with contralateral weakness, ipsilateral cerebellar (ataxia, nystagmus, dizzy, nausea and vomiting)
- **Basilar arterial occlusion**: Severe quadriplegia, coma, 'locked in'
- **Cerebellar infarct**: 'Drop attack', suddenly can't walk, vertigo, headache, nausea and vomiting, neck pain. Need MRI for diagnosis
  - Typically results in cerebral oedema causing ↓ level of consciousness
  - Need urgent operation and decompression
- **Lacunar infarct**: Pure motor or sensory deficit from occlusion of small penetrating artery
- **Arterial dissection** (internal carotid artery [ICA] or vertebral artery [VA]): Often associated with trauma, sudden head turn, hypertension, chiropractor
  - Neck pain (unilateral face pain ICA), headache (unilateral if ICA). Neuro deficit may develop over hours to days. Need CTA. Signs/symptoms of posterior circulation ischaemia or SAH

Diagnosis

- URGENT: IVC + bloods (EUC, FBC, LFT, CMP, coags, G&H if possible bleed, BSL [URGENT correction of BSL if < 3.5 or > 11]) ECG, CXR
- Imaging: Take suitable patients direct to scan
  - CT head non-contrast, perfusion and/or vascular studies
  - Determine if occlusion, large vessel occlusion and salvageable tissue
- Stroke mimics: HEMIS
  - **H**ypo/ers (glucose, electrolytes)
  - **E**pilepsy/seizure
  - **MS**/migraine
  - **I**ntracranial infection/lesion
  - **S**yncope

Management CVA—use your local pathway

- Notify stroke team pre-arrival if possible/available.
- Patient needs rapid assessment in ED to identify if suitable for interventions
  - Onset of symptoms
  - Stroke assessment; e.g. recognition of stroke in the emergency room (ROSIER) scale

- Quickly place IVC, send bloods then direct to CT scan
- CTB non-contrast to rule out bleed
- CT angio and CT perfusion if available

- Thrombolysis
  - Considered if:
    - Appropriate score on stroke scale of choice; e.g. ROSIER
    - Symptoms ≤ 4.5 hours (longer if large vessel occlusion)
    - Good premorbid function
    - No contraindications (see thrombolysis contraindications in STEMI, p. 77)
    - Informed consent
  - Alteplase 0.9 mg/kg up to 90 mg IV/hr, 10% of dose as initial bolus then rest over 1 hour
  - Must closely monitor BP, give in resus
- Endovascular clot retrieval: Will need stroke specialist
  - Used for large vessel occlusion
  - Timeframe from symptom onset/last seen well
    - Symptoms < 6 hours
    - Symptoms 6–24 hours, and salvageable tissue demonstrated on CT perfusion
    - Basilar artery occlusion can be considered up to 48 hours
  - Patients should have good premorbid function. Independent/ minimal assistance
  - Patients should have significant neurological deficit
  - All patients should receive tissue plasminogen activator (tPA)
- Not for thrombolysis or clot retrieval
  - Consider antiplatelets, anticoagulants
  - Use aspirin 100–300 mg PO/day
- All patients
  - Support
  - Monitor BP, treat cautiously ONLY if > 220/120. Use IV medications; e.g. clonidine, hydralazine (see hypertensive emergencies, p. 85). Aim to decrease BP by 10–15%
  - Multidisciplinary stroke unit

TIAs

- Calculate ABCD^2 score
  - **A**ge ≥ 60 score 1
  - **BP** ≥ 140/90 score 1
  - **C**linical
    - o Speech impaired, no weakness scores 1
    - o Unilateral weakness scores 2
  - **D**uration
    - o Symptoms lasting 10–59 minutes scores 1
    - o Symptoms lasting > 60 minutes scores 2
  - **D**iabetes scores 1
- Admit if high risk
  - ABCD^2 score > 4
  - AF
  - ≥ 2 TIAs in 1 week/crescendo
  - On antiplatelets (e.g. aspirin) already
  - Neck bruit
  - AMI ≤ 4 weeks
  - Poor social supports
  - Comorbidities (fever/sepsis, cardiac valve, unstable diabetes mellitus etc.)
- Discharge if low risk (none of above)
  - AND single event, fully resolved and sinus rhythm
  - Follow-up with LMO and neurology clinic
  - Start antiplatelet: Aspirin

Intracranial haemorrhages

Intracerebral haemorrhage

- Intracerebral bleed can look just like cerebral infarct
  - Headache, nausea and vomiting often precede neurology
  - Often have ↓ level of consciousness
- Investigations and assessment
  - Bloods: EUC, FBC, coags, G&H, LFT
  - Imaging: CT brain non-contrast; CXR
  - ECG

- Management
    - Neurosurgery URGENT consult: May need ICP monitor device; operation for decompression
    - Cease/reverse anticoagulation
    - Prevent secondary injury
        - Maintain airway, normocarbia and avoid hypoxia/hyperoxia
        - BP monitor aim sBP < 180. Some possible benefit by targeting sBP < 140
        - Elevate head of bed 30 degrees, tape don't tie tubes
        - If deterioration: Mannitol 1 g/kg IV or hypertonic saline (3%) 2 mL/kg
        - Hyperventilate to $PaCO_2$ 30–35 mmHg only if deteriorating and about to take to OT
        - Query seizure prevention (controversial) phenytoin 15 mg/kg or levetiracetam IV. Treat seizures if occur

Cerebellar haemorrhage

- Signs and symptoms: Sudden nausea and vomiting, dizzy, ataxia, can't walk, gaze palsy, ↓ level of consciousness
- Diagnosis and operation to decompress URGENTLY!

Subarachnoid haemorrhage

- Causes
    - 70% from rupture of berry aneurysm
    - Other causes: Arteriovenous malformation (AVM), mycotic aneurysm, trauma, cancer
    - Risk factors: Previous SAH, FHx, smoker, HT, Connective tissue diseases (e.g. Marfan's syndrome), polycystic kidneys, anticoagulation
- History
    - Severe (worst headache ever in 90%), sudden (thunderclap OR peak pain within 1 hour), exertional (onset with exercise, sex, cough, defecation etc.), transient level of consciousness (highly specific), nausea, vomiting, neck stiffness
    - May be history of sentinel bleed (20% have history of migraine)
    - Good response to analgesia doesn't rule out SAH!!
- Examination
    - Neck stiffness, HT, photophobia, neurological deficit
    - Often examination normal

- Investigations
  - See Headache (p. 147) for when to image/red flags
  - Always investigate sudden headache, worst-ever headache, associated LOC and neurological signs
  - CT brain non-contrast: Very specific. Sensitivity decreases with time. Very sensitive if done within 4–6 hours from symptoms
  - CT angiogram sensitive for aneurysms
  - LP: CT first—if CT is normal but performed > 6 hours, consider LP. Sensitive test if symptoms > 12 hours and < 2 weeks. Positive LP if xanthochromia. RBC > 100 000 (Beware: A bloody tap may just be really positive not traumatic!)
    - Traumatic tap: No absolute rule, but likely traumatic if blood clears by tube 3, no xanthochromia, clots seen, RBC:WBB 500–1000:1
  - ECG: May show ST and T changes, deep T inversions, wide QRS, long QT. Can look ischaemic
  - Bloods: To prep for possible operation (EUC, FBC, LFT, coags, G&H)
- Management
  - Support: Prevent secondary injury
  - ABC, monitor, maintain normal oxygenation, normal carbon dioxide levels, normal temperature, normal glucose
  - Avoid increased ICP. Head of bed 30 degrees, tape don't tie tubes, mannitol if required
  - Maintain sBP 90–140 (Note: different to other ICH)
  - Treat pain, nausea and vomiting promptly
  - Monitor Na, electrolytes, glucose
  - New evidence for prophylactic antiseizure meds indicates they may worsen outcome
  - Nimodipine prevents vasospasm use PO 60 mg QID
  - Neurosurgical urgent consult: Angiography—coil/clip aneurysm, embolisation, neurosurgery

Subdural haematoma (SDH)

- Risk factors: Trauma usually with LOC, chronic EtOH, falls (children < 2, elderly), anticoagulant medications, bleeding disorders

- Diagnosis
  - CT brain non-contrast (if chronic my need contrast CT or MRI)
  - Acute SDH on CT: Hyperdense/white, crescent shape, crosses suture lines
  - Chronic SDH on CT: Hypodense (dark)
- Management: As with ICH (p. 169)
  - Discuss with neurosurgeon
  - Identify and treat other injuries

Extradural haematoma

- Cause: Usually from blunt trauma
  - Temporal/temporal-parietal area
  - Associated with skull fracture and middle meningeal arterial dissect
  - Occasionally due to parieto-occipital trauma causing tear of venous sinuses
- Typical pattern of symptoms: Significant blunt head trauma causing LOC followed by lucent period followed by LOC (occurs in a minority)
- Diagnose on CT
  - Biconvex: Football shape, usually temporal region
- Management URGENT!! Diagnosis and surgery
  - See emergency craniotomy (p. 48) if urgent surgery unavailable
  - Herniation within hours of injury

Coma

- Differential diagnosis of coma
  - Primary CNS
    - Trauma
    - Vascular (ICH, SAH)
    - Infarct
    - CNS infection
    - Neoplasm
    - Seizure (status non-convulsive, postictal)

- Causes diffusely affecting brain
  - Encephalopathies: Hypertensive, hypoxic, CO_2 narcosis
    - Metabolic: ↑↓ BSL, electrolyte abnormal
    - Organ failure: Hepatic, uremic, endocrine
  - Toxins, overdoses, drug reaction (e.g. neuroleptic malignant syndrome [NMS])
  - Sepsis
  - Environmental (↑↓ temperature)
  - Deficiency (e.g. Wernicke's encephalopathy)
- A mnemonic to remember causes: AEIOU TIPS
  - **A**lcohol
  - **E**pilepsy
  - **I**nfection
  - **O**verdose
  - **U**raemia
  - **T**rauma
  - **I**nsulin
  - **P**sychogenic
  - **S**troke

- Investigations
  - BSL
  - VBG
  - Bloods (EUC, FBC, LFT, CMP, coagulants, drug levels/ paracetamol/EtOH), thyroid function
  - ECG
  - CXR
  - Consider
    - CT head
    - MRI for suspected basilar arterial thrombosis
    - LP

Delirium

- Differential diagnosis of precipitates
  - Infection (pneumonia, UTI, CNS, sepsis)
  - Metabolic/toxic (↓ BSL, EtOH, electrolyte abnormal, hepatic encephalopathy, thyroid disease)

- Neuro (stroke, TIA, seizure, postictal, SAH, ICH, CNS mass, subdural)
- Cardiopulmonary (CCF, AMI, PE, hypoxia, CO_2 narcosis)
- Drug related (antiemetics, antihistamine, anti-Parkinson, antipsychotic, antispasmodic, muscle relaxant, TCA, digoxin, sedatives, narcotics), withdrawal
- Also: Pain, constipation—especially in elderly

- Signs and symptoms
  - Global cognitive impairment with clouding of consciousness and fluctuating level of consciousness
  - Altered attention
  - Acute onset
  - Hallucinations (often visual)
  - **Dementia** differences
    - Disturbed cognition, short-term memory loss, no clouding of consciousness
    - Slow onset, agitation, apathy, can have delusions
    - Dementia a risk factor for delirium though
- Investigations
  - Bloods: FBC, EUC, CMP, BSL, BUN. Consider LFT, thyroid-stimulating hormone (TSH), B12, +/– syphilis, ESR, CRP, folate, Fe, +/– HIV
  - CXR
  - UA
  - CTB

Space-occupying lesion

- Symptoms and signs
  - General
    - ↑ ICP (nausea and vomiting, ↓ level of consciousness, papillo-oedema), seizures, personality changes, local effects (epistaxis, proptosis)
    - False localising neuro (from ↑ ICP; e.g. CN VI compression)
    - Localising neuro
  - Temporal lobe (seizure, hallucination, dysphasia, field defect, ↓ memory, psychiatric symptoms, fear/rage)

  - Frontal (hemiparesis, personality change, grasp reflex, dysphasia, loss smell)
  - Parietal (hemisensory loss, ↓ 2-point discrimination, ↓ stereognosis, sensory inattention, dysphasia)
  - Occipital (contralateral visual field)
  - Cerebellum (intention tremor, past point, DDK, nystagmus, ataxia)
  - Cerebellopontine angle (e.g. vestibular schwannoma) (ipsilateral deafness, nystagmus, ↓ corneal reflex, VII and V palsies, ipsilateral cerebellar signs)
  - Corpus callosum (rapid intellectual ↓, loss of communication between lobes; e.g. left hand can't do verbal command)
  - Midbrain (unequal pupils, amnesia, confabulation, somnolence)
- Investigations: Imaging CT/MRI + contrast. Avoid LP! Look for primary if brain lesions look like metastasis
- Management
  - Neurosurgery consult
  - Surgery, radiotherapy, chemotherapy
  - Seizure prophylaxis; e.g. phenytoin
  - Treat headache with analgesia
  - Cerebral oedema treatment: Dexamethasone 4 mg TDS PO/IV, mannitol if deteriorating, etc.

Nystagmus and vertigo

- Differentiating central versus peripheral causes (Table 7.3)
- HINTs test: Perform if patient has nystagmus
  - **H**ead **I**mpulse/vestibulo-ocular reflex
    - Patient fixes on examiner's nose, turn patient's head slowly one way then quickly back to centre. Repeat for other direction
    - Negative test = eyes remain fixed on nose; consider central causes
    - Positive test = eyes move with head then 'catch up'; highly likely cause is peripheral
  - **N**ystagmus
    - Examine the nystagmus for the features in Table 7.3

Table 7.3 Distinguishing features of nystagmus and vertigo

	Central	Peripheral
Causes	ICH/CVA (brainstem, cerebellar), MS, cancer, migraine, drugs	Benign paroxysmal positional vertigo (BPPV), vestibular, labyrinthitis, Ménière's disease, acoustic neuroma
Onset	Can be slow (cancer) or sudden (CVA, ICH)	Sudden
Hearing loss	Rare	Common: often ear symptoms
Caloric test	Normal	Abnormal
Vestibulo-ocular reflex	Absent	Positive
Neurology signs and symptoms	Other deficits; e.g. diplopia, sensory, motor, dysarthria, headache, neck pain	No other abnormal neurology
Other	Impaired balance	Nausea, vomiting, sweating
Nystagmus	Usually absent; vertical, doesn't fatigue, bi-directional, persists with fixation, no latency from stimulus	Usually present; horizontal +/– rotational, never vertical, fatigues, fixed direction/ unidirectional, decreases with fixation, delayed onset from stimulus

  - Test of skew
    - Alternate cover then uncover test with patient looking at examiner's nose
    - Positive test = eye has moved off nose: Central cause likely
- Hallpike: Perform if no spontaneous nystagmus. Aim is to stimulate nystagmus and examine the nystagmus for features Table 7.3
- Investigations
  - CT versus MRI
  - CT to exclude bleed, not reliable if considering cerebellar pathology, need MRI
- Management
  - If considering central cause discuss with neurology
  - Symptom control
    - Prochlorperazine 12.5 mg IV, 10 mg PO
    - Promethazine 10 mg PO

- BPPV
  - Consider manoeuvres such as Epley
- Vestibular neuronitis
  - Usually viral cause
  - Consider prednisone 12.5 mg/d for 3 days then taper

Complications of shunts

- Investigations
  - Shunt x-ray series looking for fracture
  - CT brain: Need to compare with previous images; e.g. for hydrocephalus
  - Bloods with cultures if suspected infection
- Blocked or obstructed (most common)
  - Drowsy, headache, seizure, nausea, vomiting, HT
  - Management: Operation, may need urgent reservoir puncture
- Infection
  - Most occur within 4 months from insertion
  - Fever, erythema over site, WCC > 20
  - Abdominal US: Look for pseudocyst
  - Management: Shunt needs removal, external drain, antibiotics—usually vancomycin and ceftriaxone
- Shunt nephritis
  - Can result in chronic bacteraemia
- Other
  - Overdrain
  - Abdominal: Peritonitis, hernia, migration
  - Intracerebral: Bleed

CHAPTER 8

Coagulation, anticoagulation and vascular

Deep vein thrombosis (DVT)

(See Pulmonary embolism in Chapter 4 Respiratory, p. 98)

- Signs and symptoms
  - Only ≤ 50% get symptoms: calf pain, swelling, redness, warmth
  - Signs: Increased calf diameter, tenderness, Homan's sign, can get mild fever
  - Phlegmasia cerulea dolens: Tissue ischaemia from venous occlusion. Limb is blue/dusky, can have gangrene
  - Phlegmasia alba dolens: Extensive swelling, no ischaemia due to collaterals
- Risk factors
  - Hypercoagulation: Malignancy, pregnancy and postpartum (< 4/52), oestrogen, antiphospholipid antibodies, genetic mutations (factor V Leiden, prothrombin, methylenetetrahydrofolate [MTHF] reductase, Factor VIII, protein C deficiency and protein S deficiency)
  - Venous stasis: Bed rest, cast/fixator, hospitalised, long travel
  - Venous injury: Recent surgery, recent trauma with hospitalisation
- Risk stratify: Modified Wells' score
  - Give 1 point for each of:
    - Active cancer, leg immobility, bed bound for 3/7 or major OT 4/52, local tenderness, swelling to whole leg, pitting oedema to symptomatic unilateral leg, calf diameter increased > 3 cm difference, collateral non-varicose superficial veins, PHx DVT
  - Take off 2 points if alternative diagnosis is at least as likely
  - Total score ≥ 2 DVT likely, ≤ 1 DVT unlikely
- Investigations
  - Low risk can do D-dimer
  - 2-point US in ED: Rapid test, good sensitivity and specificity

    - Duplex US (if negative but moderate–high risk still consider further investigations [e.g. D-dimer] or repeat the assessment and US)
    - If patient found to have DVT consider thrombophilia screen (especially if no precipitant identified)
        - Tests to order: Factor V Leiden, prothrombin mutation, lupus anticoagulant, anticardiolipin antibodies

          AND
        - Levels for the following: Antithrombin III, protein C, protein S, factor VIII, factor XI, lipoprotein, homocysteine
        - Usually non-urgent
- Management
    - Below knee: Treat with anticoagulation. If contraindications to anticoagulation can consider serial US every 2 weeks
    - Above knee: Anticoagulation usually for 3 months
    - Enoxaparin 1 mg/kg SC BD or 1.5 mg/kg daily
        - If platelets low seek advice before commencing
        - Adjust dose if poor renal function
    - Plus warfarin same day 5 mg/day for 2/7 then adjust per INR

      OR
    - NOAC/DOAC now recommended for treatment as outpatient.
    - NOTE: These may not be appropriate in patients with thrombophilias; check with haematologist
        - Rivaroxaban 15 mg PO BD for 3 weeks then 20 mg daily
        - Follow-up with GP in first 3 weeks
        - Adjust dose if poor renal function
    - Early ambulation, analgesia
    - Extensive iliofemoral or upper limb DVT may need vascular/haem review +/– thrombolysis
    - IVC filter for recurrent clots or unable to anticoagulate via interventional radiology

DVT/PE prophylaxis

- Most hospitals have their own guidelines
- Consider in all patients being admitted to hospital and patients at home that will have significant stasis
- Consider in all patients being discharged from ED with lower limb injuries in POP/CAM boot/non-weight bearing etc.

- Assess risk
  - In all patients
    - Compression stockings: If no arterial compromise to legs
    - Early mobilisation
    - Ensure hydration
- High risk
  - Ischaemic stroke, patient history of PE/DVT, active cancer, decompensated heart failure, acute on chronic lung disease, acute inflammatory disease, age > 60
  - Hip or knee arthroplasty, major trauma, hip fracture operation
  - Use, for example: Enoxaparin 40 mg SC daily

    OR
  - Heparin 5000 units SC BD
  - + compression stockings
- Moderate risk
  - Other clotting risk factors, age > 40, CVA, abdominal or pelvic operation, other surgery + minor risk factors
  - Consider with all operations

Superficial thrombophlebitis

- Same risk factors as for DVT + varicose veins and recent cannula
- 90% are from varicose veins
- If as a result of an IVC or varicose vein and minor with no significant risk factors can consider treating with NSAIDs topical or PO (e.g. diclofenac gel TDS), elevation and compression
- If more significant/extensive clot or spontaneous or concerning risk factors: US. Usually anticoagulate; e.g. LMWH 4/52
- If potential septic thrombophlebitis treat with antibiotics + anticoagulants

Anticoagulation reversal

Guidelines vary—use local guidelines if possible

Warfarin

- Risk of serious bleed
  - INR < 5 = low; INR 5–9 = moderate; INR > 9 = high
- Risk factors for bleeding on anticoagulants
  - Age > 65, EtOH excess, hypertension + poor control, PVD, previous bleeding, platelet dysfunction, abnormal coagulation,

cancer, drugs (aspirin, NSAIDs, natural remedies), previous CVA, elderly, cognitive impairment, renal insufficiency, recent trauma, falls

- Bleeding sites: ICH, GI, GU, pulmonary, external (epistasis, gums, bruises), intra-abdominal, intramuscular, retroperitoneal
- Investigations to consider: Coags, FBC, G&H with cross-match if evidence of acute bleeding
- Management: Consider charcoal if < 1 hour and OD
    - If no bleeding:
        - INR over therapeutic but < 4
            - Adjust dose
        - INR 4.5–10
            - Cease warfarin
            - If patient has increased risk of bleeding also give vitamin K PO 2 mg or IV 1 mg
        - INR ≥ 10
            - Cease warfarin
            - Vitamin K 5 mg PO or IV
            - If patient has increased bleed risk also give prothrombin complex concentrate (PCC) 25 u/kg IV
        - Look for precipitates of increased INR; e.g. medications
        - Remeasure INR 12–24 hours, restart at ↓ dose when INR ↓ (e.g. < 4)
    - If bleeding
        - Minor bleed
            - Cease warfarin
            - If INR > 4.5: Give vitamin K PO 2 mg or IV 1 mg + 1 unit FFP
            - Repeat INR in 24 hours and adjust dose
        - Significant bleed but not life-threatening with INR ≥ 2
            - Cease warfarin
            - PCC 50 units/kg (if PCC unavailable use FFP 300 mL)
            - Vitamin K 5 mg–10 mg IV
        - Major bleed (life-threatening) and INR ≥ 1.5
            - PCC 50 units/kg IV

          AND

            - FFP 150–300 mL (increased dose if PCC unavailable)

AND

- Vitamin K 5–10 mg IV

- Overdose; see Chapter 11 Toxicology, p. 219
  - Must consider reason for taking warfarin and risk of thromboembolism if fully reversed!

Heparin

- Adjust dose as per APTT
- If bleeding occurs then cease
- If bleeding severe use protamine: 1 mg neutralises 100 units given in last 15 minutes. Maximum 50 mg. Check black box warnings for protamine—can have severe adverse reactions; don't give if fish allergy; always give in resus
  - Give slow IV over 10–30 minutes and < 50 mg/10 min. Side effects severe anaphylaxis; heparin rebound (may need 2nd treatment)

LMWH

- Protamine (incomplete reversal), dose = 1 mg per 1 mg enoxaparin (1 mg protamine per 100 u dalteparin) given in the last 8 hours PLUS 0.5 mg protamine per 1 mg of enoxaparin given in the last 8–12 hours (see black box warnings for protamine)
- FFP, packed cells for severe bleeding

Heparin-induced thrombocytopenia (HIT)

- Patient on heparin, develops HIT: 2 types
- Diagnose with lab antibodies: Platelet factor 4—but do not await results before treating
- Cease heparin including heparin locks
- Commence danaparoid or fondaparinux
- Haematology advice
- Avoid platelet transfusions

Novel oral anticoagulants (NOACs)

Rivaroxaban and apixaban

- Test
  - Elevated PT > elevated APTT = rivaroxaban issue likely
  - Normal PT = rivaroxaban issues unlikely
  - No test for apixaban

- Mild bleeding
  - Delay next dose or cease
- Significant bleeding: Cease
  - Charcoal if less than 4 hours
  - Local haemostasis, ensure hydration
  - If bleed ongoing transfusion of packed cells and platelets (if < 50)
  - If bleed still ongoing treat as life-threatening (below)
- Life-threatening: Above measures AND
  - PCC 50 units/kg IV

    AND
  - Tranexamic acid 20 mg/kg IV

Dabigatran

- Test
  - Elevated TT and APTT = dabigatran issue likely
  - Normal TT and APTT = dabigatran issues unlikely
- Mild bleeding
  - Delay next dose or cease
- Significant bleeding: Cease
  - Charcoal if less than 4 hours
  - Local haemostasis, ensure hydration
  - If bleed ongoing transfusion of packed cells and platelets (if < 50)
  - If bleed still ongoing treat as life-threatening (below)
- Life-threatening: Above measures AND
  - Idarucizumab 2.5 g + 2.5 g (5 g total) IV over 5–10 minutes each

Aortic dissection and aneurysm

- Risk factors
  - Cardiothoracic disease, family history of aneurysm, atherosclerotic risk (↑ age, smoker, hypertension, ↑ cholesterol, diabetes mellitus), fluoroquinolones
  - For dissection
    - HT, congenital heart disease, cardiothoracic disease, pregnancy, connective tissue diseases (Marfan's syndrome,

Ehlers-Danlos), heart surgery or PCI, cocaine, arteritis (e.g. syphilis)

- Can get aneurysms at sites of previous vascular reconstruction/graft; e.g. aortic, iliac, femoral artery. Rupture leads to severe bleed

- Assessment
  - AAA: Sudden severe abdominal or back pain, syncope, shock, atypical pain (flank, groin, hip), nausea and vomiting, tender, pulsatile mass central abdomen, Cullen/Grey Turner's sign, inguinal mass, iliopsoas sign, haematemesis, melaena, haematuria may be asymptomatic
  - Thoracic AA: Compression/erode structure (oesophagus, trachea, bronchial)
  - Dissection: 95% have pain in chest, back or abdomen; in 90% pain is sudden onset; in 90% pain is severe; in 50% pain is tearing. Syncope, neurology/TIA symptoms, nausea and vomiting, sweat, AMI, tamponade
  - ↑↓ BP, unequal pulses (< 40% will have this sign), new aortic regurgitation murmur (30%), tamponade, ischaemic complications (neurology, limb, viscera), shock, heart failure
- Investigations
  - AAA +/– rupture
    - ECG
    - Point-of-care US (POCUS)/bedside abdominal US
    - CT/CTA
  - Dissection
    - CXR: Many abnormalities, 90% are abnormal in some way. Can't rely on CXR to exclude. Most common finding = unusual looking aorta. Wide mediastinum
    - ECG: Can be normal. Can look like STEMI or pericarditis. Can be evidence of tamponade
    - D-dimer: If negative dissection is very unlikely but not enough to rely on
    - Bedside ECHO: Look for tamponade, pericardial effusion, dilated aortic root
    - CT aortogram: Gold standard
    - TOE: Good at seeing proximal aorta and assessing LV function
    - MRI high sensitivity and specificity

- Management
  - Large-bore IV access, send group and cross-match, warn blood bank of potential massive transfusion
  - Ruptured AAA
    - DON'T waste time imaging for confirmation of diagnosis if it's clinically apparent!
    - If endovascular repair is available, CT may be needed to plan surgery
    - URGENT surgery/cardiothoracic surgery
    - Fluid and blood resuscitation; minimal volume resus; sBP 90
  - Dissection
    - IV beta-blocker to be given first: Esmolol 500 microgram/kg bolus then 50 microgram/kg/min or propranolol 1 mg every 5 minutes or metoprolol
    - Then give glyceryl trinitrate (GTN) 1 microgram/min, titrate (50 mg GTN in 500 mL glucose) or IV hydralazine or SNP infusion
    - Aim for sBP 100–120, HR 60–80
    - Analgesia: Morphine, fentanyl (ensure good analgesia—will decrease stress on vessels)
    - Oxygenation
    - Invasive monitoring
    - Call surgeons, call theatres
  - If tamponade, unstable and no vascular surgeons on site consider pericardiocentesis

Peripheral arterial diseases

Critical limb ischaemia with ulceration or gangrene

- Systolic foot BP usually < 50
- Management
  - Surgical review URGENT (revascularisation bypass, angio and thrombolytics may be considered by specialist team)
  - Analgesia
  - Protect limb–cage, heel pad, don't elevate
  - Maintain high to normal systolic BP
  - May need to ↓ antihypertensive
  - IVAB as per cultures. Empiric: Metronidazole + cephalexin OR amoxicillin + clavulanate forte

  - If severe/limb threat use meropenem 500 mg IV TDS or piperacillin + tazobactam

Cholesterol embolism

- Can cause: Digital ischaemia, livedo reticularis (net-like skin discolouration), claudication (intact pulses), hypertension, renal failure, TIA, stroke, ischaemic viscera
- May be spontaneous or post vascular surgery, trauma, anticoagulation, thrombolysis
- Investigations: ↑ ESR, hypergammaglobulinaemia, ↓ C3/C4, eosinophilia, renal failure
- Management: Support, treat hypertension and ARF

Inadvertent intra-arterial injection

- Drugs injected into artery by mistake
- Sudden severe peripheral ischaemia
- Check CK, renal function
- URGENT vascular consult
- Management options: Consult specialist first
  - Vasodilator (amlodipine 5–10 g PO/day)
  - Anti-inflammatory (dexamethasone 4 mg IV stat then prednisolone 50 mg PO 2/7 and taper)
  - Anti-ischaemic (papaverine 1 mg/kg slow intra-arterial inject or alprostadil)
  - Anticoagulation (heparin infusion or enoxaparin 1 mg/kg SC daily or aspirin 100–300 mg daily)

Acute limb ischaemia

- Presentation
  - New or worsening claudication symptoms, rest pain
  - Change in colour of limb
  - Change in temperature of limb
  - Decreased sensation
  - Decreased muscle power
  - Risk factors: AF, CVD, other vascular disease, valvular disease, prior revascularisation of lower limbs, direct trauma, DVT, crush injury, compartment syndrome
  - Always ask time of onset of symptoms, intensity, duration

- Classification: Rutherford classification—use to determine urgency of treatment
  - I
    - Asymptomatic, mild, moderate or severe symptoms with exertion
    - No sensory loss or muscle weakness
    - Dopplers audible both arterial and venous
    - No immediate threat to limb
  - II(a)
    - Ischaemic rest pain
    - +/– sensory loss limited to toes, no muscle weakness
    - Dopplers inaudible for arterial audible for venous
    - Threat to limb, need prompt treatment
  - II(b)
    - Ischaemic rest pain with some tissue loss
    - Sensory loss, mild to moderate muscle weakness
    - Dopplers inaudible for arterial audible for venous
    - Threat to limb, need immediate treatment
  - III
    - Major tissue loss
    - Profound sensory loss and paralysis
    - Dopplers inaudible arterial and venous
    - Irreversible injury to limb
- Examination
  - Look: Colour, asymmetry, skin lesions, ulcers
  - Feel: Cool, difference between limbs, check sensation, check pulses
  - Move: Check for muscle weakness, pain with passive movement
  - Measure
    - Ankle/brachial index = sBP ankle/sBP arm > 1 = normal, < 0.95 considered abnormal
    - Buerger's test
      - Patient supine: Lift legs at feet to 45 degrees for 2–3 minutes, look for pallor
      - Sit up patient with legs over bed, look for change in colour from pallor to pink to red (sunset foot)

    - Six Ps: Pain, Pallor, Paralysis, Pulseless, Paraesthesia, Poikilothermic
- Investigations
    - Consider US if not limb threatening. US is relatively reliable and without radiation and contrast, but it is slow
    - Consider CTA after discussion with vascular surgeons if limb threat but there is still a little time (Rutherford IIa) or if on the way to OT
- Management
    - Depends on level of threat to limb
    - Consult with vascular surgeons
    - Rutherford II(b) and III need urgent operation or interventional radiology
    - Heparin IV if no contraindications
        - Bolus: 80 units/kg IV
        - Then IV infusion: 18 units/kg/hr
        - Titrate to APTT
- **Complications post angiography: Consult with surgeons**
    - Pseudoaneurysm
        - Painful and pulsatile
    - Vessel occlusion
        - Pain, pallor, paraesthesia, AB index < 0.5
    - Haematoma, can be retroperitoneal
    - AV fistula (uncommon)
        - Bruit, tender, painful, haematoma
    - Others: DVT, bleed, pain, infection, contrast extravasation, femoral nerve injury, arterial embolisation, CVA, dissection

CHAPTER 9

Renal and urology

Acute kidney injury (acute renal failure)

- Signs and symptoms
  - Only develop symptoms when severe uraemia
    - Nausea, vomiting, drowsy, fatigued, confused, ↓ level of consciousness
  - Precipitants: Sepsis, dehydration, AMI, haematuria, urethral obstruction
  - Complications: CNS (e.g. seizures), cardiac (e.g. arrhythmias), GI (e.g. ulcers, ileus), haematological (e.g. anaemia, platelet dysfunction), infection, drug accumulation
- Identify cause
  - Calculate Ur/Cr ratio
    - Plasma urea (mmol/L) : creatinine (mmol/L)
    - If Cr given in micromol/L then divide by 1000 to get mmol/L
    - > 100 = prerenal
    - 50–100 = normal or postrenal
    - < 50 = renal
  - **Prerenal** (70% of community-acquired acute kidney injury [AKI])
    - Volume loss (bleed, vomiting and diarrhoea, diuretics, primary hypoaldosteronism etc.)
    - ↓ cardiac output (AMI, cardiomyopathy, valvular cardiac disease, beta-blockers, high-output cardiac failure etc.)
    - ↓ perfusion (renal artery and small vessel disease)
      - Malignant hypertension, embolic disease, cyclosporin, transplant rejection, haemolytic uraemic syndrome (HUS), vasculitis, ↑ calcium
  - **Intrinsic renal** (acute tubular necrosis [ATN] = 70% of hospital-acquired AKI)
    - Tubular disease (ATN, nephrotoxins, rhabdomyolysis)
    - Interstitial disease (sarcoid, SLE, infection, nephritis)
    - Glomerular disease (glomerulonephritis—Goodpasture's, SLE, post infections)

    - Vascular disease (malignant hypertension, scleroderma, HUS, PAN, renal vein thrombosis)
  - **Postrenal**
    - Urethra/bladder (benign prostatic hyperplasia [BPH], phimosis, stricture, cancer, nephrogenic bladder, clot, trauma)
    - Ureter (vesicoureteral reflux, calculi, papillary necrosis, cancer, fibrosis, stricture, AAA, pregnant, IBD, clot, trauma)
    - Infrarenal (crystals, protein casts)
  - Drugs associated with AKI: NSAIDs, contrast (new evidence suggests perhaps not), ciclosporin, ACE inhibitors, aminoglycosides, EtOH and cocaine (causing rhabdomyolysis), methotrexate, aciclovir, chemotherapy, penicillin, cephalosporins, rifampicin, ciprofloxacin, thiazides, phenytoin, furosemide (frusemide), allopurinol, cimetidine etc.
- Investigations
  - Bloods (EUC, BUN, FBC, CMP, LFT), venous gas (for K^+)
  - ECG, CXR
  - Urine (MCS, protein, casts +/– urine electrolytes, osmolality)
  - Renal US, CT of kidneys, ureters and bladder (CT KUB; look for obstruction)
- Management
  - URGENT management of fluid resuscitation and ↑ K if present
  - Carefully monitor fluids and electrolytes
  - IDC; completely drain urine from obstructed bladder
  - Monitor urine output (can get post-obstructive diuresis: > 250 mL/hr for > 2 hour)
  - DON'T use albumin, AVOID potential nephrotoxins; e.g. NSAIDs, ACE inhibitors, tetracyclines, aminoglycosides and so on
  - May consider cautious use of diuretics if overloaded—talk with specialist first
  - If cause is pigment nephropathy: May need large volume IV fluids, mannitol, $NaHCO_3^-$
- **Dialysis**: Generally, need dialysis if:
  - Volume overload
  - $K^+ > 6.5$ or rising
  - Acid–base imbalance, uncontrollable

  - HT uncontrollable
  - Urine output < 5 mL/kg/day
  - Uraemia symptomatic (pericarditis, encephalopathy, bleeding, nausea and vomiting, pruritus)
  - BUN > 100
  - Dialysable intoxications (e.g. methanol, ethylene glycol, theophylline, aspirin, lithium)
  - Na < 115 or > 165
  - Severe dysthermia
  - Cr > 1000 Ur > 30

Chronic kidney disease (chronic renal failure)

- Definition
  - Glomerular filtration rate (GFR) < 60 mL/min, more than 3 months with no reversible cause
  - ESRD = GFR < 10 mL/min, uraemia, symptomatic
- Results of chronic kidney disease (CKD)
  - Excretory failure: ↑ toxins, urea, PO_4/Na/K^+/H^+
  - **Uraemia** (contamination of blood with urine)
    - Biosynthesis failure: ↓ renal hormones, ↓ vitamin D, ↓ erythropoietin (EPO) causing anaemia, bone disease
    - Regulatory failure: Secondary ↑ parathyroid hormone (PTH; from ↓ Ca) leading to ↑ bone breakdown leading to ↑ ALP. Dyslipidaemia, abnormal sex hormones
- Causes: Diabetes mellitus most common, hypertension/renovascular, GN, cystic (PCKD), nephrotoxins (e.g. NSAIDs), reflux nephropathy
- Uraemia complications
  - Neurological (encephalopathy, dialysis dementia, peripheral neuropathy, subdural haematoma)
  - Cardiovascular (coronary artery disease [CAD], hypertension, cardiac failure, pericarditis)
  - Haematologic (anaemia, bleeding, immunodeficiency)
  - Electrolyte dysfunction (↑ H^+, ↑ K^+, ↑ phosphate, ↓↑ Ca, ↓ Na^+)
  - GI (GI bleed, anorexia, nausea and vomiting, diverticulitis, ascites)
  - Bone (metastatic calcification, ↑ PTH, osteomalacia)
  - Drug toxicities/accumulations

- Dialysis complications: Always discuss with team
  - Fistulas (should have soft compressible pulse and continuous thrill)
    - Thrombosis/stenosis
      - Absent palpable thrill
      - Vascular review, treat within 24 hours
    - Infections (usually treat with vancomycin 1 g IV + gentamicin 100 mg IV but discuss with team)
    - Haemorrhage (URGENT! Pressure, may need tourniquet, vascular review)
    - Aneurysm/pseudoaneurysm (need operation, vascular review)
    - Vascular insufficiency to distal limb (US and urgent vascular review)
    - High-output cardiac failure (↓ HR with temporary access occlusion—diagnose with US. Need surgery)
  - During dialysis
    - ↓ BP (due to ↓ volume, cardiac disease, GI bleed etc.)
    - Altered mental state
      - Dialysis disequilibrium (fluid shift, altered GCS, seizure)
      - Other (SDH, ICH, thrombotic CVA, seizure, encephalopathy)
    - Air embolism
    - Electrolyte abnormal, ↓ BSL
    - Septic shower: If contaminated equipment/infected fistula. Patient gets fevers, hypotension during dialysis
  - Peritoneal dialysis (PD)
    - Peritonitis (fever, abdominal pain, cloudy effluent—send to lab)
      - Treat with rapid exchange of fluid lavaged to ↓ inflamed cells in peritoneum
      - Add heparin 500–1000 units to dialysate and antibiotics to dialysate (e.g. cefalotin 20 mg/kg + gentamicin +/– vancomycin)
    - Infections around PD catheter
    - Abdominal wall hernia (pericatheter hernia; need URGENT repair!)

- Transplant patients: Complications that may present are listed below. Always discuss as soon as possible with transplant team and/or renal specialist
  - Rejection: Tender over transplant, decreased urine output, increased weight/oedema, malaise, fever, increased Cr
  - Infection: > 80% in their first year will get infection. CMV, EBV, varicella, mycobacteria, listeriosis, aspergillus, John Cunningham (JC) virus, etc.
  - Malignancy: Cutaneous, lymphoma, Kaposi's sarcoma, cervical
  - Cardiovascular: HT, renal artery stenosis
  - Haematological and electrolyte: Anaemia, thrombocytopenia, leukopenia, ↑ Ca, ↑ K, ↓ Mg, ↑ Ur, glucose intolerance, lipids
  - GI/surgical: Pancreatitis, peptic ulcer, ileus, hepatitis
  - Glomerulonephritis
- Questions to ask patients before talking to renal team
  - Cause of CKD
  - Dialysis (mode, schedule, any missed)
  - Dry weight, baseline bloods/Cr and BP
  - Access
  - Are they still producing urine?
  - Symptoms of uraemia
  - Native kidneys, transplants
  - Immunosuppressant used, compliance, when last taken, last drug levels

Urinary tract infection (UTI)

- Signs and symptoms
  - Dysuria, frequency, haematuria
  - Cystitis: Flank pain, no systemic features
  - Pyelonephritis: Fever, nausea and vomiting, loin pain, renal angle tenderness, rigors
- Risk groups
  - Predisposing factors: Stone, anatomical, fistula, short perineum, IDC, contaminated sexual practices, retention
  - ↑ risk pyelonephritis: ↑ age, pregnant, prolonged symptoms, ≥ 3 UTI past year, immunocompromised, poor health, comorbidities, obese, IDC, self-catheter, institutionalised

    - Diabetic patients at increased risk of emphysematous pyelonephritis
- Common pathogens: *E. coli*, *Proteus*, *Klebsiella pneumoniae*, Group B strep etc.
- Investigations
    - Urine dipstick: Nitrites good specificity, leucocytes good specificity. Positive on dipstick supports diagnosis; negative doesn't exclude
    - MSU with culture
    - Infants: 40% of infants with a fever have pyuria and no urine source of infection. Therefore, just pyuria in an infant doesn't mean definite UTI. Pyuria + nitrite positive does suggest UTI. Always send sample
    - US if suspecting obstruction, severe pain, ↓ renal function
    - For suspected pyelonephritis take bloods + blood culture
- Management
    - **Cystitis**: Trimethoprim 300 mg PO 3/7 or cephalexin 500 mg BD 5/7
        - Pregnant: Use cephalexin 500 mg BD 10/7
        - Men: Use trimethoprim for 14/7 or cephalexin 14/7, must investigate underlying cause
    - **Pyelonephritis**
        - Mild (low fever, no nausea or vomiting): Cephalexin 500 mg QID 10/7 or trimethoprim 300 mg daily for 10/7
        - Severe: Gentamicin 4–6 mg/kg renal adjusted IV daily + ampicillin 50 mg/kg (max. 2 g) IV QID
            - Can use ceftriaxone 1 g IV/day alone

Fournier gangrene

- Necrotising infection that is highly virulent. Increased risk: Alcoholism, immunocompromised, diabetes mellitus, increased age
- Note: Women can get; men:women ratio 10 : 1
- Signs and symptoms: Pain in genitals severe and disproportionate to physical examination. May find crepitus genitals or perineum, black area of skin
- Patient may be very unwell/septic. WARNING: Patients may initially look well with minimal findings on exam, but they can get very sick very quickly!

- TIP: ALWAYS look at every bit of skin in a patient with fever of unknown origin (especially elderly) and don't forget the perineum
- Treat with fluid resuscitation, broad-spectrum IV antibiotics (e.g. piperacillin/tazobactam) AND vancomycin AND clindamycin
- URGENT surgery: Specialty team—either surgery, urology or both

Male genitourinary emergencies

Scrotal abscess

- Is it localised to wall or intrascrotal?
- Need US and urology referral if not localised

Balanoposthitis

- Inflammation of glans and foreskin
- Erythema, can have red moist macular lesion; can be purulent, malodorous
- Can be fungal/candida, bacterial or contact dermatitis
- Treat: Topical antifungals, topical antibiotics, topical steroids. Ensure hygiene—clean and dry area (avoid soap). Circumcision considered if recurrent

Balanitis

- Inflammation of glans penis (or clitoris) caused by fungus/bacterial/virus/irritants
- Symptoms: Discharge, pain with foreskin retraction, tender/red/itchy glans, difficulty passing urine
- Examination: Red, swollen glans, foul odour, discharge
- Can cause phimosis, rarely can lead to sepsis
- Contributing factors: Poor hygiene, diabetes mellitus (DM), irritants, obesity
- Treatment: Topical antifungals, topical steroids, consider antibiotics if bacteria suspected. Hygiene. Control DM, and other precipitants

Phimosis

- Can't retract foreskin
- Normal in infants; 10% of boys aged 6 still persisting
- Usually not ED issue. Treat with topical steroids, may need circumcision, may need ostium dilation to relieve retention

Paraphimosis

- Can't reduce oedematous foreskin over glans. Can lead to arterial compromise and gangrene. Urological EMERGENCY!

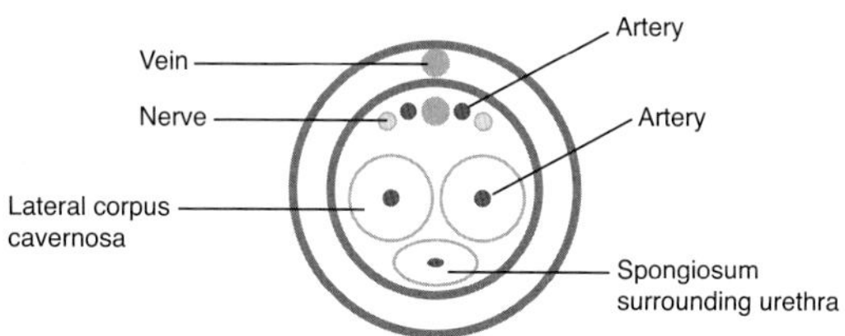

Figure 9.1 Anatomical landmarks

- Attempt to ↓ swelling of glans: Give analgesia (can use 2% lignocaine gel). Try **one** of the following then attempt reduction
  - Apply hydrocortisone cream liberally. Wait 5–10 minutes
  - Compression; tightly wrap glans for 5–10 minutes
  - Use ice pack 5–10 minutes
  - Glucose/osmotic solution. Soak gauze in 50% glucose and apply for 5–10 minutes
- May need superficial dorsal incision of the constricting band. Always use a dorsal penile nerve block first (see Fig. 9.1)

Entrapment

- Hair can get caught around penis causing hair-tourniquet. May be hard to see. Always look for in a crying infant/child when cause unknown

Penis fracture

- Tear/rupture corpus cavernosa tunica albuginea. Trauma during sex, sudden snap. Penis is swollen, tender, flaccid
- Urology referral

Priapism

- Urological EMERGENCY!
- Persistent erection > 4 hours not associated with desire
- Two types
  - Ischaemic
    - Persistent, painful erection, rigid and tender
    - Causes: Medication related (PDE5 inhibitors such as sildenafil, PGE injection, calcium channel blockers, prazosin, hydralazine, chlorpromazine, antipsychotics),

haematological (sickle cell anaemia, procoagulant), spinal cord disease

- Investigations: FBC, ESR, coags, US, cavernosal blood gas (shows acidosis, high CO_2, low O_2)
- Management
  - Urgent urological consult
  - Analgesia
  - If persistent perform corporal aspiration, adrenaline and irrigation (see below)
- Corporal aspiration
  - Dorsal penile nerve block (see Fig. 9.1, p. 196)
  - Aspiration: Use 19 G needle. Insert into lateral corpus. Aspirate 20 mL. Perform blood gas. Some patients will resolve priapism after this. Gas with acidosis, low CO_2, high O_2 = ischaemic priapism
  - Irrigate lateral corpus with 10 mL normal saline
  - Adrenaline: Administer into lateral corpus 1 mL 1 : 100,000 adrenaline every 5 minutes × 5 doses; 80% will resolve
  - Other medications that can be tried: metaraminol, phenylephrine
  - If fails: Need operation

- Non-ischaemic
  - AKA high flow. Caused by unregulated cavernous artery inflow
  - Penis is not fully rigid or painful
  - May be recent trauma
  - Cavernosal blood gas is normal
  - Management: Non-urgent
    - Ice, compression
    - Urology consult
    - May need embolisation or operation if conservative treatment fails

Epididymitis

- Symptoms: Gradual onset pain, discharge, dysuria, nausea
- Signs: Fever, tender, redness, oedema, hydrocele. Elevation of scrotum relieves the pain

- Causes: Young male (congenital abnormal reflux), 16–35 years of age (sexually transmitted infection [STI]), older male (pathogens of UTI such as *E. coli*). Older male look for stricture, BPH
- Investigations: May have pyuria on UA. Send MSU, PCR for STI on urine (must be first pass) or urethral swabs. May need US
- Management
  - Consider admission if fever, ↑ WBC, toxic, need IV analgesia
  - Scrotal elevation, ice, bed rest, NSAIDs, antibiotics, morphine
- Antibiotics; examples below
  - If UTI source, trimethoprim 300 mg 14/7 PO or cephalexin
  - If STI source, ceftriaxone 500 mg IM stat + doxycycline 100 mg BD 14/7 PO
  - If systemic toxicity, use ampicillin IV and gentamicin IV

Prostatitis

- Lower back pain, fever, genital pain, obstructive urinary tract symptoms (e.g. frequency, urgency), pyuria. Rectal exam: Prostate large, warm and tender
- Investigate for STI (swab, first-pass urine), UA, MSU
- Treat with ciprofloxacin 500 mg BD 4/52 or similar to UTI management
- Admit if severe: Stat gentamicin, IV ampicillin 2 g QID

Urethritis

- Urethral discharge purulent
- Usually STI
- Ceftriaxone 500 mg IM stat + doxycycline 100 mg BD 14/7 PO

Urethral stricture

- Risk: STIs, trauma, instrumentation
- Attempt catheter with lots of lidocaine (lignocaine) lube
  - Gentle attempt, if unable and retention get urgent urology consult
- May need urgent suprapubic/infra-umbilical-suprapubic. Seldinger technique +/– US

Urinary retention

- Look for cause: Systemic illness, medications, stricture, BPH, silent priapism
- Examine abdomen, genitals, meatus, rectal exam
- US: Bladder volume
- Catheter: IDC or suprapubic catheter (SPC) if necessary
- Can get gross haematuria; post-obstruction diuresis
- If well, discharge with IDC (if symptoms chronic must observe 4–6 hours first), urology follow-up

Testicular torsion

- Peak incidence: Neonates and puberty; can occur any age. Often recent strenuous event (trauma, exertion)
- Symptoms: Usually sudden severe pain unilateral testicular. Can be abdominal pain, loin pain, groin pain etc. Nausea, vomiting. Can have fever. Beware the adolescent with abdominal pain; always check the genitals
- Signs: Testicle involved is firm, tender, higher in scrotum, transverse lie, cremasteric reflex absent, hemi-scrotal oedema. Cremasteric reflex = stroke inner thigh downward—testicle pulls up due to cremaster muscle
- Investigations: CLINICAL DIAGNOSIS. Don't waste time with imaging. US may help only if equivocal
- URGENT Urology consult! NEED OPERATION
- Testicular detorsion: At foot of patient rotate left testicle clockwise and right counterclockwise. Pain relief = positive endpoint. If pain is increased, rotate the other way. Temporising measure only
- Torsion of appendages/appendix may get blue spot sign with illumination, usually not harmful condition. Usually point tenderness, normal testicle position. Often need operation anyway unless diagnosis is absolutely certain

Dorsal penile block

- Fig. 9.1 shows anatomical landmarks for administering a dorsal penile block
- Indications: Dorsal slit foreskin, phimosis and paraphimosis reduction, laceration or other injury repair, relief of priapism
- Contraindications: Overlying infection, suspected testicular torsion
- Preparation: Sterile procedure, aseptic technique. Analgesia for patient

- Landmarks: 2 injection sites
  - Base of penis
  - Lateral to midline on both sides
  - 2 and 10 o'clock
- Use 27 G needle
- Make small wheel of LA at site then insert needle approx. 0.5 cm directed towards centre of shaft. Aspirate to confirm not within artery/vessel
- Inject 2 mL of lidocaine (lignocaine) 1% WITHOUT ADRENALINE

Ureteric stones

- Signs and symptoms: Acute severe, episodic pain, flank–abdomen–groin. Little abdominal tenderness. Associated nausea and vomiting, sweating, writhing
- Conditions that ↑ risk: ↑ calcium, gout, infection, hyperoxaluria, congenital malformations, renal tubular acidosis (RTA), IBD, drugs
- Investigations
  - Urine (usually 85–90% haematuria +/– UTI)
  - βHCG, EUC, +/– CMP, +/– albumin, +/– urate
  - Plain x-ray KUB: can see most stones, used to monitor passage
  - CT KUB
    - Exclude AAA (especially if > 60 and male)
  - US if young patient (< 50)/can't CT. Usually don't see stone but can see hydronephrosis
- Exclude serious causes of severe abdominal pain: Examples
  - AAA (look for mass, ↓ pulses, ↓ BP): do bedside USS
  - Ectopic
  - Incarcerated hernia
  - Torsion
  - AMI
  - Pneumonia
  - PE
  - Pyelonephritis
- Exclude infected, impacted stone: Patients usually febrile, unwell, can be septic, hypotensive. Need urgent management, IVAB

- Management
  - Analgesia, opiates, NSAIDs: Indomethacin 100 mg PO/PR
  - IV fluids, for replacing deficit or maintain hydration not to increase urine flow
  - Expulsive treatment: Tamsulosin. Conflicting studies
  - Admit if: Infection, obstruction, AKI, multiple ED visits, underlying disease severe, large stone, sloughed renal papillae, elderly, comorbidities, ongoing IV analgesia required, single kidney
  - Discharge if: Young, no infection, otherwise well, hydronephrosis < 10 mm, non-transplant, normal renal function, stone < 6 mm, pain controlled, 2 normal kidneys, use strainer to catch stone. Urology or GP follow-up, return if symptoms recur/fevers/gross haematuria, give analgesia (e.g. indometacin script)
  - Bladder calculi: Dysuria, haematuria, end of micturition. Need URGENT treatment if cause obstruction or infection

CHAPTER 10
Haematology

Anaemia

- Signs and symptoms: Asymptomatic, general weakness/fatigue, SOB with exertion, palpitations, orthostatic ↓ BP, ↑ HR, pallor, angina in IHD/atherosclerosis. Signs and symptoms of cause
- Causes
  - Loss of RBC
    - Bleeding: Acute or chronic
  - ↑ Destruction
    - Inherited: G6PD, thalassaemia, sickle cell anaemia, etc.
    - Antibody mediated: Transfusion reactions, drug induced, autoimmune
    - Mechanical trauma: HUS, DIC, thrombotic thrombocytopenic purpura (TTP), heart valves
    - Infection: Malaria, clostridium
    - Toxic: Snake venom, lead poisoning
    - Sequestration: Hypersplenism
  - ↓ production
    - Inherited
    - Nutritional: B12, folate, iron
    - Renal disease: EPO deficiency
    - Immune: Aplastic anaemia
    - Anaemia of chronic disease
    - Neoplastic: Leukaemia, myelodysplastic, myeloproliferative, bone marrow lesions
  - Dilutional
- History: Ask about timeframe of symptoms, history of blood loss (trauma, GI, gynaecological), chronic illness (heart, renal, inflammation, malignancy), medications, drug and alcohol, nutrition, FHx
- Investigations
  - FBC (↓ Hb = diagnosis, normal range depends on age and sex)

- Look for cause
  - Generally, clues to cause
    - FBC differential, MCV (micro/macro/normocytic anaemia), reticulocytes
    - K (increased in haemolysis)
    - Cr (renal disease)
    - Ur:Cr (increased in GI bleed)
    - LFTs (bilirubin and LDH increased in haemolysis)
  - Specific causes: Fe, B12, folate, LFT, stool occult blood, bleeding disorder (coags), fibrinogen, urine, scopes, imaging
  - See Table 10.1 for causes of anaemia based on MCV result

Table 10.1 Types of anaemia divided by MCV

Macrocytic MCV > 100 fL	Microcytic MCV < 80 fL	Normocytic MCV 80–100 fL
EtOH	Thalassaemia	Chronic disease
B12 deficiency (pernicious anaemia, gastrectomy, malabsorption, diet, nitrous oxide). B12 deficiency also causes neuro disease, degeneration of spinal cord and peripheral neuropathy	Iron deficiency (bleeding, malabsorption, diet) ↓ serum Fe, ↓ ferritin, ↑ transferrin, ↓ haematocrit, ↓ MVC	Anaemia of chronic disease. Bloods show N/↑ ferritin, N/↓ transferrin, ↓ Fe, ↓ transferrin saturation, ↑ hepcidin, ↓ EPO
Hypothyroid	Sideroblastic	Haemolysis
Chronic liver disease	Chronic systemic disease	Congenital
Folate deficiency (diet, malabsorption, increased demands, drugs—methotrexate/trimethoprim/phenytoin etc.)		Any type of anaemia, early stages
Aplastic anaemia		Aplastic anaemia
Myelodysplastic syndrome		

- Management
  - Depends on symptoms, comorbidities, cause
  - For example: If minimal symptoms, chronic, iron deficiency anaemia—may only require iron transfusion despite very low Hb
  - Treat the cause
  - May need blood transfusion
    - For acute blood loss + shock (i.e. trauma) replace blood loss with blood
    - For anaemia Hb < 70 g/L or Hb70–100 g/L + comorbidities; e.g. IHD
    - Dose—1 unit packed RBC max. over 4 hours
    - 1 unit should increase Hb by approx. 10 g/L
    - Check fluid status in patient frequently

Transfusion reactions

Management

- Prevention
  - Always take accurate G&H! Monitor EUC, monitor fluid status, may need diuretic to prevent overload—titrated to effect; e.g. 10 mg IV furosemide after each bag
- Acute event during transfusion: Fever, ↓ BP, unwell
  - STOP TRANSFUSION: CALL LAB, consult haematology
  - Retake: EUC, FBC, coags, haptoglobin, LDH, LFT, bilirubin (unconjugated)
  - Also send remaining blood, used giving set and new G&H to lab
  - CXR
- Supportive care
  - Maintain renal blood flow and urine output, check volume status (may need fluids or furosemide), may need vasopressors

Acute reactions

Infections

- Low risk
- Sepsis: Can get bacterial sepsis from contamination during storage usually *Yersinia enterocolitica*
  - Manage as above + antibiotics
- Viruses; e.g. CMV (can use CMV-tested or leucocyte-reduced blood for pregnant, immunocompromised, premature babies, transplant patients)

Acute haemolytic reaction

- 1 in 1 million
- Usually acute and a result of human error in cross-match leads to DIC, anaphylatoxins
- Symptoms: Pain at IVC site, back pain, headache, fever, ↓ BP, APO, bronchospasm, bleeding, AKI
- URGENT cease T/F! steps as above
- Results: Haptoglobin ↓, LDH ↑

Febrile reactions

- 1 in 300
- More common
- Fever during or few hours post transfusion
- Can also get rigors, myalgia, headache, ↑ HR, SOB. Can look like haemolytic reaction or sepsis
- Investigate as above, stop transfusion
- Usually self-limiting and respond to antipyretics. Can pre-treat with antipyretic, paracetamol, if patient has had a previous febrile reaction
- Can often restart transfusion

Allergic reactions

- Urticaria, pruritus during transfusion
- Rarely result in anaphylaxis, wheeze etc.
- Stop transfusion, above management if severe
- Treat with antihistamines. Adrenaline if severe
- Can often restart transfusion if mild

Transfusion-related acute lung injury (TRALI)

- Usually FFP or platelets. Within 6 hours
- Bilateral pulmonary infiltrates on CXR, non-cardiac pulmonary oedema.
- Supportive care. Usually self resolves

Transfusion associated circulatory overload (TACO)

- APO. Carefully consider main differential diagnosis, TRALI
- Best to pre-empt and give slow transfusions in at-risk patients; e.g. elderly. Assess frequently and use frusemide between bags

Electrolyte imbalance

- Can get ↓ Ca, ↑↓ K^+ from large volumes

Delayed

Delayed haemolysis

- 1 in 1000
- Usually in spleen or liver, bone marrow
- ↑ unconjugated bilirubin. Positive Coombs' test
- Rarely fatal. Treatment supportive.

Others

- Allo-immunisation, graft versus host, iron overload

Hereditary conditions

Haemophilia

- Deficiency of factor VIII (haemophilia A) or factor IX (haemophilia B) X-linked recessive
- Factor level
  - < 1% = severe
  - 1–5% = moderate (may bleed spontaneously but mostly trauma cause)
  - 6–25% = mild (trauma related bleed)
- Bleeding usually into joints, muscles > abdomen, CNS
- Investigations: ↑↑ APTT, normal PT, ↓ factor VIII or IX
- Assessment
  - ABC
  - Imaging, CT head
  - Note: ↑ risk compartment syndrome
- Management
  - Early physio refer and treat haemarthrosis
  - Analgesia (no NSAIDs, aspirin, DON'T give anything IM)
- Factor replacement
  - As per injury site, current % factor, weight, haem A or B. Discuss with haematology as soon as possible
  - Severe patients: Will need Factor VIII (Factor IX if haemophilia B) within 30 minutes (1 unit increases factor by 2%)
  - For mild/moderate (levels > 5%) can use desmopressin/DDAVP 0.3 microgram/kg IV
  - Some patients have factor inhibitors: Very difficult to treat. Use PCC, high dose Factor VIII, activated Factor VIIIa; get haematology advice

von Willebrand disease (VWD)

- Type 1 (↓ von Willebrand factor [vWF] mild), type 2 (normal levels of abnormal vWF), type 3 (secondary ↓↓ vWF to Factor VIII ↓)
- Usually skin and mucosal bleeding, including GI and menorrhagia
- Investigate with vWF (may be normal), ↑ APTT, Factor VIII
- Avoid aspirin, NSAIDs, heparin
- Management
  - Type 1 and 2 NOT 3: Desmopressin/DDAVP (↑ vWF release) 0.3 microgram/kg (max. 20 microgram) SC or IV BD max. 4 doses (can also get intranasal)
  - vWF/FVIII concentrate used for types 2 and 3 and sometimes type 1 if severe
- Cryoprecipitate, platelets and/or FFP may be beneficial if other treatments are failing
- Can use tranexamic acid 10 mg/kg IV
- Can use aminocaproic acid

Sickle cell anaemia

- ↑ risk African, Middle Eastern, Indian
- Features: Joint pain, pulmonary infarcts, haemolytic anaemia, CNS ischaemia, CCF, cor pulmonale, abdominal pain, gallstones, jaundice, renal necrosis, splenomegaly, bone infarcts, skin ulcers
- Sickling
  - In most children and ⅓ adults: Precipitated by infection
  - Results in hypoxia, acidosis, volume depletion, vascular stasis
  - Consequences: Bone infarct, organ ischaemia, pulmonary infarction, CNS infarct/bleed, priapism, renal infarct, haem crisis, acute spleen sequestration, aplastic crisis, infection crises
- Investigations
  - FBC, reticulocyte count, LFT
  - Sickle cells, Howell Jolly bodies, increased WCC, increased platelets
  - CXR, bone x-rays
  - NOTE: CTPA can precipitate sickling
- Specific ED presentations
  - Vaso-occlusive pain crisis: Precipitants—infection, cold, altitude, dehydrated
    - Intravascular sickling, small vessel occlusion leads to infarction bone, viscera, soft tissue causing bone/muscle/joint pain

        - Treat with O_2 if hypoxic, analgesia, IV fluids/hydration, PCA, NSAIDs, +/– hydroxyurea, +/– IVAB to prevent sepsis, +/– exchange transfusion
        - Pain syndromes usually sites of infarction/infection; e.g. bone, chest, abdomen, genitourinary
    - Splenic infarction: Micro infarcts. Can lead to non-functioning spleen and infections
        - Splenic sequestration leading to sudden enlarged spleen
            - Causes acute ↓ Hb with blood volume moved into spleen resulting in ↓ BP
        - Treat with fluid resuscitation, exchange transfusion, splenectomy
        - Blood transfusions should be aimed at previous known Hb NOT to normal Hb
    - Infections: Patient may be functionally asplenic and therefore ↑ risk infections. Always vaccinate; prophylactic antibiotics

Thalassaemias

- Microcytic, hypochromic anaemia
- ↑ risk Mediterranean, Middle Eastern, African, South-East Asian
- Thalasaemia trait: Often no symptoms, mild ↓ Hb
- Thalasaemia major: Hepatosplenomegaly, jaundice, severe anaemia, marrow expansion
- Treatments
    - May need transfusions
    - May develop Fe overload: Treat with desferrioxamine

Henoch-Schönlein purpura (HSP)

- Most common vasculitis
- Presentation
    - Ages usually 2–8 years old
    - 50% have recent URTI
    - Palpable purpura, arthritis abdominal pain, renal complications (haematuria, proteinuria, hypertension)
- Examination: Check BP
- Investigations
    - Urine analysis is the only necessary investigation in unequivocal cases

  - Other investigations may be needed to exclude differential diagnosis or to look for complications
    - FBC, EUC, cultures, abdominal imaging, autoantibodies
- Management
  - Mild: NSAIDs, paracetamol
  - Moderate–severe: Steroids (decrease duration of pain but not risk of complications)
  - GP follow-up to check BP and urine
- Complications
  - Intussusception, GI bleed, bowel ischaemia/necrosis/perforation, diffuse alveolar haemorrhage, encephalopathy, ICH, nephrotic/nephritic syndrome, HT, renal failure

Acquired haemolytic anaemia

Autoimmune

- Autoantibodies against RBC
- Primary or secondary; e.g. underlying cause chronic lymphocytic leukaemia (CLL), infection with EBV or CMV, HIV
- Warm antibody autoimmune haemolytic anaemia (AIHA) = 70% of cases. Autoantibody reacts most at 37°C. Treat with steroids, transfusion, splenectomy, cytotoxic drugs
- Cold antibody AIHA. Autoantibody most strong 0–4°C. Keep patient warm, query steroids (evidence equivocal). Transfuse with warm blood

Alloimmune

- Antibodies to allogenic RBC (e.g. fetus, post transfusion). Patient has haemolytic transfusion reaction from previous sensitisation

Drug related

- Drug (e.g. methyldopa, levodopa, diclofenac, 2nd- or 3rd-generation cefalosporin) triggers autoantibodies against patient's own RBCs, resolves days–months on stopping drug
- Antibodies against drug: RBC complex e.g. penicillin, DTP vaccination (diphtheria, tetanus, pertussis). Cease drug usually stops haemolysis

Thrombotic thrombocytopenic purpura (TTP)

- Classic pentad (in minority of cases)
  - ↓ platelets, microangiopathic haemolytic anaemia, fever, renal impairment, neurological impairment (fluctuating symptoms; focal neurology, mental state changes)

- Precipitating events: Pregnancy/postpartum, infection, HIV, vaccination, SLE, cyclosporine, tacrolimus, clopidogrel, bone marrow transplant, chemotherapy
- Investigations ↓↓ Hb, ↓ platelets (< 20), helmet cells, ↑ reticulocytes, ↓ haptoglobin, ↑ unconjugated bilirubin, normal coags, normal fibrinogen, fragmented red cells, 65% anti-ADAMTs13 antibody
- Treatment
  - Plasma exchange, FFP (in congenital), steroids (in acquired)
  - Support: Packed cells, anticonvulsants, antihypertensive, dialysis. Avoid aspirin, heparin
  - ***Avoid platelets unless life-threatening bleed; they may worsen thrombosis***

Haemolytic uraemic syndrome (HUS)

- Like TTP, HUS causes microthrombi
- Presentation
  - Peak 6 months to 4 years old. Adult HUS looks like TTP
  - Often post infection
  - *E. coli* is a well-known precipitate; others: Shigella, *Yersinia*, salmonella, *Campylobacter*, *Streptococcus pneumoniae*, varicella, coxsackie, ECHO virus
  - Signs and symptoms: Fever, dysentery, oliguria, purpura, pulmonary oedema, pericardial effusion, atrial arrhythmia
- Investigations
  - Microangiopathic haemolytic anaemia: ↓ platelets < 100, ↓↓ Hb, fragmented red cells, schistocytes, reticulocytes ↑
  - ↑ Cr, blood and protein in urine
  - Coags normal or mild increased INR
  - ↓ haptoglobin, ↑ LDH, Coombs' test negative
  - Stool culture
- Treatment: Careful fluid balance and correction, correct electrolytes, support
  - More severe cases: query steroids (evidence equivocal), plasma exchange, dialysis, vitamin E, thromboxane, whole blood or FFP transfusion
  - DON'T give antibiotics or antimotilities

Pregnancy associated

(See Chapter 13 Obstetrics and gynaecology, p. 274)

- Pregnancy-associated TTP
- Pregnancy-associated HUS
- HELLP syndrome

Malignancy associated

- Widely disseminated cancer can lead to haemolytic anaemia
- Higher risk cancers = gastric, lung, breast, colon, prostate, hepatic
- May lead to DIC
- Poor prognosis from cancer
- Treat with chemotherapy

Bleeding disorders

Platelet defects/thrombocytopenia

- Severity
  - Platelet > 50×10^9/L = asymptomatic
  - 30–50 = bleeding with trauma
  - 10–30 = petechiae
  - < 10 leads to spontaneous bleed
  - ↑ risk with ↑ age, comorbid (e.g. liver disease), falls/trauma
- Assessment
  - First assess haemodynamic stability
  - Ask detailed HPI, family history, medications, recent illness
  - Look for bleeding sites
- Investigate with FBC and smear for clumping
- Causes:
  - Platelet clumping causing pseudothrombocytopenia
  - ↓ platelet production
    - Neonatal: Infection (e.g. CMV, rubella)
    - Child: Lymphoma, leukaemia, myelofibrosis
    - Adult: EtOH, medications (e.g. thiazides), B12 deficiency
    - Chemotherapy, radiotherapy

- ↑ Platelet destruction or consumption
  - Immune mediated; e.g. idiopathic thrombocytopenic purpura (ITP) (see p. 209)
  - Non-immune mediated; e.g. TTP, HUS, DIC, HELLP syndrome, pregnancy, platelet sequestration with splenomegaly, RA, SLE, hepatitis C, haematological cancers, trauma, post transfusion
  - Infection; e.g. sepsis, dengue, malaria, Ebola
  - Drugs; e.g. heparin, paracetamol, NSAIDs, phenytoin, vancomycin, furosemide, amiodarone, ranitidine
- Qualitative platelet abnormal
  - Uraemia, liver disease, DIC, cardiac bypass, AML, ALL, vWD, myeloma

Liver disease

- Abnormal/↓ synth of clotting factor (except VIII)
- Can also get ↓ vitamin K clotting factor with fat malabsorption
- Severe liver disease leads to portal hypertension which leads to splenomegaly causing platelets to be sequestered
- Investigations: ↓ platelet, ↓ fibrinogen (due to ↑ fibrinolysis), ↑ fibrin degradation products, normal ↑ D–dimer, ↓ coagulant factors, may look like DIC
- Treatment
  - If no bleeding can observe
  - If significant bleeding need urgent specialist input, RBC transfusion, PO/IV vitamin K +/– platelets, cryoprecipitate, FFP +/– desmopressin

Renal disease

- Abnormal platelet function, abnormal clotting factors. Prevent with dialysis, good nutrition
- Treat bleeding with dialysis, packed cells, desmopressin, cryoprecipitate, platelet transfusion

Disseminated intravascular coagulation (DIC)

- Activation of coagulation cascade leads to fibrin + $^{+}$fibrinolysis leading to break down fibrin, consume clotting factor
- Triggers
  - Common: Infection/sepsis especially Gram-negative, massive bleeds/trauma, venom, eclampsia, rhabdomyolysis, heat stroke, pancreatitis

  - HOTMISS
    - **H**epatic failure
    - **O**bstetric (amniotic fluid embolism, fetal death in utero, eclampsia)
    - **T**rauma
    - **M**alignancy
    - **I**mmune
    - **S**epsis
    - **S**hock
  - Others: Vascular disease, ARDs, transfusion reactions
- Result is multi-organ involvement: Renal, ARDS, hepatic injury, neurological involvement, CCF
- Signs and symptoms: Bleeding, thrombosis, purpura fulminans, organ failure, mental change, oliguria, focal ischaemia, ARDS
- Investigations: ↑ PT (> 3 sec), ↓ platelet (< 100 × 10^9/L), ↓ fibrinogen (< 1 g/L), ↑ fibrin degradation product (FDP)/D-dimer (> 30 mg/L, if < 2 DIC unlikely), ↑ LDH, ↓ haptoglobin, schistocytes on blood smear, ↓ clotting factors/protein C/antithrombin
  - Can get chronic compensated DIC most likely with malignancies
- Treatment: Support, treat cause, fluid resuscitate, packed cells, platelet (aim > 50 × 10^9/L), fibrinogen (aim > 1 g/L) and coagulant factors with cryoprecipitate (contains fibrinogen) and FFP (contains clotting factors), consider heparin if thrombosis and no bleeding

Others

- **HIV**: can present with ↓ platelet, bleeding
- **Factor VIII inhibitors**: can develop in patient with haemophilia A, SLE, RA etc.
- Antiphospholipid antibody
  - Associated with SLE, drug reaction, malignancy, HIV
  - Can result in DVT/PE, miscarriage

Idiopathic thrombocytopenic purpura (ITP)

- Antiviral antibody: Antigen complex on platelets resulting in platelet destruction

- Presentations
  - Children: Common 2–6 years old. Often 23 weeks post viral illness or vaccine. Petechiae/bleeding/bruising. Exam otherwise normal
    - If child limping, hepatosplenomegaly or lymph nodes present: Consider alternative diagnosis such as lympho-proliferative diseases
  - Adults: Usually gradual onset. Most will relapse, petechiae, epistaxis, menorrhagia
  - Precipitants: EBV, rubella, CMV, viral hepatitis
  - Chronic: Usually women of childbearing age. Autoantibodies
  - No organomegaly/nodes/pallor, normal bone marrow
- Investigations
  - Isolated platelet decrease, normal film, normal coags. Platelet-bound antibody. Increased bleeding time
- Management
  - Children
    - Usually no treatment; 80% recover
    - Observe, ensure follow-up, avoid contact sports/aspirin
    - Admit if platelets < 20 or significant bleeding or platelets 20–50 and increased risk of bleeding
    - Significant bleeding: Use IVIg high-dose steroids
    - Life-threatening bleeding: Platelet transfusion, splenectomy
  - Adults: Prednisone, rituximab, anti-D Ig splenectomy, thrombopoietin
  - Severe bleed: Transfusion platelets, IV steroids, aminocaproic acid
  - Recurrence
    - Most children need no treatment and 80% recover without recurrence
    - Most adults will have recurrence

Haematological oncology

Leukaemia

- Acute lymphoblastic leukaemia (ALL)
  - Mostly children
  - Abrupt onset

  - Presentations: Anaemia, bruising, bone pain, secondary infection, lymph nodes, splenomegaly, CNS symptoms
  - Investigations: Pancytopenia, lymphoblasts
  - Management: Need specialist input urgently, treat inter-current illness, infection, chemo, allogenic bone marrow transplant
- Acute myeloid leukaemia (AML)
  - Mean age 70 but can affect all ages, more common in men
  - Risk factors: Myelodysplasia, smoking, chemo or radiation therapy, benzene
  - Presentations: Secondary infection, bone pain, splenomegaly, anaemia, fatigue, bleeding
  - Investigations: Raised WCC with pancytopenia
  - Management: Urgent specialist input, treat infection, chemotherapy
- Chronic myeloid leukaemia (CML)
  - Adults, insidious onset
  - Presentation: Anaemia, splenomegaly, hepatomegaly, bleeding, infection, hyperviscosity, splenic infarction, weight loss, fatigue
  - Investigations: Increased WCC, blasts on film
  - Management: Hydroxyurea, stem cell transplant, imatinib
  - Complications: Blast transformation (20% per year)—very large spleen, weight loss, lytic bone lesions, lymph nodes, hypercalcaemia
- Chronic lymphocytic leukaemia
  - Adults, usually elderly, slowly progressive
  - Proliferation of a clone of incompetent lymphocytes
  - Presentation: Lymph nodes, splenomegaly, infection, pulmonary disease
  - Investigations: Increased WCC, smudge cells, secondary autoimmune TTP or haemolytic anaemia
  - Management: Discuss with specialist, monitor, chemo, bone marrow transplant

Multiple myeloma

- Plasma cell tumour, age > 40
- Presentation
  - Symptoms of anaemia (fatigue etc.), thrombocytopenia (bleed, bruise), hyperviscosity, immune suppression, recurrent infection

  - Metastasis symptoms (pain, fracture), common locations: Spine, skull, rib, pelvis. Punched out lesions on x-ray
- Investigations: ↑ protein, ↑ gamma globulin, ↑ Ca, ↑ LDH, ↑ urate, ↑↑ ESR, ↑ Cr, proteinuria, Bence Jones proteins in urine
- Management: Specialist input, support, allopurinol, prednisone, antibiotics, bisphosphonates, chemotherapy, interferon alpha, bone marrow transplant

Lymphoma

- Hodgkin's lymphoma
  - Patients usually younger
  - Presentations: Lymphadenopathy painful/painless/mass effects, weight loss, fever, night sweats, hepatosplenomegaly, paraneoplastic syndromes, chest pain, cough, SOB, back pain, bone pain
  - Investigations: Anaemia, lymphopenia, ↑ neutrophils or ↑ eosinophil, ↑ ESR, ↑ LDH, ↑ Cr, ↑ cytokines
  - Management: Specialist referral, chemotherapy, radiotherapy, local excision
- Non-Hodgkin's lymphoma
  - Patients usually older
  - Presentations: Varied. Painless nodes. Fevers, night sweats, weight loss can occur in more advanced disease. Extranodal symptoms such as GI, GU, CNS. Nodes causing obstruction such as superior vena cava (SVC) syndrome
  - Investigations: Anaemia, can have haemolysis, low platelets, leukopenia or pancytopenia, lymphocytosis of malignant cell. ↑ LDH, abnormal LFT, ↑ Ca
  - Management: Specialist referral, chemo and radiotherapy, rituximab

Malignancy-associated emergency

Pathologic fracture

- X-rays
- IV analgesia
- Immobilise
- Surgery/orthopaedics

Spinal cord compression

- Most often thoracic
- ↑↑ pain; worse supine

- Weakness, sensory change, retention, incontinence
- Need CT, MRI
- Analgesia, spinal surgical URGENT review, operation, radiotherapy, steroids

Pericardial effusion with tamponade

- Most common cancer type: Breast, lung
- Usually slow onset, can get very large, often well tolerated
- Symptoms/signs: SOB, chest pain, hoarse voice, hiccup, dysphagia, muffled heart sounds, jugular vein distension, pulsus paradoxus, low-volt QRS
- Tamponade: ↓ BP, narrow pulse pressure, shock
- Diagnose with US, and clinically
- Treat with emergency pericardiocentesis (see procedures, p. 45), urgently if tamponade. Radiotherapy, chemotherapy

Superior vena cava (SVC) syndrome

- Causes: Primary lung cancer (70%); lymphoma, metastasis, non-cancer related (aortic aneurysm, thyroid, TB, syphilis)
- Signs and symptoms: Facial swelling, venous engorgement trunk, neck and upper limb; nausea and vomiting, headache, SOB, cough, hoarse voice, stridor, dysphagia, syncope, Pemberton's sign, chest pain
- Management: Elevate head of bed, O_2, urgent oncology input
  - Query diuretics (40 mg IV furosemide), evidence questionable
  - Query dexamethasone IV 8 mg, evidence questionable
  - Radiotherapy, chemotherapy, SVC stent

Biochemical abnormalities

(See Chapter 12 Endocrine, p. 251)

- Hypercalcaemia
- Syndrome of inappropriate antidiuretic hormone (SIADH)
- Adrenal insufficiency
  - Treat stressed and steroid-dependent patient with IV steroids. Hydrocortisone 200 mg IV
  - Investigations: ↓ Na, ↓ BSL, ↑ K, ↑ eosinophils

Tumour lysis syndrome

- More common in haematological malignancies
- Can be spontaneous or post chemotherapy

- Presentations: Abdominal pain, urine symptoms, flank pain, symptoms of low calcium, symptoms of high potassium, lethargy, oedema, CCF, arrhythmia, syncope
- Causes: ↑ uric acid, ↑ PO_4, ↓ Ca, ↑ K^+, AKI, ↑ LDH
- Treatment: Urgent specialist input
  - Ensure hydration, fluid resuscitation. Usually avoid diuretics
  - $NaHCO_3^-$ (urine alkalisation) + IV fluids acetazolamide
  - Usual treatment of ↑ K but avoid calcium unless ECG changes
  - Rasburicase
  - PO_4 binders. Dialysis

Clotting

- Thromboembolism
  - Cancer leads to ↑ risk clotting
  - Treat with heparin and warfarin
- Hyperviscosity syndrome
  - Abnormal blood (e.g. plasma); rouleaux on blood smear
  - Fatigue, abdominal pain, changes in mental state, thrombosis
  - Urgent haematology review; plasmapheresis
  - If coma: 1 L phlebotomy replace with 3 L normal saline

Febrile neutropenia

- Fever > 38°C for over 1 hour or one reading over 38.5°C + neutrophils ↓ < 1.0×10^9
- Take cultures and treat before examining! Don't delay antibiotics for cultures. Cultures are important; however, they do often change management in these patients
- Look for source: May be no signs of infection on full examination; DO NOT perform rectal examination
- Investigations: FBC, cultures, EUC, LFT, CMP, urine, CXR, sputum, swabs
- LP not routine
- Give empiric broad-spectrum antibiotics
  - Gentamicin 5–7 mg/kg/day IV (as per creatine)
  - + piperacillin/tazobactam 4.5 g QID IV
  - + vancomycin 1.5 g if suspecting MRSA or line source or low BP
  - Metronidazole if suspecting intra-abdominal source 500 mg IV
- Reverse barrier nursing, treat shock, may need high-dependency unit (HDU)/ICU

CHAPTER 11

Toxicology

Overdose overview

- Assessment: Full history, corroborative history: Drug, amount, route, preparation (e.g. slow release), time, last seen, any empty packets found, co-ingestions, comorbidities
- Investigations
  - **BSL**
  - **ECG** (wide QRS > 120 ms, long QT)
  - Drug levels (**paracetamol**, anticonvulsants, aspirin, digoxin, lithium, iron, methotrexate, K^+, theophylline, alcohols)
  - Bloods: EUC, LFT, βHCG
  - VBG: Respiratory ↓ with ↑ pCO_2, acidosis
  - CXR if ↓ O_2 or suspecting aspiration
  - CTB if potential for other cause or associated possible head injury
  - Other imaging if associated trauma
  - **For every patient: Need BSL, ECG, paracetamol level**
- Management
  - ABC
  - Discuss with toxicologist
  - Note: CPR if required may be prolonged
  - Look for and treat: Seizure, electrolyte, glucose and temperature derangements
  - Replace electrolytes Mg, K, calcium (except digoxin toxicity—theoretical risk)
    - $MgSO_4$ 10–20 mmol over ½ to 1 hour IV
    - Calcium gluconate 10% 10–20 mL over 10–30 minutes IV
    - KCl 10–20 mmol over 1–2 hours IV
  - Decontamination—charcoal
    - Dose = 50 g (1 g/kg) PO or NGT
    - Consider if:
      - < 1 hour from ingestion (sometimes considered up to 24 hours; e.g. in massive paracetamol ingestions)

  - Slow-release preparations
  - Gut stasis likely with ingestion
  - Potential for bezoar; e.g. large number of tablets, salicylates
  - Some massive ingestions; e.g. paracetamol
  - Specific drugs require urgent decontamination; e.g. paraquat
- AND either
  - GCS = 15 and unlikely to drop GCS/seize

    OR
  - Intubated patient
- NOTE: Can't use charcoal in hydrocarbons, alcohols, metals, corrosives

- Decontamination—other
  - Whole bowel irrigation—consider for: Iron, slow-release K, slow-release verapamil/diltiazem, arsenic, lead, body packers, massive ingestion lithium
  - Skin and ocular decontamination
- ↑ Elimination
  - Dialysis: Toxic alcohols, methotrexate, lithium, metformin, salicylates, anticonvulsants, valproate, K, theophylline, paraquat
  - Urinary alkalinisation: Salicylates, phenobarbitone
  - Multiple dose charcoal: carbamazepine, dapsone, quinine, phenobarbitone, theophylline
- Chelation
- Consider antidotes
- $NaHCO_3^-$: Dose usually 1–2 mmol/kg; 8.4% $NaHCO_3^-$ contains 1 mmol/mL
- Sedation
- Anticonvulsants
  - Diazepam or midazolam (5 mg IV may need larger doses)
  - Can use PR (diazepam), intranasal or buccal (midazolam)
  - If continuous seizure use levetiracetam or phenobarbitone *NOT* phenytoin (Na channel blocker)
- Identify and treat aspiration pneumonitis with supportive care

Toxidromes and specific overdoses

Alcohols—methanol, ethylene glycol and isopropyl alcohol

- Risk: Potentially toxic doses
  - Methanol (100%) > 0.5 mL/kg (half this for a toddler)
  - Ethylene glycol > 1 mL/kg
  - Isopropyl alcohol > 2 mL/kg
- Assessment
  - Initially 1–2 hours looks like excess alcohol but doesn't smell like alcohol. GI upset, ataxia, confusion, CNS depression
  - Other features
    - Methanol: Vision changes, fixed and dilated pupils, papillo-oedema, cardiac failure, APO, AKI, apnoea, seizure, opisthotonos
    - Ethylene glycol: Fixed and dilated pupils, papillo-oedema, pulmonary toxicity, vascular calcium deposits, HT, CCF, APO, shock, coma, renal toxicity
    - Isopropyl alcohol: Haematemesis, acetone breath, renal failure, myopathy, haemolytic anaemia
- Additional investigations
  - Check alcohol level for co-ingestion, ECG, BSL, VBG, EUC
  - High anion gap metabolic acidosis (HAGMA), increased osmolar gap, increased lactate (these may be mild or normal in isopropyl alcohol OD)
  - Methanol: CT head for putaminal bleed
  - Ethylene glycol—urine: Fluorescent under Wood's lamp
  - Isopropyl alcohol—urine: Ketones, acetone
- Antidote (methanol and ethylene glycol)
  - Ethanol—PO/NG 2 mL/kg 50% commercial alcohol or 3 shots or 6 mL/kg IV/NG 10% ethanol
  - Followed by 1–2 mL/kg/hr IV/NG 10% ethanol or 1 shot/hr
  - Target blood alcohol of 0.1%
  - Fomepizole 15 mg/kg (may not be available)
- Other management
  - Support, resuscitation, ABC
  - Dialysis
  - Thiamine 100 mg IV
  - Methanol: Folate 50 mg (2 mg/kg)
  - Ethylene glycol: Pyridoxine 100 mg IV

Anticholinergic and cholinergic

Anticholinergic/antimuscarinic

- Examples: Antihistamines, tricyclic antidepressants (TCAs), amanita mushrooms, antimuscarinics, hyoscine, atropine, angel's trumpet, jimson weed, belladonna, nightshade
- Signs and symptoms—the saying goes like this (I did not make this up, don't blame me!): blind as a bat (dilated pupils), dry as a bone (warm dry skin), hot as a hare (increased temperature), mad as a hatter (confusion, hallucinations), red as a beet (flushed). Also ↑ HR and urine retention
- Management: Support and sedation usually required, use IV benzodiazepines
- Antidote for isolated anticholinergic agent only
    - Physostigmine 2 mg (0.02 mg/kg max. 0.5 mg in kids) or neostigmine
    - Only use if pure anticholinergic; e.g. benztaropine
    - NEVER use if not pure; e.g. TCA

Cholinergic—muscarinic

- Examples: Organophosphates, cybe mushrooms, betel nut, funnel-web spider, pilocarpine
- Signs and symptoms: DUMBELS
    - **D**efecation
    - **U**rination
    - **M**iosis
    - **B**radycardia
    - **E**mesis
    - **L**acrimation
    - **S**alivation
- Management: Support, benzodiazepines for agitation/seizures.
- Antidote
    - Atropine 1.2 mg IV
    - Dose doubled every 5 minutes until atropinised, then start infusion 10–20% of loading dose every hour
    - Pralidoxime for organophosphates

Cholinergic—nicotinic

- Examples: Insecticides, redback spider, funnel-web spider, nicotine, tobacco
- Signs and symptoms: Tachycardia, hypertension, fasciculations, paralysis

Antiepileptics

Carbamazepine

- Risk
  - 20–50 mg/kg: Mild–moderate
  - > 50 mg/kg: Significant toxicity (including CNS and Na channel blocking)
  - 1 tablet/400 mg: Significant toxicity in a toddler
- Assessment
  - Mild/moderate: Nystagmus, ataxia, delirium, mydriasis
  - Anticholinergic effects
  - Larger doses: Fluctuating GCS, coma, seizure, cardiac, VF/VT/ asystole, hypotension
  - Symptoms may be delayed 8–12 hours
- Additional investigations: Serum levels
- Management
  - Support, resuscitation
  - Charcoal for large ingestions, may need to intubate first. Multidose charcoal considered once intubated
  - Ventricular arrhythmias: $NaHCO_3^-$ 1–2 mmol/kg IV
  - Dialysis: Prolonged coma, unstable, levels remaining elevated

Phenytoin

- Risk
  - > 20 mg/kg mild–moderate
  - > 100 mg/kg significant
- Assessment
  - > 20 mg/kg: Dysarthria, ataxia
  - > 100 mg/kg: Coma, seizure, hyperosmolar, high glucose and sodium, hypotension, arrhythmia
- Additional investigations: Check levels
- Other management: Support, can use charcoal if < 4 hours

Valproate

- Risk
  - 200–400 mg: Moderate
  - 400–1000 mg: Severe
  - > 1000 mg/kg: Potentially lethal

- Assessment: Symptoms usually delayed
  - 200–400 mg: Variable decreased CNS
  - 400–1000 mg: Coma (may be delayed 12 hours), multi-organ dysfunction (MOD)
  - > 1000 mg/kg: Coma, MOD, lactate, cerebral oedema, bone marrow suppression
- Additional investigations: Levels, EUC, VBG, FBC, CMP
  - ↑ Na, ↓ BP, HAGMA, ↓ glucose, ↓ calcium, ↑ lactate
- Other management: Charcoal with repeated doses, dialysis for severe overdoses, instability or significantly elevated levels

Antipsychotics/antidepressants

Quetiapine

- Risk and assessment
  - < 3 g mild–moderate sedation and tachycardia
  - > 3 g (100 mg in children) dose-dependent sedation, coma, hypotension, delirium, seizure
  - Occurs 2–4 hours, lasts 1–3 days
  - Clinically significant prolonged QT rare
- Management: Resuscitation, ABC, don't usually give charcoal

Venlafaxine

- Risk and assessment
  - Dose-dependent seizures, serotonin syndrome if in combination with other agonists
  - Does not cause coma
  - 1.5 g: < 5% get seizures
  - > 3 g: > 30% get seizures
  - > 4.5 g almost everyone gets seizures, ↓ BP, ↑ QRS, ↑ QT
  - > 7 g cardiac arrhythmias
  - Onset can be delayed up to 12 hours
- Management: Support, early intubation
  - Charcoal if < 2 hours and > 4.5 g or intubated
  - Benzodiazepines for seizure
  - $NaHCO_3^-$ 1–2 mmol/kg IV for prolonged QRS
  - Treat serotonin syndrome

Amisulpride

- Risk and assessment
    - > 4 g: ↑ QT, torsades
    - > 8 g: Cardio-toxic, decreased level of consciousness
- Management: Support, can use charcoal

Olanzapine

- Risk and assessment: Dose-related sedation, anticholinergic effects, low BP
- Don't usually use charcoal

Phenothiazine (chlorpromazine) and butyrophenones (droperidol, haloperidol)

- Risk and assessment: Dose-related CNS depression, anticholinergic effects, prolonged QT
- Use charcoal once/if intubated

Benzodiazepines

- Risk: Not usually life-threatening unless mixed ingestion
- Antidote (DO NOT USE IN MIXED OVERDOSE): Flumazenil 0.1–0.2 mg IV (0.01 mg/kg in kids)
    - Only use if iatrogenic overdose as in excessive benzodiazepines given in a hospital setting
- Management: Supportive

Beta-blockers

- Risk: Propranolol and sotalol are potentially lethal; any dose in children can be lethal. Most other beta-blockers low risk of toxicity
    - Risk increased with co-ingestions, comorbidities, increased age
- Assessment
    - Cardiac: ↓ BP, ↓ HR, cardiac blocks, bradyarrhythmias
    - Other: ↑ K, APO, glucose ↑↓
    - Propranolol: ↑ QRS, seizure, coma, delirium—crosses blood–brain barrier
    - Sotalol: ↑ QT—beta and K channel blocker
- Additional investigations: ECG, EUC
- Antidote: High-dose insulin, 1 unit/kg IV bolus + glucose 50 mL (1 mL/kg) of 50% (10% in children) IV bolus, followed by infusion at the above doses per hour (1 u/kg insulin per hour, 1 mL/kg glucose per hour)—titrate glucose to attain euglycaemia

- Other management
  - Resuscitation and support
  - Charcoal within 2 hours, may need intubation first
  - Graduated approach to hypotension/bradycardia
    - Fluid bolus
    - Atropine 20 microgram/kg IV
    - High-dose insulin (tending to start this sooner)
    - Isoprenaline/adrenaline infusions (for dosing see inotropes p. 12 in Chapter 1 Resuscitation and trauma)
  - Propranolol: Treat like TCA OD, prolonged QRS treat with $NaHCO_3^-$ 1–2 mmol/kg IV
  - Torsades: Isoprenaline (see inotropes, p. 12), magnesium (10 mmol [0.05 mmol/kg] over 15 minutes IV), overdrive pacing (keep HR 100–120)
  - Query glucagon 5–10 mg IV (doubtful effect from recent evidence)
  - Possible use for intralipid (studies in progress)

Calcium channel blockers

- Risk: Verapamil and diltiazem (others usually low toxicity)
  - 2–3 × normal dose can give severe toxicity, > 10 tablets potentially lethal; any dose in a child is potentially lethal
  - Risk increased with co-ingestions, comorbidities, increased age
- Assessment: Onset 1–2 hours but can be up to 16 hours with extended release
  - Cardiac: ↓ BP, ↓ HR, heart block, shock, ischaemia (heart, brain, mesenteric)
  - CNS effects rare (consider co-ingestions)
- Additional investigations: EUC, CMP, VBG, lactate, CXR
  - ECG: Initial, 8 hours, if extended release ECG also at 12, 18, 24 hours
  - ↑ glucose, lactic acidosis
- Antidote: High-dose insulin, 1 unit/kg IV bolus + glucose 50 mL (1 mL/kg) of 50% (10% in children) IV bolus, followed by infusion at the above doses per hour (1 u/kg insulin per hour, 1 mL/kg glucose per hour)
- Other management
  - Resuscitation, support, early controlled intubation if potential lethal dose. Invasive monitoring

- Graduated approach to hypotension/bradycardia
  - Fluid bolus
  - IV calcium chloride 10% 10–20 mL in adult or calcium gluconate in children 10% 0.5–1 mL/kg
  - Atropine 20 microgram/kg IV: 0.6 mg in adult every 2 minutes up to 3 mg
  - High-dose insulin (tending to start this sooner)
  - Isoprenaline/adrenaline infusions (see inotropes, p. 12)
  - Cardiac pacing if ongoing bradycardia (see pacing in Chapter 2 Procedures and ultrasound, p. 47)
  - Cardiac bypass, intra-aortic balloon pump (IABP), ECMO
- $NaHCO_3^-$ 1–2 mmol/kg IV for metabolic acidosis
- Charcoal if < 1 hour or < 4 hours and extended release
- Whole bowel irrigation if < 4 hours with extended release preparations.
- Potential use of intralipid (studies in progress)

Carbon monoxide

- Risk
  - Usually good prognosis if patient survives to hospital
  - Risk of long-term issues increased if: Chronic exposure, coma, neurological dysfunction, metabolic acidosis, increased aged, fetus, cardiac ischaemia
- Assessment
  - CNS: Incoordination, coma, seizure, headache, altered
  - Cardio: ↑ HR, ↑↓ BP, ischaemia, arrhythmia, DIC, APO
  - Metabolic: Nausea, lactic acidosis, rhabdomyolysis, ↑ glucose, alopecia
- Additional investigations: VBG, lactate, EUC, trop, FBC, βHCG
  - CoHb < 10% = normal/smoker, 20% = mild, 30% = moderate
  - CoHb 40% = confusion/coma/seizure, 50% = cardio/respiratory complications and death
  - MMSE, CT/MRI
- Antidote: Oxygen, hyperbaric oxygen
- Other management: Remove from source, ABC, resuscitation
  - High-flow oxygen
  - Hyperbaric oxygen considered if: Pregnant, other risk factors

Colchicine

- Risk
  - < 0.5 mg/kg: GI effects
  - 0.5–0.8 mg/kg: Systemic effects
  - > 0.8 mg/kg: Severe, highly lethal
- Assessment
  - 2–24 hours: Nausea, vomiting, diarrhoea, severe fluid loss resulting in haemodynamic instability
  - 2–7 days: Bone marrow suppressed, pancytopenia, rhabdomyolysis, renal failure, metabolic acidosis, ARDS, cardiac arrhythmia
  - > 7 days: Rebound leucocytosis, alopecia
- Additional investigations: VBG, EUC, FBC, CXR
- Management: Resuscitation, IV fluids for hypovolaemia, manage acid–base and electrolyte abnormalities, protect airway
  - Charcoal 50 g (1 g/kg) ASAP if > 0.5 mg/kg. Consider multidose charcoal
  - All need admission

Corrosives

- Alkali, acids, plus others (paraquat, phenols, permanganate, etc.)
- Risk: Local injury, airway burns. Acid/alkalis no systemic effects
  - > 60 mL of HCl potentially fatal from perforation
- Assessment: Mouth pain, abdominal pain
  - Laryngeal oedema: Stridor/hoarse/distressed
  - Perforation: Chest pain, SOB, subcutaneous emphysema, rub, strictures, peritonitis, multi-organ dysfunction
  - Immediate airway threat: Stridor, dysphonia, SOB, hoarse, drooling, respiratory distress
  - Lack of oral burn does not exclude serious injury
- Additional investigations: Endoscopy, CXR, AXR, VBG, FBC, saliva pH
- Other management: Decontaminate—rinse mouth with water
  - ETT, don't use NGT
  - Analgesia, NBM
  - Endoscopy and/or operation
  - Antibiotics if suspect perforation

Cyanide

- Risk: PO, inhaled potentially lethal
    - ALWAYS THINK OF IN FIRE/SMOKE INHALATION VICTIMS especially if remain unconscious or lactate ↑↑
- Assessment: Inhaled—LOC within seconds to minutes
    - PO: ½–1 hour nausea, vomiting headache, SOB, ↑ RR, ↑ BP, ↑ HR, seizure
    - Leading to ↓ HR, ↓ BP, ↓ RR, coma, tetany
    - Delayed neuro-Parkinsonism
- Additional investigations: EUC, HAGMA, lactate correlates with severity—a lactate > 10 suggests significant cyanide toxicity
    - Cyanide levels confirm diagnosis, don't change management
        - > 20 micromol/L = symptoms, > 40 = toxic, > 100 = lethal
- Antidote: Hydroxocobalamin 5 g (50 mg/kg) preferred antidote OR
    - Sodium thiosulfate 12.5 g (400 mg/kg in a child) OR
    - Dicobalt edetate EDTA 300 mg (7.5 mg/kg in a child) IV followed immediately by glucose infusion 50 mL 50% (2.5 mL/kg 10% in kids)
- Other management: Remove from source, resuscitate, immediate intubation, 100% oxygen
    - Decontamination: Wash with soap and water, bag clothes
    - Charcoal once intubated

Digoxin

Acute

- Risk: Potentially lethal, consider antidote
    - Dose: > 10 mg in an adult, > 4 mg in a child
    - Digoxin level > 15 nmol/L, K > 5.5 mmol/L
- Assessment
    - 2–4 hours onset, peak 6 hours
    - GI upset: Nausea, vomiting, etc.
    - Cardiac: Bradycardia, heart blocks, hypotension, slow AF, VT, SVT with AV block, ectopics
    - CNS: Lethargy, confusion, delirium
- Additional investigations
    - Level at 4 hours then every 2 hours
    - ECG, EUC, VBG, CMP, BSL
    - Note: ↓ Mg exacerbate toxicity

- Antidote: Digoxin immune Fab (1 vial = 40 mg)
    - Indicated if life-threatening arrhythmia, potentially lethal dose or level (see above), or K > 5.0 mmol
    - Approximately 1 vial Fab binds 500 microgram (0.5 mg) digoxin
    - Dose (in number of vials) = dose ingested (mg) × 0.8 × 2. With this formula, large doses of DigiFab used
    - Some recommendations suggest empiric treatment with 2 vials, repeated if needed and titrated to clinical effect (HR and ECG)
    - In cardiac arrest: 5–10 vials IV, repeat if required
- Other management
    - Standard ALS, support
    - If digoxin immune Fab not available
        - Treat high K with $NaHCO_3^-$ 1 mmol/kg up to 100 mmol and insulin 10 units (0.1 u/kg in children) and 50 mL 50% glucose (2.5 mL/kg of 10% glucose in children)
        - Treat AV block with atropine 0.6 mg (20 microgram/kg in children)
        - Treat VT with lidocaine (lignocaine) 1 mg/kg (max. 100 mg) IV
    - Charcoal if within 1 hour of ingestion
    - ECG monitoring for 12–24 hours
    - Ingestion unsure: Monitor for 6 hours
    - Theoretical risk if use calcium in digoxin toxicity

Chronic

- Risk
    - Level > 1.9 nmol/L: Likely symptomatic
    - Level > 3.2 nmol/L: Toxic
- Assessment: Insidious onset. Features as above + vision change (yellow haloes and colour change, decreased acuity)
- Additional investigations: Levels, ECG, EUC, CMP, BSL
- Antidote: Digoxin immune Fab considered if clinical features and levels elevated
    - Number of vials = serum digoxin level × weight/100
    - Empiric = 1–2 vials repeated at 30–60 minutes if no effect

- Other management: As above
    - No charcoal
    - Correct electrolytes
    - Correct hypovolaemia

Hydrocarbons

- Essential oils, kerosene, benzene, camphor, toluene etc.
- Risk
    - Petroleum > 1–2 mL/kg or eucalyptus oil > 10 mL is significant
    - In children > 5 mL of essential oil can cause rapid coma
- Assessment
    - Respiratory: Immediate aspiration, cough, haemoptysis, wheeze, pneumonitis
    - Cardiac: Arrhythmia
    - Neurological: Profound decreased GCS within 2 hours
    - GI: Nausea, vomiting
    - CCl_4/toluene/benzene: Renal and hepatotoxic
- Additional investigations: ECG, FBC, LFT, VBG, CXR
- Management: Resuscitation, support monitoring, ALS, intubation likely. Hyperventilation, oxygen, correct electrolytes (K and Mg in particular)
- Don't use inotropes if possible

Hydrofluoric acid (HF)

- Risk: Any dermal exposure likely to cause tissue injury, any amount inhaled likely to cause pulmonary injury
    - Systemic toxicity risk if > 100 mL oral with 6% HF, any amount PO at higher concentrations, dermal exposure TBSA 2.5% and 100% HF, TBSA 8% HF 70%, TBSA 11% HF 23%
- Assessment
    - Inhaled: Immediate irritant, cough, SOB, wheeze, APO
    - Dermal: Gradual severe constant pain, pallor/blanching over hours
    - Ingested: Vomiting, pain, dysphagia
    - Systemic: ↓ Ca, ↓ Mg, tetany, ↑ QT, arrhythmia, arrest
    - Cardiac arrest may be without any warning ½ hour to 6 hours post exposure
- Additional investigations: Serial ECG, calcium, endoscopy

- Antidote
  - Skin exposure: Calcium gluconate. DO NOT USE calcium chloride
    - Topical gel: Can make by mixing calcium gluconate 10 mL of 10% with 30 mL of lubricant gel
    - Local injection/subcutaneous if topical unsuccessful
    - Bier's block if unsuccessful. Get expert help
    - Intra-arterial as last resort. Get expert help
  - Systemic
    - Calcium gluconate IV 10% 1 mL/kg up to 60 mL
    - Calcium chloride can be used IV ONLY and ADULTS ONLY, 10% 20 mL, CANNOT BE GIVEN INTO TISSUES
  - Inhalational: Can give nebulised calcium gluconate
- Other management: Decontaminate, remove clothes, irrigate with water
  - Analgesia, don't use nerve blocks. Ongoing pain means continued toxicity, need more antidote
  - Arrhythmia: ALS, intubate, hyperventilate
  - $NaHCO_3^-$ 1–2 mmol/kg IV
  - $MgSO_4$ 10 mmol (0.05 mmol/kg)

Hyperthermic syndromes—NMS, SS, MH

Neuroleptic malignant syndrome (NMS)

- Precipitating drugs: Dopamine-blocking antipsychotics and antiemetics; e.g. haloperidol, metoclopramide, prochlorperazine
- Presentation
  - Onset: Days to weeks
  - Hyperthermia, hypertension, acute severe Parkinsonian symptoms and signs. Muscle rigidity, bradykinesia, autonomic instability, CNS↓
  - WCC elevated, CK usually > 1000, myoglobinuria, renal dysfunction, abnormal LFTs, metabolic acidosis
- Antidote
  - Bromocriptine 2.5 mg PO 8-hourly
- Other management
  - ABC, fluid resuscitation, supportive, active cooling
  - Prevent secondary complications: Rhabdomyolysis, electrolyte disturbances etc.

  - Sedation, IV benzodiazepines
  - Withdrawal from offending drugs: Abrupt withdrawal may precipitate NMS

Serotonin syndrome (SS)

- Precipitating drugs: Serotonin agents, e.g. antidepressants (SSRI, TCA, MAOI); analgesics (tramadol, fentanyl, pethidine); illicit (amphetamines); others (St John's Wort, metoclopramide)
- Presentation
  - Fast onset: Usually hours, within 24 hours
  - Hyperthermia, hyperreflexia, tremor, clonus (ocular, ankle), increased tone, HT, diarrhoea, mydriasis, agitation, coma, ↑ HR, sweating, delirium, ↑ CNS, seizure
- Antidote
  - Cyproheptadine 8 mg PO/NGT
  - Chlorpromazine 12.5–50 mg IV
- Other management
  - ABC, fluid resuscitation, supportive, active cooling
  - May require paralysis and intubation
  - Prevent secondary complications: Rhabdomyolysis, electrolyte and glucose disturbances, renal failure, DIC, HT etc.
  - Sedation, IV benzodiazepines
  - Withdrawal from offending drugs

Malignant hyperthermia (MH)

- Precipitating drugs: Volatile anaesthetics, succinylcholine
- Presentation
  - Onset: Within minutes
  - Hyperthermia, muscle rigidity, HT, tachycardia, metabolic acidosis
- Antidote
  - Dantrolene 2.5 mg/kg IV bolus, may need to be repeated. Maintenance 1 mg/kg IV 4–6-hourly
- Other management
  - ABC, fluid resuscitation, supportive, active cooling
  - Prevent secondary complications: Acid–base disturbances, electrolyte disturbances etc.
  - Sedation, IV benzodiazepines

Insulin

- Risk: Subcutaneous insulin overdose causes unpredictable hypoglycaemia. Not dependent on insulin preparation or dose. Determined by erratic release at subcutaneous site
- Assessment: Onset usually within 2 hours, can last days
  - Features of hypoglycaemia
  - Autonomic: Nausea, vomiting, sweating, tachycardia
  - CNS: Agitation, tremor, confusion, seizure, coma,
- Additional investigations: BSL every 15 minutes then 1–2-hourly when stable, EUC, CMP. ↓ K, ↓ phosphate, ↓ Mg
  - Insulin and C-peptide levels rarely needed to confirm intentional overdose versus endogenous
- Antidote: 50 mL of 50% glucose, then 100 mL/hr of 10%
  - In children 2 mL/kg 10% glucose (don't use 50%)
- Other management: ABC. May need invasive monitoring. Often need central access

Iron

- Risk: Elemental iron < 20 mg/kg asymptomatic, 20–60 mg/kg GI effects, 60–120 mg/kg systemic toxicity, > 120 mg/kg potential lethal
- Assessment (may not clinically follow these stages)
  - 1–6 hours: GI, corrosive, fluid losses; GI symptoms under 6 hours = potentially lethal ingestion
  - 6–12 hours: Symptoms appear to resolve
  - 12–48 hours: HAGMA, hepato-renal failure, vasodilation, 3rd-space losses
  - 2–5 days: Hepatic failure, coma, coagulopathy, ↓ glucose
  - 2–6 weeks: Cirrhotic liver, GI stricture
- Additional investigations: If iron levels at 4–6 hours > 90 micromol/L then systemic toxicity likely
  - VBG, AXR (confirms ingestion), glucose, FBC (elevated WCC)
- Antidote: Desferrioxamine 15 mg/kg/hr
- Other management
  - Resuscitation, fluid bolus, serial fluid assessment and replace losses
  - Decontamination: Whole bowel irrigation (if > 60 mg/kg or ingestion evident on x-ray), operation, endoscopic removal

Lithium

- Risk:
  - < 25 g benign
  - > 25 g causes GI effects
- Assessment
  - Large overdose: GI effects, fluid losses, ST changes on ECG, tremor
  - Chronic toxicity: Causes include ↓ renal function, ↓ Na, dehydration, drug interactions
    - Grade 1: Tremor, hyperreflexia, ataxia
    - Grade 2: Stupor, rigid, ↓ BP
    - Grade 3: Coma, seizure, clonus
- Additional investigations: Lithium levels, EUC, TFT, FBC, AXR, decreased AG metabolic acidosis
- Management
  - Resuscitation, rehydration, urine output aim > 1 mL/kg/hr, replace Na, monitor electrolytes and fluid balance
  - Dialysis considered

Local anaesthetics

- Risk: Usually secondary to accidental intravascular drug delivery rather than overdose
  - Dose-related toxicity
  - Methaemoglobinaemia not dose related, more likely in children, more likely with prilocaine and lidocaine (lignocaine)
  - Cardiac toxicity more likely with bupivacaine
  - Maximum doses of local anaesthetics (toxicity can occur at lower doses intra-vascularly)
    - Bupivacaine: 2 mg/kg
    - Lidocaine (lignocaine): 3 mg/kg, 7 mg/kg with adrenaline
    - Prilocaine: 7 mg/kg
    - Ropivacaine: 3 mg/kg
- Assessment
  - Early symptoms: Tinnitus, perioral numbness, confusion, dizziness
  - CNS: Seizure, coma

  - Cardiac: ↓ pulse rate, ↓ BP, arrhythmias, collapse, arrest
  - Methaemoglobinaemia: Blue mucous membranes, CNS and cardio effects
- Additional investigations: EUC, FBC, serial ECG (Na channel blocking effects), methaemoglobin concentration
- Antidote: Intralipid 20%, 1 mL/kg IV bolus, can repeat at 5 minutes. Infusion 0.25–0.5 mL/kg/min
  - Methylene blue for methaemoglobinaemia
- Other management: Resuscitation, support
  - $NaHCO_3^-$ 1–2 mmol/kg IV repeated for ventricular arrhythmias
  - Fluids and inotropes for hypotension

Methaemoglobinaemia

- Causes: Nitrites, phenols, spider bites, sulfur, local anaesthetics, glyceryl trinitrate (GTN), vitamin K, hydroxychloroquine, dapsone, well water, preserved meat
- Assessment: Onset 30 minutes to 1 day
  - Dark chocolate lips, tongue
  - No respiratory distress
- Additional investigations: VBG—methaemoglobin concentration
- Antidote: Methylene blue 1 mL/kg IV
- Other management: NAC if G6PD

Metformin

- Risk: Usually benign; however, can cause severe lactic acidosis
  - Life-threatening lactic acidosis usually secondary to renal failure, sepsis etc.
- Assessment: Asymptomatic, GI upset, ↑ HR, ↓ BP, shock, coma
  - ↓ glucose usually minimal or not present
- Additional investigations: EUC, VBG, lactate
- Management: ABC
  - $NaHCO_3^-$ 1–2 mmol/kg IV for severe acidosis
  - Charcoal if within 2 hours
  - Dialysis rapidly corrects

Mushrooms and toxic plants

Mushrooms

- Risk: Most cause GI toxicity which resolves
  - If GI symptoms *are delayed* past 6 hours THIS IS CONCERNING FOR CYCLOPEPTIDES (amatoxin, phallotoxin, virotoxin)
  - Therefore, early symptoms are actually a good sign
- Assessment
  - Early onset symptoms
    - GI, cholinergic (muscarine)
    - Hallucinogen (psilocybin)
    - Disulfiram (coprine)
    - Glutaminergic, pneumonic (dried spores)
    - Epileptogenic (gyromitrin)
  - Delayed: Amatoxin, phallotoxin, virotoxin
    - 6–24 hours: GI symptoms, hepatotoxic
    - 18–36 hours: Transient improvement
    - 2–6 days: Fulminant hepatic failure, pancreatitis
  - Very delayed: Nephrotoxic, rhabdomyolysis
- Investigations: EUC, Cr, LFT, coags, FBC
  - If possible, a mycologist should look at the mushrooms
- Antidote
  - Amatoxin potential antidotes: NAC, silibinin 5 mg/kg IV over 1 hour, benzylpenicillin 1 million units/day
  - Atropine for cholinergic symptoms
  - Pyridoxine for *Gyromitra*
- Other management
  - Resuscitation, support for coma, seizure, electrolyte derangements
  - Charcoal 1 g/kg PO if delayed symptoms

Toxic plants

- Table 11.1 gives a broad overview of some of the more common ingestions of toxic plants and their potential effects

Opioids

- Risk: Children—1 tablet or 1 mouthful of methadone can cause respiratory arrest

Table 11.1 Toxic plants and their effects

Toxin	Plant	Effects and antidote
Oxalates	Lily	AKI, airway obstruction
Amygdalin, cyanide	Pits/seeds	Cyanide effects (neuro, cardiac, coma, seizure) Antidote: Hydroxocobalamin
Glycoside	Foxglove, lily, oleander	GI, cardiac, ↑ K Antidote: DigiFab
Anticholinergic	Angel's trumpet, belladonna, mandrake, nightshade	Tachycardia, delirium, retention, Antidote: Physostigmine
Nicotinic	Hemlock, coniine, tobacco	↓ BP, tachycardia, tremor, sweat, GI
Psychotropic alkaloids	Morning glory	Psychosis, hallucinations
Hypoglycin	Ackee	Glucose ↓, acidosis
Ricin	Bean of castor plants	Multi-organ failure
Colchicine	Glory lily, crocus,	GI, multi-organ failure
Pyrrolizidine	Comfrey	Jaundice, abdominal pain
Aconite	Asian herbs	Paralysis, cardiac

- Assessment: ↓ CNS, ↓ respiratory, miosis, ↓ airway reflexes,
  - Complications: Hypothermia, skin necrosis, compartment syndrome, rhabdomyolysis, hypoxic brain injury
- Additional investigations: ECG, BSL. Investigate for complications,
- Antidote: Naloxone 100–400 microgram (10 microgram/kg) IV
  - Use only the amount needed to reverse symptoms, can precipitate severe withdrawal
  - Note: If duration of action 1–2 hours must monitor patient for repeat episodes, especially with long-acting opioids such as methadone
  - Buprenorphine overdose may need increased dose (up to 10 times)
  - Some new street opioids require very large naloxone doses
- Other management: Resuscitation, support
  - Charcoal not routine

Organophosphates and carbamates

- Risk: All intentional overdoses or ingestions in children potentially lethal
- Assessment: Staff should wear PPE
  - Minutes–hours; may note garlic smell
  - Muscarinic: DUMBELS + nicotinic
  - CNS: Coma, agitation, seizure
  - Respiratory: Pneumonitis, APO
  - Delayed: Neuropathy, neuropsychiatric
- Additional investigations: Red cell cholinesterase levels (correlate with severity), plasma and mixed cholinesterase levels
  - ECG: ↑ QT, ↑ ST, T inversion, ↑ PR interval, arrhythmias
- Antidote: Atropine 1.2 mg (20 microgram/kg) double dose every 5 minutes until secretions dry
  - Pralidoxime 2 g IV (not in carbamates—they don't age)
- Other management: Decontaminate (remove clothes, wash with soap and water) while resuscitating
- Intubate, fluids, benzodiazepines for agitation/seizure, inotropes

Paracetamol

- Risk
  - > 10 g or 200 mg/kg (children)
  - > 6 g or 150 mg/kg per day over 2 days
  - > 4 g or 100 mg/kg per day over 3 days
  - > 30 g = massive ingestion
- Assessment
  - Phase 1 (24 hours): Usually asymptomatic or GI upset
  - Phase 2 (2–3 days): RUQ pain, elevated AST, ALT and INR
  - Phase 3 (3–4 days): Hepatic failure
  - Phase 4: Recovery
  - Massive ingestions can cause coma
- Additional investigations
  - Take level at ≥ 4 hours, correlate whether treatment indicated on paracetamol nomogram. Repeat at 8 hours if initial result close to treatment line
  - Treatment line on nomogram is 1000 micromol/L at 4 hours, 500 at 8 hours, 250 at 12 hours

- If slow-release preparation, take levels at 4 and 8 hours
- If time unknown take 3 levels and calculate $T_{1/2}$. If $T_{1/2} > 4$ = toxicity
- If ingestion over 8 hours ago, check LFTs
- Other investigations: LFT, BSL, EUC, ECG, VBG

- Antidote: N-acetylcysteine (NAC)
  - Start if level > treatment line on nomogram, massive ingestion, hepatotoxicity, time > 8 hours (and significant ingestion)
  - 150 mg/kg in 200 mL of 5% glucose IVI over 60 minutes
  - Then 50 mg/kg in 500 mL of 5% glucose over 4 hours
  - Then 100 mg/kg in 1 L of 5% glucose over 16 hours
    - Or if massive ingestion 150 mg/kg over 24 hours (varies—consult poisons info)
    - Or if level on nomogram is more than double consider 200 mg/kg (consult poisons info)
  - Child dose = adult dose but use less fluid depending on weight (see nomogram)
  - Monitor closely for anaphylactoid reactions. If occur, halt or slow IVI and treat with antihistamines, bronchodilators, adrenaline if severe. Recommence when symptoms settle. Seek advice if concerned
- Other management
  - Decontaminate: Charcoal, if time from ingestion < 2 hours or < 4 hours if massive or extended release (these may benefit from multiple doses up to 24 hours—consult poisons). Do not use charcoal in liquid paracetamol OD as very rapidly absorbed so nothing in the gut for charcoal to bind
  - Massive ingestions likely need resuscitation, may need intubation

Paraquat

- Risk
  - < 30 mg/kg (10 mL): GI upset
  - 30–150 mg/kg (10–20 mL): Multi-organ failure, death
  - > 150 mg/kg: Fulminant death
  - In children as little as 5 mL can be fatal
- Assessment: Initially well or corrosive injury
  - Within hours: Multi-organ failure, ↑ HR, ↑ RR, metabolic acidosis, ↑ lactate, ↓ K, cardiac collapse, death usually within 24 hours

  - A moderate ingestion: Delayed pulmonary fibrosis progressing to death in days to weeks
- Additional investigations: FBC, EUC, LFT, pulmonary function, VBG, CXR
  - Serum paraquat level: Very good for prognosis
  - Urine paraquat levels qualitative confirms ingestion
- Other management
  - DECONTAMINATION IS A PRIORITY
    - At scene: Give patient food or soil to eat
    - In ED charcoal ASAP 50 g (1 g/kg) PO
  - ETT if airway threatened (rare)
  - DON'T GIVE OXYGEN unless sats < 90%
  - Urgent haemodialysis within 2 hours
  - Usually NAC and vitamin C 10 mg/kg given as well, benefits not clear

Salicylates

- Risk
  - 150–300 mg/kg: Mild/moderate
  - > 300 mg/kg: Serious
  - > 500 mg/kg: Potentially lethal
- Assessment
  - GI upset, erosions/ulcers/bleeding, ↑ LFT
  - Respiratory: ↑ RR, pulmonary oedema, bleeding, bronchospasm
  - CNS: Tinnitus, confusion, seizure, tetany
  - Other: ↑ HR, temp, nephrotoxic
- Additional investigations
  - VBG: Initial respiratory alkalosis, lactic acidosis +/– metabolic alkalosis from vomiting
  - EUC (low K), LFT, ECG, BSL
  - Salicylate levels poorly correlate with toxicity. Take serial levels to identify delayed absorption/bezoar
- Antidote
  - $NaHCO_3^-$ 1–2 mmol/kg IV
  - Aim for urinary alkalinisation, urine pH > 7.5

- Other management
  - Charcoal; repeat dose if levels elevated at 4 hours
  - Support, resuscitate, may need intubation, may need to hyperventilate
  - Treat seizures, abnormal potassium and glucose
  - Dialysis

Sulphonylurea

- Risk
  - 1 tablet in a non-diabetic can induce significant ↓ glucose, increased dose can cause increased and more prolonged ↓ glucose
  - 1 tablet in a child potentially lethal
- Assessment: Onset may be delayed up to 8 hours, up to 48 hours if extended release
- Additional investigations: BSL serials
- Antidote: Octreotide (only use if hypoglycaemic) 50 microgram (1 microgram/kg) IV bolus then 25 microgram/hr (1 microgram/kg/hr) IV infusion
- Other management
  - Charcoal if within 1 hour or 4 hours for extended release
  - IV glucose used initially while antidote takes effect
    - 50 mL of 50% glucose IV, then 100 mL/hr of 10%
    - In children 2 mL/kg 10% glucose IV (don't use 50%)

Sympathomimetics—cocaine and amphetamines

- Risk
  - In a child: Any dose potentially lethal
  - In an adult: Any dose of amphetamines can cause harm, 1 g cocaine potentially lethal
- Assessment
  - CNS: Euphoria, agitation, psychiatric, seizure
  - Cardiac: ↑ HR, HT, arrhythmia, ↑ QT, AMI, APO
  - Other: Hyperthermia, rigidity
  - Complications: Renal failure, dissection, ICH, ischaemic colitis, rhabdomyolysis, dehydration
  - Amphetamines: Above + hyponatraemia, SIADH, cerebral oedema

- Additional investigations
  - EUC, ECG, CK, trop, CXR (dissection), CTB, BSL
- Management: Support, may need intubation
  - Charcoal in cocaine body packers
  - VT: 100 mmol $NaHCO_3^-$, defibrillation, lidocaine (lignocaine)
  - ACS: Aspirin, nitrates, PCI
  - SVT: Benzodiazepines, adenosine, verapamil, DCCV
  - HT/tachycardia: Benzodiazepines, GTN
  - DON'T USE BETA-BLOCKERS: Classic teaching says this will result in unopposed alpha
  - Seizure/delirium: Benzodiazepines
  - Hyperthermia: Benzodiazepines, cooling
  - Amphetamines: Above + if hyponatraemia and Na < 120 and seizure or altered CNS 3% saline 2 mL/kg

Tricyclic antidepressants

- Examples: amitriptyline, dosulepin (dothiepin), doxepin, nortriptyline, imipramine
- Risk
  - 5–10 mg/kg: Drowsy, anticholinergic effects
  - > 10 mg/kg: Potential for all major effects, can be lethal in a child
  - > 30 mg/kg: Severe toxicity
- Assessment: Effects usually rapid (within 1–2 hours)
  - CNS: Sedation, seizure, coma, delirium
  - Cardiac: ↑ HR, ↑↓ BP, broad complex arrhythmia
  - Anticholinergic
- Additional investigations
  - ECG: ↑ HR, ↑ QRS, large terminal R in aVR, ↑ R/S in aVR, QT—if QT > 100 seizure likely, > 160 VT likely
  - BSL
- Antidote: $NaHCO_3^-$ 100 mmol (2 mmol/kg) IV
- Other management
  - ABC, resuscitation, support
  - Close monitor ECG at least 6 hours
  - If GCS < 12, ETT

- VT/VF: $NaHCO_3^-$ every 2 minutes until corrected, lidocaine (lignocaine) 1 mg/kg when pH > 7.5
- DON'T USE AMIODARONE OR BETA-BLOCKERS OR PHENYTOIN
- If low BP: Fluid bolus, $NaHCO_3^-$, inotropes/adrenaline/noradrenaline
- Seizures: Benzodiazepines
- Intubated patients: Hyperventilate. Aim pH 7.5–7.55
- Charcoal once airway is secured

Envenomation

Snake bite

- First aid
  - Pressure immobilisation bandage (PIB): From bite site to cover entire limb. Splint limb, absolute rest
  - Mark where the bite site is on the bandage
  - ALS
- Assessment
  - Signs and symptoms
    - Local effects can be minimal; pain, swelling
    - Systemic: Nausea and vomiting, headache, abdominal pain, collapse
    - Organ effects: Venom-induced consumptive coagulopathy (VICC), neurotoxicity (flaccid paralysis, blurred vision 1st, respiratory paralysis), myotoxicity, renal damage (secondary to rhabdomyolysis)
- Evidence of envenomation
  - Examination: Bleeding, neurology, rhabdomyolysis
  - Investigations: EUC, FBC, CK, coags
    - +/– LFT, LDH, CK, trop, fibrinogen/FDP
- Management in ED
  - PIB: Splint (mark where the bite site is on the bandage)
  - Call toxicologist: 13 11 26
  - Leave PIB until investigations normal or started antivenom
  - Venom detection kit (VDK) can be used to determine which antivenom to use NOT to diagnose if systemic envenomation
    - Sample: Cut hole in PIB and swab bite site. Can use urine. Preferably don't use plasma

- If systemic envenomation (organ effects and/or severe non-specific systemic effects) use antivenom
- Antivenom
    - Determine which type based on region, exam findings and investigation results including VDK if available
    - Use polyvalent (more risk of adverse reaction) if: Can't get monovalent, more than 3 possible snakes, severe symptoms and no time to wait for VDK, monovalent not available
    - Monovalent: Less severe adverse reactions. Can use 2 different monovalents rather than polyvalent
    - Dose: 1–2 ampoules IV in 100 mL normal saline (same dose antivenom but with 10 mL/kg normal saline in children)
    - Must give in resuscitation room, have equipment ready to treat anaphylaxis etc.
    - If antivenom causes anaphylaxis: Cease antivenom, give adrenaline, need urgent specialist consult but likely need to treat anaphylaxis and then continue antivenom at slower rate)
    - Serum sickness (fever, rash etc.) usually 5–10 days post antivenom: Treat severe cases with prednisone 25–50 mg PO/day 7/7. Warn all patients about the possibility of serum sickness

- Support/manage complications
    - VICC
        - Causes bleeding gums/bite site/IVC site/ICH etc.
        - Give FFP, cryoprecipitate may benefit
    - Rhabdomyolysis
    - Neuromuscular paralysis
- Treat complications
    - Bleeding, thrombotic, microangiopathy: Give fibrinogen/blood products
    - Rhabdomyolysis, neuromuscular paralysis: Discuss with haematology and renal
- If patient is well: Steps to discharging home
    - Leave PIB until investigations normal
    - If patient well and investigations normal, ensure patient has an IVC first then remove PIB and repeat investigations/examination at 1, 6 and 12 hours

- At any point, if symptoms develop give antivenom and reapply PIB
- If patient and serial investigations remain normal can discharge (don't discharge overnight)

Specific snakes—additional information to above

- Mulga: not east Australia or Tasmania
  - Very painful, extensive swelling
  - Almost all cause systemic symptoms
  - Usually rhabdomyolysis within 6 hours
  - Coagulopathy is mild, non-consumptive, fibrinogen is normal
  - 15% get mild paralysis
- Red bellied black snake: South-eastern Australia, not Tasmania
  - Minor symptoms, systemic envenomation rare
- Brown snake: All of Australia except Tasmania
  - 50% dry bite
  - Systemic symptoms: VICC, thrombocytopenia, thrombus, microangiopathic haemolytic anaemia (MAHA)
  - Neurology is rare, AKI rare, no rhabdomyolysis
  - Investigations: ↑ INR, ↑ D-dimer, fibrinogen undetectable, ↓ platelets, AKI, MAHA (↑ LDH, fragmented red cells)
  - Management: Antivenom, FFP, cryoprecipitate, plasmapheresis
- Death adder: All Australia except Victoria and Tasmania
  - Pain at bite site
  - Systemic symptoms within 6 hours: Progressive symmetrical descending flaccid paralysis (ptosis, blurred vision, dysphagia, diplopia), leading to hypotension, respiratory failure, arrest
  - No coagulopathy, no renal effects
  - Investigations: Spirometer/peak flow, usually bloods normal
- Tiger snake: East Australia INCLUDING Tasmania
  - Pain at bite site in 50%
  - Systemic symptoms: Rapid VICC, collapse and arrest. Initially looks just like brown snake bite. After 1–2 hours develop paralysis, later develop rhabdomyolysis and ARF which can be massive
  - Investigations ↑↑ INR, ↑↑ D-dimer, undetectable fibrinogen

- Taipan: Tropical North Australia and inland
  - Minimal pain at bite site
  - Systemic symptoms: Within minutes, collapse, paralysis within 1–2 hours (more rapid than tiger), rhabdomyolysis (more rapid than tiger), ARF. MAHA is rare
  - Investigations: For VICC, Cr, CK
- Sea snake: All coast except Tasmania
  - Bite site small and painless
  - Systemic symptoms: Symmetrical descending flaccid paralysis, rhabdomyolysis
  - Investigations: CK
  - Antivenom: If specific antivenom unavailable can use tiger snake antivenom
- Note: Tasmania sounds like a good place to live!

Spider bite

Funnel-web

- Presentation: Usually patient sees a big black spider with large fangs
- Local: Severe pain, no erythema, visible bite marks
- Only 10–20% of bites lead to envenomation
- Non-spec systemic effects
- Envenomation: From 30 minutes up to 2 hours.
  - Autonomic ↑ (piloerection, ↓↑ BP, ↓↑ HR)
  - Neuromuscular ↑ (fasciculations, spasms, ↑ tone)
  - Abdominal pain
  - Nausea and vomiting, headache
  - Cardiac (APO, ↑ trop)
  - CNS (coma, anxiety, paralysis, oral paraesthesia)
  - Sweat, salivate, lacrimate
- Management
  - **PIB**
  - If arrest: Give *at least* 4 vials of antivenom, more if available as IV push
  - Non-arrest: 2–4 vials antivenom, remove PIB post antivenom if symptom free and reapply if develop symptoms. Give a further 2 vials antivenom for ongoing symptoms
  - Atropine can help dry secretions: 20 microgram/kg IV

- ADT
- Admit all envenomed patients; patients without features of envenomation can be discharged after 4 hours of observation (do not discharge overnight)

Redback

- DON'T bandage—worsens pain
- Severe pain 5–10 minutes post bite
- Pain, sweating and piloerection: Consider redback
- Regional sweating, lymphangitis, fasciculations
- Radiating pain, pain doesn't have to be at bite site
- Systemic symptoms approx. 20% (nausea and vomiting, chest pain, abdominal pain, hypertension, fever, paraesthesia, spasms, paralysis)
- Management
  - ICE
  - NO PIB
  - Analgesia PO or IV if required
  - ADT
  - Antivenom if local symptoms not relieved by analgesia or patient has systemic symptoms. Give 1–2 ampoules IV or IM. If IV give in 100 mL (10 mL/kg in a child) of normal saline and give over ½ an hour. Give in resus room with adrenaline ready to treat anaphylaxis if it occurs
- Note about controversies with antivenom: Recent study in patients with painful bites suggested not to give antivenom and to use analgesia alone. One study also suggested IM better than IV as less anaphylaxis.

Marine venom

- First aid
  - Bluebottle, all jellyfish not mentioned, stonefish, catfish, stingray, sea urchin: Hot water at 45°C after washing sting site
  - Box jellyfish: Vinegar, BLS, prolonged CPR
  - Irukandji: Vinegar post wash site
  - Sponges: Wash site
  - Sea snakes: PIB
  - Blue-ringed octopus: PIB + BLS/EAR (expired air resuscitation)
- Symptoms and signs
  - Bluebottle: Immediate burning pain, linear elliptical red welts
  - Box jellyfish: Immediate severe pain, crosshatch tentacle marks, collapse, arrest, arrhythmia within minutes

- Irukandji: Minimal local symptoms, within ½–2 hours systemic effects of severe pain, impending doom, agitation, dysphonia, sweating, HT, tachycardia. Can develop cardiomyopathy, cardiogenic shock, pulmonary oedema, ICH
- Blue-ringed octopus: Painless bite, no local effects. Rapid progressive descending flaccid paralysis within minutes. Ptosis, blurred vision, diplopia, dysphagia, paralysis. Spontaneously resolves after 24 hours
- Stonefish: Immediate severe pain, swelling/bruise/puncture site, nausea, vomiting, dizziness. Collapse/APO/hypotension rare
- Stingray: Penetrating trauma, venom—pulmonary oedema, necrosis, bleeding, salivation, nausea, vomiting, arrhythmia, paralysis, seizure, hypotension

- In hospital
  - Box jellyfish: If arrest give all available antivenom up to 6 vials as an IV push and 10 mmol of magnesium. Collapse or arrhythmias give 3 ampoules antivenom. Morphine/analgesia
  - Irukandji: IV analgesia (fentanyl preferred) + promethazine IV 25 mg; for HT give GTN infusion 1 microgram/kg/min titrate to sBP < 160. Support treatment if APO
    - Investigations: ECG, CXR, FBC/EUC/troponin/CK, echo
  - Blue-ringed octopus: PIB, support
  - Penetrating marine injury
    - Treat trauma as usual, ADT, analgesia, immediate irrigation
    - Hot water immersion 45°C for 30–90 minutes for stingray and stonefish
    - Stonefish has specific antivenom
    - Clean wounds thoroughly, remove foreign body, leave lacerations open. May need surgical debridement
    - Consider antibiotics to cover water-associated trauma; e.g. doxycycline. Stingray high risk of secondary infection

Specific marine poisoning

- **Ciguatera**
  - Ingested ciguatoxins from tropical fish (cod, red bass, snapper, moray eel, mackerel, sea bass, barracuda). Not destroyed with cooking or freezing
  - Cause nausea and diarrhoea, abdominal pain, myalgia, neurological symptoms (ataxia, paraesthesia, weakness, temperature inversion), pruritus, rash
  - Treat with support, antihistamines, analgesia

- Tetrodotoxin
  - Blue-ringed octopus, puffer fish
  - Neurology: Perioral numbness, distal limb numb, ataxia, weakness, respiratory paralysis, coma, ↓ BP, arrhythmia
  - Observe for 24 hours if mild to moderate
  - Severe: ALS, ventilate/intubate, atropine 0.5–1.5 mg IV bolus for bradycardia
- Scombroid
  - Poorly preserved or refrigerated fish—high concentration histidine, not destroyed by cooking: Histamine release, can't distinguish from allergy. Rash, GI, wheeze, SOB, ↓ BP
  - Management: Antihistamines (promethazine 10–25 mg IV), bronchodilators, fluids, adrenaline, airway control

CHAPTER 12

Endocrine

Diabetes mellitus

- ↓ insulin or ↓ action of insulin causing ↑ BSL

Type 1

- ↓ insulin secretion from pancreas by autoimmune destruction of β cells, genetic link. Require treatment with insulin to live. Prone to diabetic ketoacidosis (DKA)

Type 2

- Insulin resistance leading to ↑ insulin and eventually β cell failure. Genetic link and risk ↑ with lifestyle, diet, obesity
- Can present with hyperosmolar hyperglycaemic non-ketotic state, microvascular (retinopathy, nephropathy, neuropathy), macrovascular (heart disease, CVD). Can be prevented/delayed

Type 3

- Secondary diabetes mellitus; e.g. pancreatitis, cystic fibrosis (CF), acromegaly, endocrine tumours, medications (steroids, thiazides, levothyroxine), infection, congenital (e.g. Down syndrome)

Type 4

- Gestational diabetes mellitus

All forms

- End result is ↑ BSL; chronic ↑ BSL leads to micro- and macrovascular complications

Signs and symptoms

- Type 1 can present with DKA, type 2 with hyperglycaemic hyperosmolar non-ketotic syndrome (HHNS) or complications
- Polyuria, polydipsia, fatigue, ↓ weight, ↓ wound healing, infections, blur vision

Diagnosis

- Fasting BGL < 6.1 mmol/L = normal
- Fasting BGL 6.1–7.0 or 7.8–11.1 oral glucose tolerance test (OGTT) = impaired glucose tolerance
- Fasting BGL ≥ 7 or ≥ 11.1 OGTT = diabetes mellitus

Acute hyperglycaemia

- Look for cause; e.g. infection, medications, IHD, CVS, PID, non-compliance
- EUC, venous blood gas, FBC, LFT, CRP
- Treat with IV fluids, IV/SC insulin, monitor EUC, CMP

Other causes for a diabetic to present to ED

- Retinopathy, glaucoma
- Nephropathy: Microalbuminuria
- Neuropathy: Peripheral and autonomic (GORD, gastroparesis, neurogenic bladder, impotence, orthostatic ↓ BP, incontinence)
- Infections: e.g. UTI, rhinocerebral mucormycosis (severe, invasive fungal infection sinuses), malignant otitis externa, cholecystitis, pyelonephritis and abscess
- Diabetic foot disease and ulcers
- Hypoglycaemia

Hypoglycaemia

- Definition: ↓ BSL and symptoms and resolves with treatment if not prolonged (hypoglycaemic coma poor prognosis)
- Causes: Diabetic medications, EtOH, medications (iron, salicylates, paracetamol), sepsis, ↓ food or ↑ exercise, OD, hepatic disease, insulinoma
- Beta-blockers may mask warning symptoms
- Symptoms
  - CNS dysfunction: Neuroglycopenic (hunger, confusion, coma, seizure)
  - Sympathetic: Adrenergic (pale, sweat, shaking, palpitations, anxiety)
- Diagnosis
  - DON'T ever forget glucose!
  - Bedside and formal BSL
  - Lower limit of normal BSL: adults < 4.0 mmol/L, children < 3.3 mmol/L, neonates < 48 hours old controversial but treat if < 2.6 mmol/L
- Management
  - Look for and treat cause
  - If conscious and cooperative: sugary food (e.g. fruit juice, jellybeans, breastmilk) then carbohydrate food (e.g. sandwich)

  - Severe: URGENT treatment with glucose
    - Adults: 50% glucose 25–50 mL IV through cubital fossa cannula or IM 1 mg glucagon. Follow with IVI maintenance normal saline + 5% dextrose
    - Children: 10% glucose 2 mL/kg then maintenance with normal saline + 5% dextrose as per weight. Glucagon IM 0.5 mg if under 25 kg
  - At home use 1 mg glucagon SC/IM (0.5 mg if < 25 kg)
  - Monitor BSL 1–2-hourly
  - If associated with seizure may take hours to recover. Need supportive care
  - Toxicology causes such as sulphonylureas, insulin (see Chapter 11 Toxicology, pp. 234 and 242)
- Investigations
  - Insulin level ↑, C peptide low (not usually performed)
  - Tests in children/critical blood tests. Take pre-treatment but don't delay treatment. Bloods (insulin, cortisol, GH, ACTH, free fatty acids, ketones), urine (organic and amino acids), newborn screening card
  - Monitor EUC especially K^+
- Admit if:
  - Moderate- or long-acting insulin
  - Continued mental change
  - Continuous ↓ BSL
  - Require ongoing glucose IV fluids
  - Precipitate requires admission; e.g. sepsis
  - OD
  - No carer/supervisor/outpatient follow-up
  - Very young or very old
  - Comorbidities

Diabetic ketoacidosis (DKA)

- Pathophysiology
  - Associated with type 1 diabetes mellitus
  - Body's response to cellular starvation
  - ↓ insulin leads to ↑ catabolic hormones causing ↑ BSL resulting in: Osmotic diuresis, prerenal azotaemia, ketones, wide AG metabolic acidosis

- Causes/precipitates: Missed insulin doses, stress, infection, stroke, AMI, trauma, pregnancy, PE, operation, steroids, pancreatitis, ↑ thyroid, type 1 diabetics new diagnosis
- Signs and symptoms
  - Hyperglycaemia (diuresis, polyuria, polydipsia)
  - Volume depletion
  - Acidosis (↑ RR), ketotic breath
  - Kussmaul respiration, ↑ HR, ↑ RR
  - Nausea and vomiting, abdominal pain, ↓ weight
  - Confusion (correlates with osmolarity [OSM] > 320), coma, weakness
- Investigations
  - BSL, urine ketones, ECG
  - ↑ blood ketones, blood gas shows ↓ pH, ↓ CO_2
  - ↑ AG, EUC, CMP
  - Look for cause: CXR, cultures, UA, FBC etc.
  - Definition: BGL > 11 or known DM, HCO_3 < 15, ketones urine ≥ 2 or blood ≥ 0.6, pH < 7.3
  - Corrected Na (cNa) = measured Na + ([glucose – 5]/3)
  - Note: $ETCO_2$ > 36 essentially excludes DKA in children
- Differential diagnosis: Metformin causing lactic acidosis, uraemia, methanol, salicylate, other wide AG ↓ pH causes etc., EtOH
- Management
  - Fluid resuscitation: Don't replace too quickly as may lead to cerebral oedema especially in children, elderly, cardiac or renal patients
    - o Monitor heart and vitals, may need CVC with CVP monitor
    - o Example of fluid strategy in adults: 1 L bolus normal saline, then 1 L for 1 hour; 1 L over 2 hours
    - o Children: If hypoperfusion/severe dehydration give 10 mL/kg IV normal saline bolus. May repeat with caution. Get expert guidance. Ongoing fluids—for paediatrics see p. 326
    - o Give dextrose in maintenance fluids once glucose < 16
    - o Decrease ↓↓ fluid rate if cNa > 150

- Insulin: IV short-acting infusion. DON'T load
  - Dose: 0.05–0.1 units/kg/hr
  - To prepare solution 100 units regular insulin in 100 mL normal saline—discard first 25 mL
- Potassium: Usually total body K^+↓↓ but 1st K^+ level can be normal; with therapy level may ↓↓ rapidly
  - Check K^+ levels, ECG
    - Rough rule of thumb (in adults): If result not back and ECG normal, add 10 mmol/hr K^+ after 1st hour IV fluids
  - If $K^+ < 3$ mmol/L give (in an adult) 20 mmol/hr, closely monitor. May need CVC
- Other electrolytes
  - PO_4 may be low: No need to replace in ED
  - Mg may be low if severe and symptoms (↑ reflexes, Chvostek's and Trousseau's signs) give PO or IV $MgSO_4$
  - HCO_3 in adults: Only give HCO_3 if severe ketoacidosis pH < 7 or HCO_3 < 5. Aim to ↓ cardiac risk not to normalise pH
    - $NaHCO_3^-$ 8.4% 70–100 mL IV over 30 minutes
- Monitor
  - BSLs: When BSL < 15, halve the insulin rate, change IV fluids to 5% glucose. Monitor EUC venous gas
  - Identify cause and treat; e.g. AMI, infection
  - Identify and treat complications: Electrolyte abnormality, ARDS, cerebral oedema, thrombosis, insulin AB
  - Nurse head-up: Prevent cerebral oedema
- Cerebral oedema
  - Risk factors: 1st presentation, age < 5, poorly controlled DM, initial cNa > 160
  - Features: Headache, behaviour change, ↓ HR, ↓ RR, HT, thermal instability, no ↓ Na with ↓ glucose, ↓ level of consciousness
  - Management: Mannitol immediately 20% 0.5 g/kg over 20 minutes. Decrease fluids. Nurse head-up

Alcoholic ketoacidosis

- Usually associated with very high chronic alcohol use with high use preceding days and acute decrease of EtOH
- Pathophysiology: EtOH metabolism with ↓↓ glucose source causes ↑ ketoacids resulting in metabolic acidosis

- Signs and symptoms: Heavy drinking then acute ↓↓ EtOH with ↓ food intake and vomiting, nausea and vomiting, abdominal pain and tenderness, anorexia. Dehydrated, acetone smell, ↑ RR, ↑ HR, Kussmaul respiration, patients are non-toxic in appearance, can have other EtOH Cx; e.g. pancreatitis, GI bleed, withdrawal
- Investigations
  - EtOH normal or can be ↑
  - HAGMA +/– metabolic alkalosis from vomiting; therefore, pH can be normal or even increased. Rely on AG for diagnosis
  - Will have ↑ AG
  - Ketones (check blood βHB; dipstick may be negative)
  - ↓ phosphate, ↓ Na, ↓ K^+, ↑ bilirubin and LFT from chronic EtOH
  - EUC, ↑ Cr (dehydrated), ↑ CK, ↑ lactate mild, mild ↓↑ BSL, FBC
- Management
  - Give thiamine 300 mg IV pre-glucose
  - Volume resuscitation + glucose (need the glucose to terminate ketogenesis)
  - Use 5% glucose in normal saline (not as bolus)
  - Consider Mg and multivitamin PO phosphate
  - Manage withdrawal and other concomitant conditions
  - Monitor electrolytes

Hyperglycaemic hyperosmolar state (HHS)

- Usually type 2 diabetes mellitus associated
- Pathophysiology and definition
  - ↓ insulin use + ↑ hepatic gluconeogenesis and glycogenolysis + impaired renal glucose excretion
  - ↑↑ BSL > 33, hyperosmolar (> 320), HCO_3 (> 15), pH (> 7.3) normal or mild ↑ ketones. Can get acidosis due to ↓ perfusion, ↑ lactate etc.
- Signs and symptoms: Abnormal vitals, mental changes, weak, anorexia, fatigue, cough, SOB, abdominal pain
  - Look for precipitates: UTI, pneumonia, non-compliance, AMI, gastroenteritis, steroids, stroke, EtOH
  - Usually elderly, poor control of diabetes mellitus, comorbidities

  - CNS signs: ↓ level of consciousness, tremor, clonus, hemiplegia, sensory defect, seizures
  - Can look like CVA, and CVA can precipitate!
- Investigations
  - BSL, EUC, FBC, LFT, CMP, VBG
  - AG and ketones normal
  - Septic screen: CXR, UA, cultures
  - LFT, lipase, trop, CK, TFT, coags
  - ECG, CT head, ABG
  - Can have acidosis, alkalosis or normal pH
  - Na can be ↑↓ normal; correct for dilutional effect of hyperglycaemia
  - Corrected Na (cNa) = measured Na + ([glucose – 5]/3)
- Management
  - IV fluids. With care if comorbid/cardiac etc.
    - Resuscitation fluids; e.g. normal saline bolus end point BP and HR normal
    - Estimate deficit and correct over 2–3 days; usually 20–25% (8–12 L) deficit
    - Give dextrose in fluids once glucose < 15
    - May need to make IV slower in cardiac failure
    - Monitor urine output with IDC
  - Monitor electrolytes
    - Na: Don't decrease Na by more than 10 mmol in 24 hours
    - Glucose: Don't decrease by more than 3 mmol/hr
    - K: Monitor and replace
    - Magnesium, phosphate and calcium
  - Insulin
    - Insulin infusion as with DKA low dose 0.05 units/kg/hr, ½ dose once BSL < 15 and give with glucose IV
  - Treat precipitants/cause
  - VTE prophylaxis

Hyperthyroid

- Causes
  - Primary: Graves, goitre, ↓ iodine
  - Central: Pituitary adenoma

  - Thyroiditis: Postpartum, radiation
  - Ectopic thyroid tissue
  - Drug induced: Lithium, iodine, amiodarone, thyroxine
- Signs and symptoms: Heat intolerance, palpitations, ↓ weight, sweat, tremor, nervous, weak, fatigue, eye signs in Graves (exophthalmos, chemosis, lid lag). Careful when palpating the thyroid can cause thyroid storm
- Investigations: ↑ T_4, ↓ TSH, autoantibodies, normal TSH essentially rules out Graves. Normocytic anaemia, high Ca, low albumin, elevated AST, ALP
- Management: Beta-blockers, propylthiouracil (PTU), carbimazole, radioactive I^-, thyroidectomy. Identify cause
- Thyroid storm
  - Undiagnosed or poor treatment hyperthyroidism or/+ precipitant: Infection, trauma, DKA, AMI, CVA, PE, OT, ingest or withdrawal thyroid hormone, iodine, palpation of gland
  - Signs and symptoms: Fever, SVT, ↑ HR, confusion, GI symptoms, tremor, ↓ weight, heat intolerance, palpitations, hypertension, wide pulse pressure, sweats
  - Investigations not usually helpful, can't differentiate hyperthyroidism from storm. Identify precipitants
    - ↑ WCC, ↑ BSL, ↑ bilirubin, CXR, ECG
  - Diagnosis: Temperature > 37.8°C, ↑ HR 120–200, CNS change (90%)
    - Differential diagnosis: Sepsis, heat stroke, MH, NMS, phaeochromocytoma, sympathetic cause
  - Management
    - ABC, O_2, IV fluids, monitor ECG, support, monitor electrolytes and glucose
    - Decrease fever, cool, DON'T give aspirin
    - Beta-blockers: Propranolol IV 0.5–1 mg over 5–10 minutes. May need to repeat. Aim HR < 100
    - PTU 900 mg load PO then 300 mg 6-hourly PO
    - Iodine IV or PO, Lugol's iodine
      - Can also use cholestyramine, plasmapheresis, lithium (if iodine allergy)
    - Steroids: Hydrocortisone 100 mg QID
    - Other: Dialysis, plasmapheresis, charcoal haemoperfusion

Hypothyroidism

- Causes
    - Primary: Autoimmune, post OT/ablation/radiation, iodine deficiency, congenital, thyroiditis, tumour
    - Secondary: Pituitary issue causing decreased TSH
    - Tertiary: Hypothalamus issue causing decreased thyrotropin-releasing hormone (TRH) and medications (amiodarone, lithium, iodine, PTU, carbimazole)
- Signs and symptoms: Fatigue, ↑ weight, cold intolerance, depression, muscle cramp, ↓ temperature, hoarse, ↓ HR, periorbital puffiness, peripheral neuropathy, menstrual abnormality, goitre
- Investigations: ↓ T_4, ↑ TSH, autoantibodies
- Management: Thyroxine 50–100 (25 in elderly) microgram/day ↑ over 3–6/12 to max. 200 microgram/day. Monitor. Look for cause

Myxoedema coma

- Longstanding hypothyroid patient and undiagnosed presents with life-threatening decompensation. Mostly elderly
- Signs and symptoms: ↓ mental state, ↓ temperature, ↓ HR, ↓ RR, periorbital oedema, non-pitting oedema, delayed tendon reflexes, ↓ BSL, ↓ Na, retention, seizure
- Precipitants: Infection, cold, drugs, trauma, CVA, CHF, inadequate thyroxine
- Investigations
    - Usually markedly elevated TSH, low T3/4 ↓ Hb, ↓ Na, ↓ BSL, ↑ CK, ↑ LDH, ↑ transaminases, ↑ cholesterol, abnormal ABG (↓ pO_2, ↑ pCO_2)
    - ECG: ↑ QT, T inversion, CXR effusion
- Management
    - ABC, support
    - Thyroxine T4 300–500 microgram slow IVI then 50–100 microgram daily (slower onset), can use T3 10 microgram IV (rapid)
    - Hydrocortisone 100 mg IV TDS
    - Treat hypothermia, warm
    - Fluids, water restrict if low Na
    - Monitor EUC, BSL
    - Treat precipitate

Adrenal insufficiency and crisis

Adrenal insufficiency types

- Primary
  - Causes: Autoimmune (Addison's disease), infection (e.g. HIV, TB), infiltrate (e.g. amyloid, sarcoid), haemorrhage or thrombosis (DIC, sepsis), metastases
  - 90% adrenal must be destroyed for symptoms causing ↓ glucocorticoids, ↓ androgen and ↓ mineralocorticoids
- Secondary
  - Causes: Steroid therapy exogenous (some call primary or tertiary), infiltrate, tumours, postpartum, head trauma, pituitary OT
  - Due to ↓ corticotropin and/or ACTH

Presentation

- Chronic
  - Fatigue, nausea and vomiting, abdominal pain, diarrhoea, anorexia, ↓ weight, ↓ BP
  - Primary adrenal insufficiency causing ↑ ACTH leading to hyperpigmentation
  - Signs and symptoms of cause; e.g. pituitary tumour
    - If secondary adrenal insufficiency may find visual field defect
    - Primary adrenal insufficiency may cause ↑ K^+, ↓ aldosterone
    - Both cause ↓ Hb, ↑ lymphocytes
- Adrenal crisis
  - Life-threatening; emergency
  - ↓ BP not responsive to catecholamines and IV fluids can lead to ↓ level of consciousness and ultimately death
  - GI symptoms, lethargy
  - Usually precipitated by stress, other precipitants: Operation, AMI, low glucose, trauma, psychiatric, etc.
  - Investigations
    - Even in crisis all investigations may be normal: ↓ Na, ↓ Cl, ↓ glucose, non-anion gap metabolic acidosis (NAGMA), ↑ K, ↑ Ca, BUN
  - Diagnosis
    - Usually not available: Plasma cortisol ↓↓ (< 83 nmol/L)
    - Short Synacthen test etc.

- Management
  - Fluid resuscitation
  - Monitor and treat electrolytes and glucose
  - Hydrocortisone 200 mg IV then 100 mg QID IV
  - Patients on steroids + acute stress should get hydrocortisone IV 50–100 mg depending on severity of stressor

Calcium

↓ Ca (< 2.15 mEq/L)

- Post surgical hypoparathyroidism is often considered the most common cause
- Other causes: Pancreatitis, medications, AKI, ↑ phosphate, malabsorption
- Serum total Ca varies with albumin, ½ plasma Ca bound to albumin; therefore, a low Ca may be a spurious result if albumin low
- Signs and symptoms: Tetany, muscle irritability, Chvostek's sign (tap CN II causes mouth twitch), Trousseau's sign positive (BP cuff arm causes carpal spasm), paraesthesia hands/feet/mouth, seizure, colicky pain, fasciculation, stridor, laryngospasm
- Treatment for acute/severe
  - Calcium chloride 10% 5 mL IV over 10–20 minutes then slow IVI or calcium gluconate 10% 10 mL IV (don't use CaCl in children—necrosis if extravasation)
  - Monitor CMP. Correct ↓ Mg with TDS 500–1000 mg Mg, give vitamin D, ongoing oral calcium

↑ Ca (> 2.55 mEq/L)

- Causes: Most common cause malignancy and primary hyperparathyroidism
  - Other causes: Sarcoid, vitamin D intoxication, vitamin A intoxication, milk alkali syndrome, thiazides, thyrotoxicosis
  - Spurious result: High albumin, venous stasis
- Signs and symptoms: Nausea and vomiting, mental ↓, coma, muscle weakness, thirst. The saying goes: Bones (pain), stones (renal), groans (abdominal pain, nausea, vomiting), moans (psychiatric symptoms, mania, behaviour change, neurological change)
- Treat only if severe and symptoms, Ca > 3.5
  - Rehydration with normal saline, avoid Hartmann's solution, monitor heart function

- IV pamidronate 30–90 mg over 2–4 hours or zoledronic acid 4 mg/15 min
- If life-threatening can use calcitonin 100 units BD IV/IM
- If refractory and due to cancer, sarcoid IV hydrocortisone 100 mg BD
- Extreme cases: Dialysis
- Careful use of furosemide to enhance elimination

Potassium

↓ K^+: $K^+ < 3.5$ mEq/L

- Causes: K^+ shift (catecholamines, insulin, alkalosis, periodic paralysis, verapamil, B12), ↓ intake, GI loss, renal loss (diuretics), drugs/toxins
- Signs and symptoms: Weakness, muscle pain, tetany, paralysis, ileus, rhabdomyolysis, ↑↓ BP, potentiate digoxin toxicity, renal
  - ECG: Flat T, U, ST↓
- Treatment
  - Treat cause
  - K^+ replacement PO, IV 10 mmol/hr KCl in 100 mL normal saline peripherally, up to maximum 40 mmol/hr (0.5 mmol/kg/hr) centrally, cardiac monitor if > 15 mmol/hr
  - Correct Mg and fluid status

↑ K^+: $K^+ > 5.5$ mEq/L

- Causes: False (haemolysis of sample, very high WCC, sample taken near fluids with K), K^+ shift (acidosis, hypoaldosteronism) exercise ++, K^+ exogenous, drugs, ARF, ↓ excretion (e.g. RTN, K sparing diuretics, renal impairment, ACE inhibitors), K^+ release (rhabdomyolysis, hyperthermia, suxamethonium, digoxin)
- Signs and symptoms: ECG
  - 6.5–7.5: Tall, peak T; short QT; ↑ PR
  - 7.5–8.0: QRS wide, flat P
  - 10–12: QRS degrade to sine wave VF, asystole, complete cardiac block
- Management: If no ECG change then repeat sample. Identify and treat cause
  - Protect heart/stabilise membrane if K > 7 or ECG abnormal
    - $CaCl_2$ (10%) 5–10 mL IV (don't use peripherally in children) or

    - Calcium gluconate (10%) 10–20 mL (0.5 mL/kg) IV over 2 minutes if unstable or 20 minutes if stable
    - **(Take care if digoxin toxic, theoretical risk of stone heart)**
- Move K^+ into cells
    - Salbutamol neb 5–10 mg over 20 minutes (2.5 mg if < 25 kg)
    - Insulin 10 units IV/SC (0.1 units/kg children) + glucose 50 mL of 50% (10% dextrose in children 5 mL/kg unless hyponatraemic): Keep close eye on BSLs for 4 hours following this
    - $NaHCO_3^-$ if pH < 7.2; 100 mL 8.4% or 100 mmol (1–2 mmol/kg); **can't give at same time as calcium**
- Remove K^+
    - Query Resonium (Na polystyrene) PO, PR 15–30–60 g PO/PR: New evidence suggests not worth adverse risks, minimal benefit.
    - Haemodialysis
- Monitor ECG and K^+; treat the cause

Sodium

↓ Na: < 135 mEq/L

- Causes/diagnosis: Step 1 check fluid volume, step 2 urine Na. Fig. 12.1 can be used to assist in identifying a cause
- Signs and symptoms: Depend on how quickly Na has changed. Mental change, lethargy, seizure, neuromuscular excitation
- Management
    - Treat cause
    - If dehydrated, IV fluids with normal saline
    - If euvolaemic or oedematous, volume restriction
    - If associated with seizure use hypertonic saline 3% 1–2 mL/kg (100 mL adult)
    - Monitor Na and EUC
    - Must not ↑ Na by > 1–2 mmol/hr if acute or 0.5 mmol/hr if chronic

SIADH

- Causes: Tumour (lung, pancreatic, thymoma), neurological (trauma, infection, GBS, SLE, SAH), pulmonary (infection, TB, COPD), drugs (fluoxetine, paroxetine, tramadol, haloperidol, omeprazole)

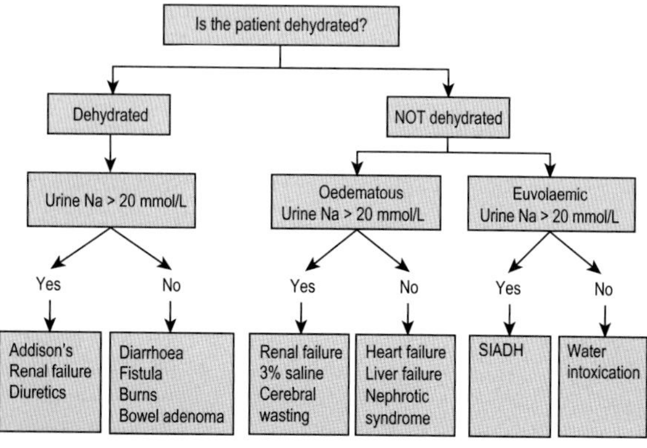

Figure 12.1 Causes of hyponatraemia sorted by clinical and lab assessment of patient

- Diagnosis criteria: Low Na, hypotonic, serum OSM > 275, urine Na > 20, normal diet, euvolaemic, urine OSM > plasma OSM, no renal water affecting medications (e.g. diuretics), no renal/heart/hepatic/thyroid disease
- Symptoms: Anorexia, nausea, malaise, confusion, seizure, coma
- Treat with water restriction; e.g. 500 mL/day
    - Severe: Frusemide can be used. Use with IV normal saline. Get expert advice
    - Must ↑ Na slowly 0.5 mEq/L/hr
    - With < 15 mEq ↑ in 1st 24 hours
    - Can use demeclocycline with expert guidance 300–600 mg BD PO

↑ Na > 150 mmol/L

- Causes
    - ↓ total body water, water loss > Na (impaired thirst, insensible loss, diarrhoea and vomiting, fistula, renal loss—diabetes insipidus [DI], sickle cell; drugs, skin loss/burns/sweating)

- Excess Na (hypertonic saline, ingestion seawater drowning, steroid excess e.g. Cushing's syndrome, peritoneal dialysis)
- Diabetes insipidus
  - Failure of central or peripheral antidiuretic hormone (ADH) response
  - Serum OSM > 290, urine OSM < 150, urine Na < 145, polyuria
  - Causes: Neurogenic (tumour, pituitary operation, trauma, infection), nephrogenic (familial, renal disease, drugs), gestational

- Signs and symptoms: Irritable, seizure, coma, brain haemorrhage and thrombosis from brain shrinking and tears vessels. If slow onset, brain adapts
- Treatment
  - Desmopressin in DI
  - Fluid resus with normal saline
  - Do not exceed Na correction of 10–15 mEq/L per day
  - Can correct Na more rapidly if onset was rapid

CHAPTER 13

Obstetrics and gynaecology

Per vaginam (PV) bleeding (non-pregnant)

- Differential diagnosis
  - **Ovulatory bleeding** (regular periods, dysmenorrhoea. Causes: Hormonal, polyps, cervicitis, fibroids, malignancy, endometriosis, PID, bleeding dyscrasias)
  - **Anovulatory** (menorrhagia secondary to anovulation: Menopause, perimenarcheal, endocrine, PCOS [polycystic ovaries syndrome], OCP, liver disease, renal disease)
  - **Non-uterine** (abnormal coagulants, ITP, VWD, malignancy, polyps, lacerations, foreign body, urethral source)
  - **Abnormal/dysfunctional uterine bleeding** (irregular uterine bleeding without any pelvic pathology, medical diagnosis or other causes)
- History/examination: Menarche age, menstrual history, last menstrual period (LMP), pattern of bleeding, PV discharge, dysmenorrhoea, pregnancy, STIs, sexually active, other signs and symptoms of abnormal coagulation, pain description, urine/GI/musculoskeletal symptoms, fever, syncope
  - Vitals, abdomen, lymph nodes, speculum, bimanual PV
- Investigations: βHCG, FBC, coags if indicated, TSH, prolactin (if potentially endocrine cause), US
- Management
  - If significant blood loss may need resus
    - Tranexamic acid 10 mg/kg IV up to 1 g, q8hourly until bleeding stops
  - Management of abnormal/dysfunctional uterine bleeding with acute bleeding
    - Tranexamic acid 1 g PO TDS
    - Norethisterone 5–10 mg TDS 5 days
  - Rule out trauma, bleeding, dyscrasia, infection, foreign body. Then if stable and bleeding mild can have outpatient investigations

Abdominal pain (non-pregnant)

- Differential diagnosis
  - **Ovarian cyst** (rupture, torsion, haemorrhage, infection): Sudden unilateral pelvic pain can be post activity. On examination tender +/– peritonism if ruptured
  - **Adnexal torsion**: Sudden unilateral pelvic pain +/– post activity +/– patient history cyst/tumour. On examination tender +/– peritonism
  - **PID**: Low abdomen/pelvic pain, bilateral, PV bleed, discharge, urine symptoms, fever. Tenderness on examination
  - **Endometriosis**: Dysmenorrhoea, chronic pelvic pain. On examination can be tender or normal
  - **Adenomyosis**: Dysmenorrhoea/menorrhagia
  - **Leiomyomas**: Pelvic pain/mass
  - **Tubo-ovarian abscess**: Fever, unilateral pain, PV bleed, discharge, adnexal tender
  - **Non-gynaecological**: Appendicitis, diverticulitis, incarcerated hernia
- Investigations: βHCG, FBC, urine, CRP, STI—urine PCR for chlamydia and gonococcal (first-pass urine—needs to have been several hours since last wee and wee directly into pot, i.e. not midstream), swabs (patient can take their own). Pelvic US, laparoscopy
- Management
  - *Rule out pregnancy*
  - Analgesia
  - Specific treatments for cause

Pelvic inflammatory disease (PID)

- Signs and symptoms: Lower abdominal pain, PV discharge or PV bleed, postcoital bleed, dyspareunia, dysuria, fever, malaise, nausea and vomiting. Can be asymptomatic
  - On examination: Lower abdomen tender, cervical motion tender, adnexal tender
  - No peritonism
- Investigations: βHCG, UA, urine PCR for chlamydia/gonorrhoea on first-pass urine (first-pass urine—needs to have been several hours since last wee and wee directly into pot, i.e. not midstream) or swabs (patient can take their own) +/– US
  - Consider in more severe cases FBC, CRP, LFT (Fitz-Hugh–Curtis syndrome)

- Management
  - Remove intrauterine device (IUD) if present
  - Antibiotics for sexually acquired PID
    - Azithromycin 1 g PO single dose then repeat dose with GP in 1 week

      OR
    - Doxycycline 100 mg BD for 14/7
    - + metronidazole 400 mg BD for 14/7
    - + ceftriaxone 500 mg IM/IV single dose
  - Antibiotics for non-sexually acquired PID
    - Amoxicillin with clavulanate forte
    - + doxycycline 100 mg BD for 14/7
    - +/– roxithromycin
  - Severe cases: Use IV antibiotics ceftriaxone 2 g daily OR cefotaxime 2 g 8hourly + azithromycin 500 mg daily + metronidazole 500 mg BD
  - Treat contacts

Ectopic pregnancy

- Signs and symptoms
  - Abdominal pain
  - PV bleed/spotting: Can be mistaken as a period
  - Amenorrhoea
  - Hypovolaemic shock (initially just tachycardic)
  - Pain of rupture: Lateral, sudden, sharp, severe
  - Shoulder pain
  - Early pregnancy symptoms
  - Peritonism
  - Adnexal mass
  - Tenderness if ruptured
- Assessment
  - Risk factors: Previous infections/PID, history of tubal surgery, IUD, previous ectopic, assisted reproduction, abnormal anatomy (septate uterus, tumour, adhesions etc.), increased age, endometriosis

    - History: Approximately 90% of patients with ectopic pregnancy have abdominal pain, 75% have abnormal bleeding but 10% have neither
- Investigations
    - *All female patients of childbearing age get βHCG*
    - Consider the need for FBC, blood group and cross-match
    - Change in βHCG (guide only)
        - An increase of > 50% in 2 days = pregnancy likely
        - An increase of < 50% in 2 days = consider ectopic
        - A decrease of > 35% in 2 days = miscarriage likely
        - A decrease of < 35% in 2 days = consider ectopic
    - Ultrasound
        - If βHCG > 1500 should expect to see fetus on US (transvaginal)
        - If βHCG > 700 and US shows empty uterus = ectopic likely
        - If US demonstrates intrauterine pregnancy, it is still possible to have an ectopic as well especially if fertility assisted. This is very rare
- Management
    - If ruptured: Resuscitation, urgent operation
    - Not ruptured
        - Operation
        - Can consider medical treatment; e.g. methotrexate if very early in pregnancy, no rupture, asymptomatic, no fetal heartbeat, βHCG < 3500

Pregnancy

- Physiology
    - Heart: 50% ↑ blood volume, 40% ↑ cardiac output, 20% ↑ HR, 20% ↓ SVR, BP ↓ slightly in first trimester then normalises
    - Respiratory: SOB common, 40% ↑ tidal volume, ↓ TLC/FRC/RV/ERV. ↑ MV. Vital capacity and RR should not change
    - GI: ↓ motility, reflux, ↓ oesophageal sphincter tone, ↑ ALP, ↑ risk gallstones
    - Renal: ↑ kidney size, ↑ renal blood flow, ↑ GFR, ↓ Cr, ↓ BUN
    - Haematology: ↑ blood volume (therefore ↑ plasma volume, ↑ RBC), Hb ↓ (not < 110), ↓ leucocyte function but can have

slight neutrophilia, slight ↓ platelets, ↑ clotting factors and ↑ D-dimer

- Endocrinology: Postprandial ↑ BSL, thyroid hyperplasia
- Uterus: ↑ uterus size/weight. Approximations:
  - Fundal height—1 cm above pubic symphysis for every week over 12 weeks
  - Fundus at the umbilicus = 20 weeks, xiphisternum = 40 weeks

- Syncopes
  - Common: Palpitations, dizzy, presyncope, syncope
  - Exclude anaemia, electrolyte imbalance, dehydration, PE, arrhythmia
- Medications
  - NEVER USE: ACE inhibitors, amphetamines, tricyclic antidepressants, barbiturates, carbamazepine, ciprofloxacin, chloramphenicol, diazepam, gentamicin, iodide, lithium, lorazepam, methotrexate, metronidazole, misoprostol, paroxetine, phenytoin, propylthiouracil (PTU), salicylates, sulfonamides, streptomycin, tamoxifen, tetracyclines, trimethoprim, valproic acid, warfarin
  - DON'T use if breastfeeding: Tetracyclines, isoniazid, sedatives, barbiturates, benzodiazepines (BZDs), metronidazole, nitrofurantoin, ketorolac, lithium, chemotherapy, iodine, chloramphenicol, moderate–high dose prednisone
  - Safe in pregnancy: Cephalosporins, erythromycin, azithromycin, penicillins, nitrofurantoin, paracetamol, promethazine, prochlorperazine, metoclopramide, ondansetron, lidocaine (lignocaine), doxylamine, adenosine, heparin, verapamil, loratadine
  - Vaccines: DON'T give live vaccines (measles, mumps and rubella [MMR], varicella, polio) while pregnant or 3/12 pre-conception
    - Can give inactivated (influenza, tetanus toxoid +/– diphtheria)
    - Can give immunoglobulins (tetanus, hepatitis, rabies, varicella)
- Signs and symptoms needing investigation:
  - Change in fetal movement pattern
  - Fevers, chills
  - Refractory emesis
  - Visual change

- Abdominal pain
- Significant headache
- Oedema
- Dysuria
- PV bleed
- PV fluid loss
- Abnormal PV discharge

Emergencies in pregnancy

Septic abortion

- Miscarriage complicated by pelvic infection
- Usually secondary to non-professional termination or retained products
- Presentation: Pelvic pain, PV bleeding, offensive discharge fever, sepsis
- Investigations: FBC, CRP, blood cultures
- Management
    - Resuscitation
    - Operation: Dilation and curettage (D&C)
    - IVAB: Ampicillin, gentamicin and metronidazole

Bleeding in early pregnancy

- Loss of pregnancy at < 20/40
- Terminology for miscarriage
    - Threatened: Any PV bleeding without cervical dilatation
    - Inevitable: PV bleed + cervical dilatation
    - Complete: All products passed
    - Incomplete: Not all products passed
    - Failed pregnancy/miscarriage on US: Crown–rump length (CRL) > 6 mm on US with no cardiac activity, gestational sac > 20 mm with no fetal pole, sac > 12 mm and no yolk, or no embryo with fetal heartbeat 2 weeks after sac shown
    - Failed pregnancy will either progress to complete or incomplete miscarriage or not progress (sometimes called missed abortion)
- Assessment
    - Unless cervical shock/significant bleeding no need to perform speculum examination

    - FBC, blood group, UA, βHCG
    - US to exclude ectopic: Will need full bladder
- Management
    - If continued profuse bleeding and/or hypotension
        - Resuscitation if required
        - Exclude cervical shock (clot in cervical canal causing vasovagal stimulation usually hypotension with bradycardia). Perform speculum examination. Ensure good lighting, long forceps and lots of gauze. Remove clot(s) if seen. Patient usually recovers rapidly
        - Tranexamic acid (TXA), ergotamine
        - D&C
    - Rho(D) immunoglobin if patient is Rh factor negative, discuss with gynaecology registrar. Some evidence suggests not needed if < 12/40
    - For most patients management is expectant
    - Offer counselling

Gestational trophoblastic disease

- Molar pregnancy: Choriocarcinoma with metastases
- Signs and symptoms: PV bleed, hyperemesis, hypertension
- ↑ βHCG abnormally high, ↑ uterus size
- US, discuss with obstetrics and gynaecology (O&G), will need D&C

Nausea, vomiting

- Common 1st 12 weeks
- If abdominal pain present must consider other diagnosis; e.g. ectopic, gall bladder disease (↑ risk with pregnancy)
- Hyperemesis gravidarum: Intractable vomiting, ↓ weight, dehydration, ↓ K or ketonaemia
- Management of ketonaemia/severe: IV thiamine, 5% dextrose in normal saline
- Diet and lifestyle modifications; e.g. smaller frequent meals, increased rest, avoid spicy foods
- Antiemetics
    - Ginger tablet 250 mg PO QID
    - Pyridoxine 25 mg PO TDS
    - Doxylamine 25 mg PO nocte

- Metoclopramide 10 mg PO/IV TDS
- Ondansetron 4 mg PO/IV BD/TDS (Note: Can cause constipation which may already be a problem)
- Persistent hyperemesis despite above. May consider steroids; e.g. methylprednisolone (seek specialist advice)

- Admit if: Severe dehydration, PO fluids not tolerated, significant electrolyte abnormalities, ketosis, infection
- Discharge if: Reversed ketonuria and passed trial of fluids. Always check urine. Discharge with antiemetics

Antepartum haemorrhage

- Bleeding in later pregnancy > 20/40
- Differential diagnosis: Placental abruption, placenta previa, preterm labour, genital lesion

Placental abruption

- Risks: HT, smoking, EtOH, trauma, short cord, fibroids, increased age, cocaine
- Assessment: Dark blood (blood can be concealed), severe pain and tenderness, contracted uterus
- Complications: Fetal distress and death, maternal death, DIC

Placenta praevia

- Risks: Previous caesarean section (C-section), increased age, multiple pregnancies, smoker, terminations, cocaine
- Assessment: Bright sudden blood loss, soft non-tender uterus, no fetal distress
- Complications: Premature delivery, shock

Vasa previa (rare)

- Risks: Placenta praevia, in-vitro fertilisation, usually diagnosed when in labour
- Assessment: Small amount of blood, no pain, fetal distress, mum okay
- Complications: Fetal death

Assessment/investigations

- DON'T EXAMINE/PV UNTIL PLACENTA PRAEVIA EXCLUDED
- FBC, coags, FDP, cross-match
- Kleihauer test
- US
- CTG

- Management
  - Urgent O&G involvement
  - Monitor mum and baby, resuscitation
  - Steroids: Betamethasone 11.4 mg IM (depending on gestation)
  - Anti D if needed

Hypertension—preeclampsia, HELLP and eclampsia

- Risk factors: Nulliparity, age > 40, pre-pregnancy hypertension, CKD, African American, diabetes mellitus, multiple gestation, gestational trophoblastic disease, obesity, previous history

Preeclampsia

- Definition
  - Pregnancy > 20 weeks gestation or up to 3 months post delivery

    AND
  - Hypertension: BP > 140/90 severe > 160/110

    AND
  - End-organ dysfunction: Proteinuria, renal impairment, liver involvement, neurological involvement, IUGR, ↓ platelets DIC, haemolysis
- Symptoms: Headache, vision change, oedema, abdominal pain
- Investigations: Urine (protein), LFT (↑ AST, ↑ ALT, ↑ bilirubin), ↑ uric acid, ↓ creatinine clearance, ↑ Cr, ↓ platelet, DIC, ↑ INR, ↓ fibrinogen, ARDS on CXR
- Management
  - Left lateral position, monitor mum and baby
  - $MgSO_4$ 4 g IV/15–30 min (50% solution in normal saline)
  - Anti-HT: Aim BP < 140/90. Examples: labetalol 10 mg IV, hydralazine 5–10 mg IV, nifedipine 10 mg PO
  - Call urgently O&G and neonatologist
  - Cautious fluids
  - Steroids—betamethasone 11.4 mg IM repeat in 12 hours
  - Delivery if > 37/40, can't control BP, abnormal CTG, abruption, significant end-organ effects
  - Look for neurology—consider secondary stroke
  - Must monitor Mg levels and signs Mg toxicity (e.g. reduced reflexes); can be hazardous if severe renal imp (give ½ dose) or ↓ Ca, myasthenia gravis, heart disease. Antidote if develops

toxicity (loss knee jerk, ↓ RR, slur speech, paralysis, arrest) CaCl or Ca gluconate 10 mL of 10% solution over 3 minutes

HELLP syndrome

- Haemolysis, ↑ LFT, ↓ platelets
- Complication of preeclampsia. Microvascular thrombi. Initially liver then CNS, kidneys. End-organ damage, DIC, hepatic rupture (RUQ/ epigastric pain), ascites
- ↓ haptoglobin, ↑ bilirubin, ↑ LDH
- Treatment—as for preeclampsia: Dexamethasone prepartum 10 mg BD and postpartum 5 mg BD

Eclampsia

- Preeclampsia with coma or seizure
- Complications: Abruption, premature delivery, neurological injury ICH, peripheral oedema
- Management
  - As for preeclampsia
  - IV $MgSO_4$ 4 g/15–30 min (50% solution in normal saline) or IM (2 g each buttock) then infusion 1 g $MgSO_4$ (50% solution) per hour
  - Consider midazolam
  - Must monitor. Check CMP levels; can be hazardous if severe renal impairment (give ½ dose) or ↓ Ca, myasthenia gravis, heart disease, antidote if develops toxicity (loss knee jerk, ↓ RR, slur speech, paralysis, arrest) CaCl or Ca gluconate 10 mL of 10% solution over 3 minutes
  - NEVER use ACE inhibitors!
  - IV hydralazine 5–10 mg titrate and repeat, other options: labetalol, methyldopa, GTN
  - URGENT delivery! Steroids if < 34/40 weeks' gestation

Postpartum presentations

- Can get **eclampsia** even up to 3 months
- **Peripartum cardiomyopathy**
- **Thromboembolic disease** ↑ risk with LSCS
- **Postpartum haemorrhage** (see below)
- **Postpartum infection** (see Septic abortion, p. 271)
  - Fever, profuse bloody discharge, abdominal pain. If unwell, toxic or history of C-section must admit for IVAB
  - Get O&G consult

- **Ruptured uterus**
  - Risks: Obstructed labour, malposition, large infant, prior C-section
  - Assessment: Abdominal pain, PV bleed, tachycardia, hypotension, fetus palpable through abdominal wall
  - Management: URGENT resuscitation and delivery

Postpartum haemorrhage

- Any bleed that could cause haemodynamic instability, > 500 mL in 24 hours, > 1 L post C-section, massive = 50% of blood volume in 3 hours
- Causes (the 4 Ts): Atonic uterus, trauma, tissue retained, thrombin
- Risks: Multiple pregnancy, coagulopathy, large baby, abnormal uterus, long labour, instrument use, previous PPH
- Management: Team approach, call for help
  - Resuscitation, activate massive transfusion protocols, IVC large bore, cross-match
  - Remove clots, bimanual compression, uterine massage
  - Empty bladder: IDC
  - Syntocinon 10 U IM or 5 units slow IV then infusion 10 U/hr (40 U in 1 L normal saline over 4 hours)
  - Consider ergometrine 250 microgram slow IM or slow IV over 1–2 minutes
  - Consider misoprostol 800–1000 microgram PR
  - Identify cause: Speculum, look for trauma, assess for coagulopathy
  - Rotational thromboelastometry (ROTEM)/thromboelastography (TEG) if available to guide blood products
  - Tranexamic acid 1 g IV bolus then 1 g q8hourly
  - URGENT O&G review
  - Operation, embolisation

Emergency delivery

- Preparation
  - May be no time—may need to grab delivery kit: Towels, clamps, scissors, cord clamp
  - If time to prepare (e.g. Bat call), prepare 2 resuscitation bays—1 for mum, 1 for baby

  - Baby
    - Resuscitaire: Prewarmed
    - Check NeoPuff: Pressures, gas supply (start on air)
    - Check suction
    - Have equipment ready: Blades (size 0), tubes (2.5, 3.0), umbilical catheter, umbilical tape, syringes, 3-way tap
    - Have drugs ready: Adrenaline, saline
    - Pulse oximetry with attachment for baby
  - Mum
    - Check intubation equipment
    - Check IVC equipment
    - Ready for G&H/cross-match
    - Delivery kit: Towels, clamps, scissors
    - Monitoring: ECG, sats, BP, CTG
    - US
    - Drugs: Syntocinon, analgesia
- Call everyone! O&G, paeds/neonatologist, midwife
- If fully dilated, wanting to push, crowning then deliver in ED
- Delivery (stage 2)
  - Have patient on bed, lithotomy position
  - Examine PV, determine the presenting part—hopefully it's the head
  - Place sterile pad on inferior perineum to support and other hand on head. Control descent of head
  - Deliver head, look for cord around neck, free cord, if can't free cord then cut cord
  - External rotation—baby is now lateral
  - Deliver anterior then posterior shoulder with support to head and minimal traction
  - Place baby on mum
  - Clamp cord
    - If baby is term and no resuscitation required, delay cord clamp 2–3 minutes
    - Otherwise or if unsure clamp cord immediately
    - First clamp approximately 10 cm from baby
    - Place umbilical clamp 1–2 cm from abdomen

    - Always palpate to check for other babies
    - Syntocinon 10 U IM once baby delivered and pre-placenta birth
- Deliver placenta (stage 3)
    - Look for signs of separation—cord lengthens, PV gush of blood, uterine shape change
    - Gentle traction down and backward with one hand and place other hand suprapubic to guard uterus
    - Deliver placenta
    - Massage uterus
    - Check placenta intact
- After care
    - Monitor mum and baby
    - Baby can stay with mum if well
    - Call O&G and paeds (should already be there)

Abnormal presentations

Shoulder dystocia—get HELP!

- Baby shoulder caught on pubic bone. Look for the signs: Turtle sign
- Position mum with McRoberts manoeuvre: Extreme lithotomy with legs hyperflexed, held by assistants
- Make more room
    - Drain the bladder with IDC
    - Episiotomy
- Assistant apply suprapubic (NOT fundal) pressure
- Insert hand behind shoulder and rotate
- Corkscrew manoeuvre: Twist, rotate shoulders to free
- Aim to time these manoeuvres with contractions and urging mum to push ++
- If fails: Urgent C-section

Cord prolapse—get HELP!

- Position mum in Sims position: Knees to chest
- Push presenting part back up
- Replace cord
- Fill bladder with 500 mL normal saline
- Urgent delivery PV if possible, otherwise C-section

Breech—get HELP!

- Go to C-section immediately if at all possible
- Only deliver these if it's absolutely necessary and baby is coming like it or not! Otherwise WAIT
- If you see a foot: DON'T PULL IT
- NO traction should be used at all to prevent baby extending head
- Place hand behind baby's thigh
- Gentle pressure behind baby's knee then deliver leg then other leg
- Maternal push: Deliver to umbilicus
- If traction at this stage is needed it must be gentle: Use a dry towel and wrap around baby's hips NOT abdomen
- Assistant should apply pressure at fundus. This keeps baby's head flexed
- Maternal push: Deliver to clavicles
- Rotate 90 degrees, deliver anterior arm, rotate 180 degrees the other way and deliver other arm
- Rotate baby to be chest down
- Assistant keeps fundal pressure. Baby's head should be kept flexed
- Place hand on maxillary prominence with arm down chest and other hand on back then deliver head

CHAPTER 14

Psychiatry and substance abuse

Control of patient at risk

- Patient is risking themselves or others in the ED
- Always attempt to deescalate situation
  - Provide calm reassurance. Be empathetic
  - Explain exactly what the process is and why. Make reasonable claims from the beginning; e.g. telling a patient they will be seen and sent home within an hour is unlikely to happen and while it may settle someone immediately, it will likely eventually cause anger
  - Offer food/drink
  - Offer to contact or allow patient to contact friend or family member
  - Minimise language and cultural barriers, ensure hearing aids in etc.
- Take a full history if possible and collateral, be sure to ask:
  - Medication history, current drugs (e.g. EtOH, narcotics)
  - Co-existing-existing medical illness, heart disease, asthma, diabetes etc.
- Offer oral sedation: 'You seem anxious; can I offer you a medication to help you calm down?'
  - Diazepam 5–10 mg PO, repeat interval 30 minutes. Max. 60 mg in 24 hours. Note: Patients have varying tolerance to benzos
  - Olanzapine 5–10 mg PO, repeat interval 60 minutes. Max. 30 mg in 24 hours. Use caution if patient already taking serotonin agents
  - Risperidone for elderly 0.25–0.5 mg PO, repeat interval 8-hourly, max. in 24 hours 1 mg; or quetiapine 12.5–25 mg, max. 100 mg in 24 hours
- Be prepared
  - Call security
  - Get IVC ready + medications + resuscitation trolley available
  - Prepare monitoring equipment

- Show of strength
  - Make security visible and calmly explain to patient what will happen and why
- If necessary, can use mental health room but must not stay there once sedated. **Never seclude sedated patients**
  - Tell nursing unit manager (NUM) and psychiatric clinical nurse consultant (CNC)
  - Schedule
- Restrain patient: 5-point immobilisation. Never restrain prone! Use security +/– police
- IV or IM sedation choices: Aim for rousable drowsiness + IV fluids
  - Current preference is initially use IM droperidol, less chance needle stick and onset action 15 minutes IV or IM
  - Droperidol 5–10 mg repeat interval 20 minutes, max. in 24 hours 20 mg
  - Midazolam 2.5–5 mg, repeat interval 5 minutes, max. in 24 hours 20 mg
  - ½ doses in elderly, unwell or intoxicated patients
  - NOTE: Diazepam dangerous if extravasates so avoid or if must be used, be cautious. Slow IV in antecubital fossa vein
- Monitor: RR and sats, BP, HR, level of consciousness. Must have pulse oximetry + ECG, monitor vitals
  - Ensure hydrated
- Notes
  - Extreme cases may require RSI in resus
  - Patient on psychostimulants: ↑ risk hyperthermia, arrhythmia, rhabdomyolysis, electrolytes abnormal
  - Send bloods: EUC, FBC, LFT, CMP, drug levels. Must check BSL
  - Dystonic reactions (see Drug induced under Movement disorders, p. 155): Use benzatropine (Cogentin) 1–2 mg IV

Suicide risk

- High-risk patients
  - Hopelessness, serious ideation, plan, previous attempt, males, Indigenous, in custody, adversity, sex abuse history, recent change in relationships, psychiatric diagnosis (depression, anxiety, psychosis etc.)

- Lethal factors
  - Consider IMOP: **I**ntention, **M**otivation, **O**pportunity, **P**lan
  - Increased risk if violent method for suicide and precautions taken against rescue
- SAD PERSONS/modified SAD PERSONS index
  - **S**ex male, **A**ge over 45 or under 19, **D**epression
  - **P**revious attempt, **E**tOH, **R**ationality lost, **S**ocial support lost, **O**rganised plan, **N**o spouse, **S**ickness (changed to '**S**tates future intent' in modified version)
  - Modified score: < 5 = low risk, > 9 = high risk

Eating disorders

- Signs/symptoms
  - Anorexia: Body weight > 15% below expected, BMI < 17.5, menstrual changes, image distortion, over-exercising, diuretic use, vomiting/purging
  - Bulimia: Preoccupation with eating, overeating, vomiting/purging, morbid fear of being overweight
- Indications to admit
  - Medical: HR < 40, BP < 90/60, K < 3, temperature < 36°C, dehydration, symptomatic hypoglycaemia, Na < 130, phosphate < 0.5, prolonged QT
  - Weight: < 75% of expected, > 1 kg of weight loss per week, patient can't eat independently. NGT is required
  - Psychiatric: Co-existing psychiatric conditions, outpatient treatment failure
- Investigations
  - Bloods: EUC (↓ K, ↑ Ur), CMP (↓ Ca), LFT (↓ albumin), FBC (↓ Hb, ↓ platelets, ↓ WCC), iron deficiency
  - ECG: T inversion, ↓ ST, ↑ QT, VT
- Complications
  - Osteoporosis, stress fractures, short stature
  - Abnormal coagulation, immune suppression
  - Amenorrhoea, miscarriage, low-birth-weight babies
  - Renal calculi
  - Hypotension, bradycardia, arrhythmia, heart failure, MV prolapse

Substance abuse

EtOH (alcohol)

- Overdose
  - Average lethal blood alcohol concentration (BAC) 0.45–0.5%, can be lower especially if mixed OD
  - Investigations
    - IVC + BSL
    - +/– EUC +/– BAC (don't actually need BAC, should not change management, patient will be treated clinically)
    - + FBC, LFTs and coags if chronic EtOH with liver disease
  - Supportive treatment
    - IV fluids, monitor level of consciousness and sats
    - If chronic use watch for withdrawal
    - EtOH overdose can cause ↓ BSL, metabolic acidosis
- Withdrawal
  - Increased risk of withdrawal
    - > 8 drinks/day (male), > 6 drinks/day (female)
  - Example: Alcohol withdrawal scale (AWS) (max. score 27)
    - Tremor (0–3)
    - Sweating 0–4)
    - Hallucinations (0–4)
    - Anxiety (0–4)
    - Agitation (0–4)
    - Axillary temperature (0–4)
    - Orientation (0–4)
  - NOTE: This is one example; other AWS systems exist. Use the AWS for your hospital
  - Other signs and symptoms: Nausea, vomiting, tactile/auditory hallucinations, visual disturbances, headache
  - Symptoms usually 6–24 hours post last drink
  - Example management as per AWS: Use your hospital guidelines
    - Score < 4: Mild; diazepam 5–10 mg PO 6–8-hourly
    - Score 5–14: Moderate; diazepam 10–20 mg PO 1–2-hourly until score < 5
    - Score > 15: Severe; diazepam 5 mg IV in large antecubital vein (be aware of extravasation risk) ½-hourly, monitor in ICU

    - Other management
        - Give thiamine 300 mg IV stat (see Thiamine deficiency, p. 155)
        - Give thiamine BEFORE glucose if hypoglycaemic (giving glucose with thiamine deficiency may precipitate Wernicke's encephalopathy)
        - Ensure hydration
- Delirium tremens
    - Severe withdrawal; ~72–96 hours post last drink
    - Gross tremors, seizure, fluctuating agitation, hallucinations, impaired attention, +/– fever, ↑ HR
    - Medical emergency
    - Usually associated complications: Infection, anaemia, metabolic, head injury
    - Treatment: Supportive, use AWS and thiamine as above

Opiates

- Overdose: See toxicology
- Withdrawal
    - Agitation, sweating, muscle pain, abdominal cramp, nausea and vomiting, diarrhoea, seizure, goose flesh
    - Peak 2–3/7, resolve 5–7 days
    - Not life-threatening
    - Treat symptoms: e.g. diazepam 5–20 mg PO QID, loperamide, metoclopramide, paracetamol

Benzodiazepines

- Overdose: See Chapter 11 Toxicology, p. 225
- Withdrawal
    - Variable anxiety, insomnia, palpitations, seizure
    - Treat with diazepam
    - Supportive care

CHAPTER 15

Dermatology

General

- Examination
  - Look at all skin and mucosal surfaces, hair, nails, scalp
  - Describe
    - Distribution (location)
    - Pattern (functional, anatomical)
    - Arrangement (symmetry)
    - Configuration (applies to the single lesion's individual features or multiple lesions' relationship to each other; examples of terms—annular, confluent, linear, reticular, dermatomal, circular, discoid)
    - Morphology (erosion, fissure, ulcer, macule, petechiae, purpura, cyst, pustule, bulla, plaque, vesicle etc.)
    - Nikolsky's sign: Apply pressure with finger to skin and slide. Epidermis will separate if Nikolsky's sign positive
- Any patient with a rash, look for the following
  - Fever: Consider serious bacterial causes; e.g. meningococcal, necrotising fasciitis
  - Area of necrosis/black (often start very small) and/or subcutaneous emphysema: Consider necrotising fasciitis
  - Rashes that look like burns (e.g. deep colour, severe, peeling). Consider scalded skin syndrome, Stevens-Johnson syndrome (SJS), toxic epidermal necrolysis (TEN), toxic shock syndrome (TSS), Kawasaki disease etc.
  - Blisters: Consider pemphigoid, pemphigus, herpes etc.
  - Mucous membranes affected: Consider SJS, TEN etc.
  - Organ involvement (e.g. abnormal LFT, Cr elevated): Consider TEN, TSS, DRESS etc.
  - Patients with immune-compromise; e.g. DM: Consider serious causes
  - Signs of anaphylaxis: Breathing compromised, facial swelling, hypotension etc.
- Treatments: Extreme generalisation warning!
  - Initial treatment of rashes: 'If it's dry wet it; if it's wet dry it'

  - Corticosteroids: Urticaria, angio-oedema, allergic dermatitis. May need topical or systemic steroids
  - Antihistamines: To control pruritus
  - Antimicrobials, antifungals

Soft tissue and skin infections—cellulitis

- Assessment
  - Localised: Pain, shiny, swelling, erythema, pits
  - Note: Cellulitis doesn't extend to ear pinna or nose as there is no subcutaneous tissue here
  - Systemic features: Fever, rigors, vomiting, unwell
- Investigations
  - Usually not needed
  - Bloods: FBC, EUC, blood cultures if septic (rarely change management), +/– CRP
  - Imaging: X-ray if traumatic, US if possible foreign body
- Management: Always check latest guidelines for your area (constantly changing)
  - Mild/moderate
    - Flucloxacillin PO 500 mg QID (12.5 mg/kg child) for 7/7

      OR
    - Cephalexin PO (dose same as above)

      OR
    - If allergy use clindamycin
  - Severe
    - IV flucloxacillin QID (or cefazolin TDS) 2 g (50 mg/kg child)
    - If allergy use clindamycin 600 mg (15 mg/kg child) TDS
  - Severe and not responding
    - Consider MRSA and use vancomycin IV 1.5 g or piperacillin/tazobactam 4.5 g IV TDS usually after discussion with infectious diseases specialist
  - Treating patients from home
    - Criteria: No systemic features, stable, no severe comorbidities, can manage at home, not IVDU, safe for nurses to visit
    - Use 2 g IV, cefazolin + 1 g PO probenecid (if no renal impairment)

- Management in special circumstances
  - Periorbital cellulitis
    - PO amoxicillin with clavulanate 875/125 mg BD (22.5 mg/kg/3.2 mg/kg child)
  - Orbital cellulitis: See Infections in Chapter 16 Ophthalmology, p. 301
  - Diabetic foot
    - Amoxicillin with clavulanate

      OR
    - Cephalexin and metronidazole

      OR
    - Piperacillin/tazobactam if severe
  - Bites
    - Prophylactic antibiotics: Amoxicillin with clavulanate. Ensure wound well cleaned
    - If established infection: Operation, ceftriaxone and metronidazole, or piperacillin/tazobactam
  - Water-related wounds:
    - Flucloxacillin 1 g (25 mg/kg) QID PO *AND either*
      - If fresh water: Ciprofloxacin 400 mg (10 mg/kg child) PO; OR
      - If saltwater: Doxycycline 100 mg BD PO (ceftriaxone child)
    - If needing IV antibiotic usually flucloxacillin and ciprofloxacin
  - Cutaneous abscess
    - US, drainage, consider wick
    - No antibiotics required usually unless, for example, immunocompromised, systemic features, surrounding cellulitis, endocarditis prophylaxis required and so on

Necrotising fasciitis

- Examination
  - Can look like cellulitis
  - Specific signs: Blisters, pale or darkened skin, oedema, crepitations, odour, pain > findings, oedema beyond the area of skin changes, skin tense, impaired sensation, persistent ↑ HR, ↓ BP, rapid change—always outline redness

- Risk factors: Immunocompromise, diabetes mellitus, alcoholism, chronic disease, IVDU, trauma, surgical procedure, local infection (e.g. perianal)
- Investigations
  - Bloods: FBC (↑↑ WBC, haemolysis, ↓ Hb), blood gas (↓ pH, ↑ lactate), EUC, LFT (renal/hepatic dysfunction, ↓ Na), CRP, blood cultures, CK
  - Imaging: CT/x-ray—free gas
- Management
  - Resuscitation
  - URGENT surgery, debridement
  - TRIPPLE IVAB: Vancomycin 1.5 g (15 mg/kg) AND clindamycin 600 mg (15 mg/kg) AND meropenem 1 g (25 mg/kg) (or piperacillin/tazobactam)
  - ADT
  - IVIg for strep, antitoxin for clostridial infections
  - Hyperbaric oxygen (rarely something we arrange)

Erythema multiforme (EM) spectrum, Stevens-Johnson syndrome (SJS) and toxic epidermal necrolysis (TEN)

- Spectrum from localised papular skin eruption to severe multisystem disease with widespread vesiculobullous lesions + erosions of mucous membrane. SJS and TEN considered variations of the same entity. EM is divided into major and minor
- Precipitates: Infection (especially mycoplasma, HSV), drugs (especially antibiotics, anticonvulsants) and malignancies

Erythema multiforme minor

- Lesions vary: Usually maculopapular hands/feet/limbs progressing to target lesions, no epithelial loss.
- Treatment
  - Identify and cease precipitant
  - Treat symptoms: Antihistamine, analgesic, topical steroids can be useful, PO steroids sometimes used (controversial)
  - Aciclovir in HSV associated EM

Erythema multiforme major

- Target lesions or papules. Can have epidermal detachment but < 10% total body surface area
- Involves 1 or more mucous membrane

- Treatment
  - Identify and cease precipitant. Consider all meds started in the prior few months
  - Symptomatic care: Antihistamines, analgesics, skin care, ocular lubricants etc.
  - Burns care dressings
  - Topical betamethasone, PO/IV steroids controversial
  - Other suggested treatments: Dapsone, azathioprine, antivirals (prophylaxis for herpes-associated EM with recurrence). Note: In herpes-associated EM, antivirals started after rash comes out, don't change course of illness

Stevens-Johnson syndrome

- Widespread rash, maculopapular, blistering
- Minor form of TEN with epidermal detachment < 10% TBSA
- SJS/TEN overlapping syndrome if epidermal detachment 10–30% TBSA
- Involves 1 or more mucous membrane
- Treatment
  - Identify and cease precipitant ASAP
  - Manage same as severe burns. Usually in ICU or burns centre. Burns dressings.
  - Fluid resus and ongoing replacement. Electrolyte monitoring and replacement
  - Prevent and treat secondary infection
  - Supportive and symptomatic treatment including analgesia
  - Other suggested but controversial treatments: Steroids, IG, plasma exchange.

Toxic epidermal necrolysis

- Most common in elderly females. Drugs more likely the cause
- 2/52 prodrome post exposure then tender erythema, bullae progressing to exfoliation
- Full thickness, epidermal necrosis, Nikolsky's sign positive, epidermal detachment > 30% TBSA, large bullae, desquamation, mucous membrane involvement
- Often LFT and amylase abnormal
- Treatment
  - Identify and cease precipitant ASAP
  - Admit to burns unit, ICU. Isolation. Burns dressings

  - Fluid resus and ongoing monitoring volume/electrolytes. Need central access and IDC
  - Prevent temperature loss
  - Prevent and treat secondary infection (no prophylactic antibiotics due to resistance)
  - Analgesia, PCA
  - Can get airway epithelium sloughing may need tube
  - Nutrition enterally via NGT usually needed. Parenteral nutrition if required.
  - Controversial therapies: Steroids, IG, plasma exchange, cyclosporin

Toxic infectious erythemas

Staph toxic shock syndrome (TSS)

- Due to an enterotoxin produced by *Staphylococcus aureus*
- Infection entry points: Tampon use, nasal packing, postop wounds, skin wounds etc.
- Desquamation erythroderma, shock, MOD, CNS dysfunction
- Treatment
  - Resuscitation, shock management
  - Identify infection source; e.g. foreign body removal
  - IVAB; e.g. cefazolin or flucloxacillin 2 g (50 mg/kg)
  - Consider IVIg, clindamycin (inhibits exotoxin), hyperbaric oxygen therapy
  - Vancomycin if suspect MRSA

Strep TSS

- Develops post severe soft tissue infection with GAS leading to necrotising fasciitis, shock
- *Treat* with urgent AB: Penicillin G IV, IV immunoglobulins. Aggressive and prompt debridement of infection site

Scalded skin syndrome

- Staph, exfoliative toxin
- Usually children < 6 years old
- Often begins with staph infection; e.g. conjunctiva, nasopharynx, umbilical
- Tender erythroderma diffuse then exfoliate stage, large fluid filled bullae then desquamation

- Nikolsky's sign positive, NO mucosa involved, NOT full-thickness skin involvement, patient NOT toxic
- Investigations: WCC often normal, elevated ESR, PCR for toxin, culture bullae
- Management
  - Fluid resus, correct electrolytes
  - Identify and treat source of toxigenic staph flucloxacillin 2 g PO or IV 6-hourly (50 mg/kg)
  - Clindamycin
  - Burns dressings

Viral infections

Viral exanthems

- Many viral infections associated with generalised cutaneous eruptions
- Erythematous macules and papules occasionally petechiae or vesicles. Usually develop centrally spreading to palms and soles. Usually blanching
- Treat symptomatically

Herpes zoster/shingles

- Reactivated dormant virus
- ↑ risk in immuno-suppressed
- Usually prodrome 2–3 days with pain and itch
- Rash: Dermatomal, discrete clusters. Halts at midline/unilateral
- Can get pain without rash
- Involvement of the tip of the nose should prompt corneal examination
- Complications: Immunocompromised may develop disseminated infection, Bell's palsy, trigeminal neuralgia, transverse myelitis, Ramsay Hunt syndrome, varicella ophthalmicus, aseptic meningitis, neuronal deafness, postherpetic neuralgia
- Treatment
  - Analgesia
  - Antivirals if:
    - Ophthalmic involvement, > 50 years old, complications, within 72 hours of 1st eruption
    - Aciclovir 400–800 mg PO 5× a day

      OR
    - Famciclovir 500 mg PO TDS

- Steroids 50 mg/day prednisone, decreases pain
- Disseminated or ophthalmic involvement: Admit, IV antivirals

Herpes simplex

- Usually only localised
- Can disseminate: Neonates, malignancy, immunosuppressed, HIV
- Treatment
    - Genital: Always give aciclovir 400 mg PO TDS or valaciclovir 500 mg BD
    - Gingivostomatitis: Give aciclovir
    - Neonatal/encephalitis: Aciclovir 10 mg/kg IV TDS
    - Pregnancy: Primary maternal infection give aciclovir PO

Other dermatology emergencies

Disseminated gonococcal infection

- Fever, arthralgia, multiple papular vesicular or pustular lesions on extensor surfaces (wrist, hands, ankles, feet). Initially small macules progress to necrotic centre then develop haemorrhagic petechiae
- Test urine PCR, Gram stain fluid from lesion, blood culture
- Treatment: Ceftriaxone 1 g IV daily

Purpura fulminans

- Widespread ecchymoses, haemorrhagic bullae and epidermal necrosis associated with DIC and vascular collapse, or protein C or S deficiency
- Treat cause

Bullous disease

- Bullous pemphigoid
    - Erythema, urticaria, plaques, itch, usually elderly
    - General mucocutaneous blistering. Nikolsky's negative
    - Tense blisters, don't expand or rupture when pressed
- Pemphigus vulgaris
    - General mucocutaneous autoimmune blistering eruption
    - Tense blisters, easily rupture. Nikolsky's sign positive
    - Often mucosal involved. Often secondary infection
    - Poor prognosis

- Treatment
  - Dermatology consult
    - Admit, correct fluid and electrolytes
    - Prednisone, azathioprine, as per dermatology team

Urticaria

- Transient erythematous and/or oedema swellings of dermis or subcutaneous tissues which may be itchy or painful
- Causes: Most common is infections (mostly viral URTI), drug allergy, food reaction, contact allergen
- Ensure not associated with anaphylaxis
  - Throat/tongue swelling
  - Airway involvement
  - Hypotension
- Treatment
  - Antihistamines
    - Loratadine 10 mg PO daily (child 2–5 years use 5 mg)
      OR
    - Cetirizine 10 mg (0.25 mg/kg for children over 6 months) PO daily
  - If poor response can increase dose with specialist advice
  - Remove precipitate

Angio-oedema

- Cause
  - Idiopathic
  - Allergic (angiotensin-converting enzyme inhibitors [ACE inhibitors], ARB, nuts, strawberries)
  - C1 esterase inhibitor deficiency (genetic or acquired—sepsis, DIC), chronic (Hashimoto's disease)
- Signs and symptoms: Usually worsen over 24 hours
  - Acute oedema subcutaneous tissue. Commonly periorbital, lips, tongue, face
  - 80% have abdominal pain
  - Diarrhoea
  - Exclude anaphylaxis

- Investigations
  - If chronic or recurrent: TFT, C4, US (thick bowel wall, ascites)
- Management
  - Analgesia, antiemetic
  - Icatibant: Use if severe, airway threatened. NOT IF PREGNANT
    - 30 mg SC
  - C1 esterase inhibitor concentrate: Use if severe, pregnant
  - Others: Aminocaproic acid

CHAPTER 16

Ophthalmology

Exam

- Fig. 16.1 shows the structures of the eye
- Acuity with Snellen chart at 6 metres
  - If can only read top line = 6/60, if can read to bottom line = 6/4
  - Test with distance glasses. Test with pinhole (cardboard and 19 G needle holes); this will correct acuity the same way glasses do
- External eye exam: Evert lids with cotton bud and wipe with second cotton bud if any concerns of foreign body presence
- Check pupils. Check also for afferent pupillary defect with swinging torch
- Eye movements and visual fields
- Slit lamp: Look at anterior chamber and use fluorescein dye with cobalt blue light (this is NOT the green light on the slit lamp)
- Fundoscopy: Red reflex
- Drops that can be used for examination
  - Fluorescein when examining cornea
  - Anaesthetic drops: Tetracaine (amethocaine) 0.5%
  - Mydriatics (make pupils bigger): Antimuscarinic
    - Tropicamide 1%
    - May precipitate acute glaucoma; warn patient to report eye pain, patient must not drive post. Take ~15 minutes to dilate

Trauma

Lid laceration

- Consider orbital CT if suspected foreign body or fracture
- If superficial: Irrigate with saline, consider repair in ED
- Refer to ophthalmology if: Associated ocular trauma requiring OT, foreign body, laceration is nasal or near to upper or lower lid punctum, distortion of anatomy, full thickness, involves lid margin, significant contamination (e.g. bite)
- Remember to give ADT if needed

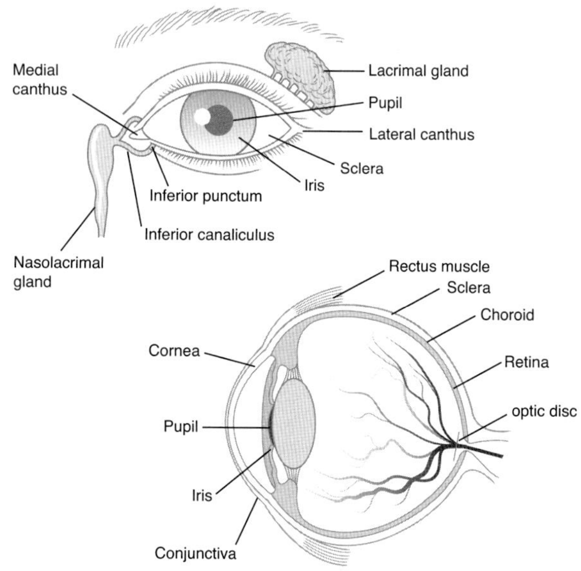

Figure 16.1 Structures of the eye

Corneal foreign body

- Tetracaine (amethocaine) or tetracaine 1% drops to aid assessment
- Ensure lids checked and everted for foreign body
- To remove: Hold head very still, oblique approach, use cotton bud first, if unsuccessful can use 25–30 G bevelled needle with caution. Anchor hand by resting on patient's cheek, needle always angled away from patient. Needle should lightly scratch cornea ONLY. Otherwise refer to ophthalmology
- Fluorescein to assess defect after removal
- Topical antibiotic QID chloramphenicol
- No need to pad eye
- Follow-up eye clinic or GP. Don't wear contact lens until healed

Ocular trauma

- If all examinations normal, eye clinic follow-up
- Any suspicion of penetrating eye injury = URGENT referral
- If suspected fracture need CT orbits
- Penetrating trauma: Management same as globe rupture below

Globe rupture

- Ocular emergency
- Acuity may be normal
- Pupil distorted, dark exposed tissue
- Subconjunctival haemorrhage, swelling, chemosis
- Seidel test: Use fluorescein drops, look with slit lamp and cobalt blue light, look for a clear band in the green fluorescein stain (this is aqueous fluid leaking out). Only perform if unsure. If you know there is a rupture, don't examine any further
- Management
  - Urgent ophthalmology review
  - Analgesia, antiemetic, NBM
  - Bed rest, may require sedation
  - IVAB (e.g. cefazolin 1 g, ciprofloxacin 400 mg)
  - Eye shield
  - ADT

Chemical burns

- LA drops for comfort during irrigation and assessment
- Irrigate with normal saline (with Morgan Lens if available) at least 30 minutes. Continue until pH ~7.5 (universal indicator paper)
- Contact Poisons Information 13 11 26 for specific information on offending agent
- Ophthalmology follow-up, preferably same day

Flash burns

- Causes: Welding etc.
- Topical antibiotics QID chloramphenicol +/– PO analgesia
- Eye clinic follow-up

Orbital fracture

- Mechanical (e.g. squash ball, punch)
- Symptoms: Pain especially with eye movement, tender, diplopia, lid swelling, epistaxis, ptosis, eyelid crepitus, infraorbital nerve dysaesthesia

- CT orbits + CTB
- Antibiotics (e.g. amoxicillin with clavulanate)
- Ice packs, don't blow nose, discuss with ophthalmology

Red eye—painless

- Usually non-urgent

Blepharitis

- Eyelid inflammation
- Treat with hygiene and lubrication

Ectropion

- Lids turn outwards
- Treat with lubrication

Entropion

- Lids turn inwards
- Can cause corneal abrasion

Conjunctivitis

- Usually painful

Pterygium

- Fleshy overgrowth of conjunctiva
- Treat with sunglasses to protect from UV; lubrication; eventually surgery

Subconjunctival haemorrhage

- Ensure vision normal, check BP and coags if indicated (e.g. on warfarin), exclude fracture (if associated trauma), hyphaema, globe rupture

Red eye—painful

Herpes

Herpes keratoconjunctivitis

- Primary HSV infection
- Dendritic ulcer, enhances with fluorescein
- Treat with PO aciclovir 800 mg PO 5× daily

  OR
- Valaciclovir 1 g TDS
- Must seek ophthalmology involvement

Herpes zoster ophthalmicus

- Classic lesions in the area. Lesion on the tip of the nose should raise suspicion of HZO (V1 dermatome)
- Can get conjunctivitis, scleritis, optic neuritis, keratitis, etc.
- Look for and treat secondary bacterial infection
- Must treat with antivirals (e.g. valaciclovir 1 g TDS)
- Steroids reduce pain. Don't give if immunosuppressed, diabetic
- Must seek ophthalmology involvement
- Often requires admission

Corneal ulcer

- Increased risk: Diabetic, immunocompromised, contact lens wearer (usually pseudomonas)
- Treat with antibiotics (e.g. ciprofloxacin 750 mg BD PO)
- Remove contact lens!
- Ophthalmology review and follow-up
- Do not patch

Corneal erosion

- Abrasion without trauma
- Dryness causes lid to adhere to cornea
- Painful, photophobia, tearing
- Requires ophthalmology review and follow-up
- Topical NSAIDs and antibiotics

Chalazion/stye

- Warm compress
- Topical antibiotics (not always required if minor)
- May need PO antibiotics if severe

Conjunctivitis

- Diffuse conjunctival infection
- Viral: Highly contagious, one eye first then spreads to other eye, recent URTI, profuse watery discharge; treat with lubricants +/– antibiotic drops, good hygiene, refer if ↓ acuity, chronic
- Allergic: Extremely itchy and atopic history, treat with lubricant
- Bacterial: Purulent discharge, treat with topical antibiotics and hygiene, refer if abnormal vision, and > 5/7
- Dry eyes

Acute angle-closure glaucoma

- Increased risk: Increased age, anticholinergic use, mydriatics, beta agonists, female, shallow anterior chamber, family history etc.
- Cornea hazy, irregular semi-dilated pupil, non-reactive pupil, very tender tense eye, headache, nausea, vomiting
- IOP > 30 mmHg (normal is 10–20)
- URGENT referral to ophthalmology
- Management
  - Constrict the pupil: Pilocarpine drops
  - Decrease aqueous humour production
    - Timolol drops (beta-blocker)
    - Acetazolamide
    - Brimonidine
  - Increase aqueous humour outflow
    - Latanoprost

Episcleritis versus scleritis

- Episcleritis: Less painful, usually younger, no systemic association
  - Self-limiting
- Scleritis: Extremely painful, usually elderly
  - Redness or red/blue discolouration
  - Photophobia
  - Associated with RA, systemic vasculitis etc.
  - Treat with topical steroids, cycloplegics
- Conditions with anterior chamber involved
  - **Iritis**: Associated with collagen vascular disease
    - Pain/ache, photophobia, decreased vision
    - Pupil can be small, normal or irregular
    - Manage with steroids (topical, oral), dilate pupil
  - **Hypopyon**: Visible accumulation of white cells anterior chamber can be secondary to iritis, infection, ulcer etc.
  - **Hyphaema**: Blood anterior chamber
    - Management: Bed rest, head of bed 30 degrees, rest eyes, cycloplegics, acetazolamide
    - Complications: Glaucoma, iron stain, re-bleed (day 3–5 usually)
- All require URGENT discussions and review with ophthalmology

Infections

Orbital cellulitis

- Features: Lid oedema, proptosis, globe displacement, decreased vision, toxic, photophobia, pain with eye movement, pupil dilation, afferent pupillary defect
- Imaging: CT
- Need ophthalmic consult URGENTLY
- Treat with ceftriaxone AND flucloxacillin, both 50 mg/kg (max. 2 g)

Dacryoadenitis

- Inflammation, enlargement lacrimal gland
- Severe pain, redness, pressure, swollen upper lid. Unilateral
- Supratemporal
- Treat with IVAB, need ophthalmology review

Dacryocystitis

- Infection, obstruction nasolacrimal duct
- Can be congenital or secondary to trauma or stone
- Severe pain, redness, swelling, excessive tears
- Inferomedial
- Treat with IVAB, need ophthalmology review

Acute vision change

TIA—amaurosis fugax

- Monocular vision loss, lasts seconds–hours then returns. Usually fundus normal
- Assess as per stroke/TIA
- Must discuss with neurology

Central retinal vein occlusion

- Sudden painless vision loss over minutes, no floaters
- Acuity and RAPD variable
- Increased risk: Glaucoma, hypertension, diabetes mellitus, ↑ age
- Fundoscopy: Abnormal red reflex; fundus—large areas haemorrhage, 'thunderstorm', 'tomato sauce'
- Need ophthalmology

Central retinal artery occlusion

- Sudden painless vision loss
- Acuity < 6/60, marked RAPD
- Thrombotic or embolic
- Fundoscopy: Abnormal red reflex, pale retina, cherry red spot
- URGENT ESR and CRP query GCA
- URGENT ophthalmology referral
- TIA workup

Vitreous haemorrhage

- Associated with trauma, DM, coagulopathy
- Floaters, visual haze
- Fundoscopy: Bleeding seen, cobwebbing
- Urgent referral

Valsalva haemorrhage

- Capillary rupture
- Sudden unilateral decrease acuity
- Increased IOP
- Fundoscopy: Blood seen with fluid level
- Good recovery

Posterior vitreous detachment

- Sudden painless vision loss, floaters
- US
- Fundoscopy: Weiss ring (blue haze)
- Need ophthalmology: Treat with laser, bed rest

Optic neuritis

- Vision loss over days usually unilateral
- Cause mostly idiopathic, other: MS etc.
- Female > male, middle age. Can be bilateral (especially in children)
- Pain with eye movement. RAPD, ↓ acuity, ↓ colour vision, ↓ fields, swollen optic disc
- Bloods: ESR
- URGENT refer eye registrar, steroids

GCA/ischaemic optic neuropathy

- Headache, scalp tender, jaw claudication, ↓ vision, tender temporal artery +/– RAPD
- URGENT ESR/CRP
- URGENT ophthalmology

Lens dislocation or subluxation

- Blurred vision, may have minimal symptoms
- Increased risk Marfan's syndrome, post surgery
- Ophthalmology referral, URGENT if glaucoma developing

Retinal detachment

- Increased risk: Trauma, short sighted, cataract removal, vitreous disease
- Painless vision loss over hours
- Flashes, floaters, dark shadow, grey veil
- ↓ acuity, abnormal/asymmetric red reflex, partial visual field loss
- Bed rest, URGENT eye registrar, laser treatment

CHAPTER 17

Ear, nose and throat (ENT)

Ear

Tinnitus

- Perception of sound without external stimulus
- Objective (examiner can hear): AV malformation, arterial bruits, enlarged Eustachian tube, stapedial muscle spasm
- Subjective: Sensorineural hearing loss, hypertension, conductive hearing loss, head trauma, labyrinthitis, medications, TMJ disease, depression, MS acoustic neuroma, Ménière's disease, Cogan syndrome
- Treatment depends on underlying disease/cause

Sudden hearing loss

- Causes
  - Sensorineural examples
    - Infection: Mumps, EBV, herpes, CMV, labyrinthitis
    - Haematology: Leukaemia, sickle cell, polycythaemia
    - Vascular: Cerebral aneurysm,
    - Autoimmune: Wegner granulomatosis, Cogan syndrome
    - Other: Diabetes, Ménière's disease, tumour, MS, trauma
    - Medications (see below)
  - Conductive examples
    - Acute otitis media (AOM), OE, foreign body, tumour, otosclerosis, trauma
  - Idiopathic sensorineural: Majority of cases
    - Treat with early steroids. Prednisone PO 1 mg/kg/day max. 60 mg for 7–14 days

Ototoxic medications

- Loop diuretics, salicylates, NSAIDs, quinines, aminoglycosides, erythromycin, vancomycin, chemotherapy (cisplatin, carboplatin, vinblastine, vincristine), topical agents (propylene, ethanol, neomycin)

Infections

Otitis externa

- Commonly pseudomonas and staph
- Other causes: fungal (candida), contact dermatitis, psoriasis
- Ex: Swelling, purulent discharge, tender pinna
- Tx: Analgesia, cleansing external canal, topical antibiotic +/– steroid (e.g. framycetin and dexamethasone TDS for 5/7). If treatment fails or TM is perforated use ciprofloxacin drops. Can use wick or gauze in canal if significant oedema present. If systemic symptoms or pinna involved, use PO AB (e.g. flucloxacillin)
- Follow-up if ↑ symptoms or no resolution in 1 week
- **Malignant otitis externa**: Begins as simple otitis externa then spreads to deep tissues (↑ risk, immunocompromised, elderly, diabetes mellitus, HIV). Usually pseudomonas. Can progress to base of skull and cause death!
- Suspect in patient with persisting otitis externa, look for parotitis, TMJ involvement, CN IX, X, XI signs, facial paralysis, exposed bone in canal
- Mx: CT, URGENT ENT review, IVAB gentamicin and either ceftazidime 2 g or ciprofloxacin 400 mg

Otitis media

- Commonly strep pneumoniae, haemophilus, *Moraxella*. Often mixed virus and bacteria. No bacteria found in ~25%
- Examination: Immobile eardrum, bulging TM, cloudy TM, erythema
- Treatment: 85% will improve without AB, increased to 95% with AB. AB don't reduce rate of perforation, recurrence, hearing loss
  - Amoxicillin 15 mg/kg TDS (500 mg adult)
  - If treatment fails: Amoxicillin with clavulanate 22.5 mg/kg (875/125 mg in adult)
- Complications
  - TM perforation, effusion, hearing loss
  - Severe complications requiring URGENT ENT review
    - Facial nerve paralysis
    - Acute mastoiditis
      - Examination: Fever, otalgia, ear displaced down and forward, posterior auricular erythema, swelling and tenderness, mastoid erythema and fluctuance
      - Investigation: CT
      - Mx: IVAB e.g. ceftriaxone + vancomycin, +/– OT

    - Intracranial complication: Meningitis, brain abscess
    - Lateral sinus thrombosis
        - Hx/Ex: Headache, papillo-oedema, CN VI palsy, vertigo
        - Investigations: CTA/MRI
        - Mx: IV penicillin + ceftriaxone and metronidazole, may need anticoagulants
    - Cholesteatoma
        - Erosive, expanding growth
    - Petrous apicitis
        - Infection spreads to temporal bone leading to pus extradural
        - History/eamination: Otorrhoea, abducens palsy, retroorbital pain
        - Investigation: CT
        - Mx: IVAB, OT

Bullous myringitis

- Painful bulla formation on TM and deep external ear canal. Blood-filled blisters. Middle ear effusion. Occasional otorrhoea with bulla rupture
- Causes: Virus, mycoplasma
- Manage with analgesia and warm compresses. Macrolide AB if suspected mycoplasma. ENT review and follow-up

External ocular trauma

- Will usually require discussion with ENT unless minor to prevent long-term deformity. Haematomas need draining

Insects in ear

- Drown first if alive with olive oil or 2% lidocaine or viscous lidocaine then remove. Complete examination post removal. ENT follow-up

Nose

Epistaxis

- 90% anterior; mostly from Little's area
- Anterior bleeds, usually unilateral, patient doesn't feel blood in throat
- Posterior bleeds, more profuse, difficult to control often bilateral (blood reflux to unaffected side), flows to throat

- Hx: Previous epistaxis, trauma, head/neck Cancer/OT, radiation, bleeding, discharge, anticoagulant use, NSAIDs, HT
- While patient awaits review (if not severe): position patient seated, leaning forward. Pinch elastic areas of nose together, 10–15 minutes on the clock (tell patient not to stop, and check tissues every few minutes!) ×2 attempts
- Always check vitals especially BP
- Examine nose: Aim to identify bleeding site
  - Set up first: Ensure good light source (head lamp if possible), gauze, saline, silver nitrate sticks, suction, nasal tampons, vaso-constricting sprays (e.g. Co-Phenylcaine)
  - Suction clot
  - Use vasoconstrictors (e.g. Co-Phenylcaine as spray and/or soaked gauze and apply direct pressure)
- Management
  - Do not lie flat (or if required, lie flat at the last minute)
  - Pressure (as above). If fails, try again with vasoconstrictor applied first
  - Silver nitrate stick: Apply to area of bleeding on one side of septum only. Beware—can perforate septum
  - Nasal pack/nasal tampon; e.g. rapid rhino—choose appropriate size (e.g. ant/post/double) and inflate balloon as per instructions (careful not to overinflate)
  - Alternative options: Gauze soaked in either lignocaine/adrenaline or tranexamic acid (5 mL of 100 mg/mL), then placed in affected side and apply pressure
  - If severely hypertensive, will likely need to control BP in order to ease bleeding
  - Antiemetic
  - Antibiotic PO (e.g. amoxicillin with clavulanate) if nasal pack in situ
- **Severe bleeds**
  - Stabilise in resuscitation room
  - Monitor vitals, IVC and bloods with G&H and coags, FBC, EUC
  - Examine as above, nasal packing, may need bilateral rhinos
  - Can use Foley catheter
  - Usually need analgesia. Very uncomfortable
  - Discuss with ENT

- Packed noses: If packing in situ and patient develops significant pain, always remove. Packing can cause: Arrhythmia, hypoxia, aseptic necrosis, arrest, AOM, sinusitis
- Disposition
  - Discharge home if: Stable, no bleed in the last few hours, definitive treatment (cauterised), follow-up arranged
  - Discuss with ENT if: Severe bleed, packing required
  - Patient advice: Avoid hot drinks, use saline nasal sprays to keep passages moist and regular Vaseline, can use over-the-counter vasoconstrictors (e.g. Drixine) (provided not contraindicated)

Nasal fracture

- Swelling, tender, crepitations, ecchymosis, deformity, epistaxis, rhinorrhoea
- Examination: Head, neck, neuro, nasal mucosa with otoscope for mucosal defects, septal haematoma (bluish fluid filled sac overlying septum) and bony displacement
- Usually no imaging required, CT if concerned serious/complicated fracture (e.g. cribriform plate fracture)
- Fracture cribriform plate can cause torn meninges and CSF rhinorrhoea
  - Diagnose by: Putting drop of rhinorrhoea fluid (suspected CSF) on filter paper—clear area central blood stain
  - CT head
  - CSF rhinorrhoea may be delayed so warn patient to return if rhinorrhoea
- Treatment: Delayed reduction if required by ENT, within 14 days or within 7 days in children

Nasal foreign body

- Prepare with vasoconstrictor and anaesthetic spray
- Remove with curette, suction, forceps, etc.
- Can use positive pressure: Patient blows their nose with normal nostril covered or carer gives puff of air into child's mouth with normal nostril covered
- If removed no follow-up required

Sinusitis

- Symptoms > 1 week, purulent nasal secretions, pain increased bending forward or sneezing
- Different sinus involved lead to pain/tenderness in different locations
  - Maxillary (90% of sinusitis): Pain/tender upper teeth, cheek
  - Ethmoidal: Pain behind eye, tender central face, root of nose

  - Frontal: Frontal pain/tender (note: children under 12 don't have a frontal sinus)
  - Sphenoid: Headache, poorly localised
- Investigation note: CT can show mucosal thickening; 40% of normal patients have this on CT
- Manage
  - AB usually don't change outcome
  - Give AB only if severe, symptoms prolonged (> 10 days), relapse, immunocompromised
  - AB (e.g. amoxicillin with clavulanate 10 days)
- Complications/extensions of infection
  - Frontal bone OM (oedematous doughy forehead), frontal
  - Brain abscess, subdural and epidural collections
  - Orbital/periorbital cellulitis
  - CNS infections, meningitis
  - Cavernous, venous sinus thrombosis
  - Extensions more likely with non-maxillary involvement
  - If suspect extension, urgent CT, IVAB and review (ENT, neurology, ophthalmology, neurosurgery depending on location of extension)

Face

Salivary glands

Viral parotitis

- Mumps (and other viruses), prodrome (fever, malaise, arthralgia, anorexia 3–5 days) then develop salivary gland swelling usually bilateral, can be unilateral
- Treatment: Supportive, usually self resolves
- Complications: Orchitis, oophoritis, mastitis, pancreatitis, thrombocytopenia etc.

Suppurative parotitis

- Potentially fatal bacterial infection. Usually unilateral
- ↑ risk—recent anaesthesia, ↑↓ age, dehydration, sialolithiasis, oral cancer, duct strictures, duct foreign body, tracheostomy, medications (diuretics, antihistamines, tricyclic antidepressants, phenothiazines, beta-blockers, barbiturates), chronic disease (HIV, hepatic and renal failure, diabetes mellitus, Sjögren's syndrome, CF, anorexia, ↑ uric acid)
- Rapid onset, skin over parotid gland is red and tender

- Massage the parotid gland to express pus into mouth. Duct opens usually upper cheek opposite 2nd molar. Swab and culture pus
- Treatment: Hydration, massage and heat to gland. Usually require admission, give IV flucloxacillin 2 g QID. Always discuss with ENT

Sialolithiasis

- Salivary calculi. Unilateral pain, swelling, tenderness, ↑ with meals. May palpate stone in duct. Gland is firm, can perform US
- Treat with analgesics, massage and monitor for causes (e.g. infection). Discuss with ENT

Submandibular infection—Ludwig's angina

- Risk factors: Poor hygiene, dental/oral procedures, dental infection (especially molar), mandible #, peritonsillar abscess, sialadenitis
- History/examination: Facial swelling, pain, erythema, fever, malaise, nausea and vomiting, sepsis, woody induration, dysphagia, dysphonia
  - Imminent obstruction to airway: Can't protrude tongue, trismus, drooling, stridor, obstruct airway with neck flexion
- Investigations: CT scan only if patient safe and airway not compromised!
- Complications: Airway obstruction/compromise, sepsis, extension (retropharyngeal, mediastinal, pericardial, mandible, carotid sheath, subphrenic)
- Management: Sit patient up
  - ETT if needed, perform fibreoptic with OT backup—often lots of swelling, distortion of anatomy and trismus
  - HDU/ICU
  - IVAB; e.g clindamycin monotherapy OR benzylpenicillin + metronidazole

Temporomandibular joint dysfunction

- Acute; e.g. direct blow causing # or can be chronic
- Usually pain localised to muscle of mastication (e.g. masseter), ↓ ROM, clicking, tender, areas of rigidity and swelling
- Panoramic x-ray or CT mandible
- Refer to ENT/maxillofacial surgeon

Dislocated mandible

- Anterior most common; can be acute, chronic recurrent or chronic
- Can have posterior and lateral dislocation

- Severe pain, ↓ speaking and swallowing ability, sensory change chin or mouth
- Anterior can be caused by laugh, yawn, vomit, large bite, GA, oral sex
- Panoramic x-ray or CT
- Consult ENT if associated #, chronic, other complicating factors
- If none of the above relocation in ED
  - Traditional technique
    - Patient sits upright facing the doctor
    - Place both thumbs in patient's mouth (wears gloves), thumbs placed over lower back molars
    - Doctor curves fingers around patient's mandible
    - Doctor pushes thumbs down and back; mouth should be kept open
    - Don't get bitten!
  - Syringe barrel technique
    - Place a 5 or 10 mL syringe barrel in patient's mouth, as far towards molars as possible, having the patient bite down on it
    - Patient then rolls the syringe back and forth
- Discuss with ENT if unable to relocate. Relocation with muscle relaxation, OT

Teeth

- For dental blocks see Face/dental block, p. 62
- Fig. 17.1 shows the usual layout of adult teeth.

Bleeding socket

- Ask patient to bite down on gauze for 10–20 minutes
- If ongoing, soak gauze in lidocaine (lignocaine) with adrenaline and continue with pressure
- If ongoing soak gauze in 1 g tranexamic acid and continue with pressure
- If ongoing inject with lidocaine (lignocaine) with adrenaline
- If ongoing can try silver nitrate stick to bleeding source
- If ongoing loose suture over gauze pack
- Start PO amoxicillin with clavulanate, ensure dental follow-up
- If severe consider bleeding diathesis

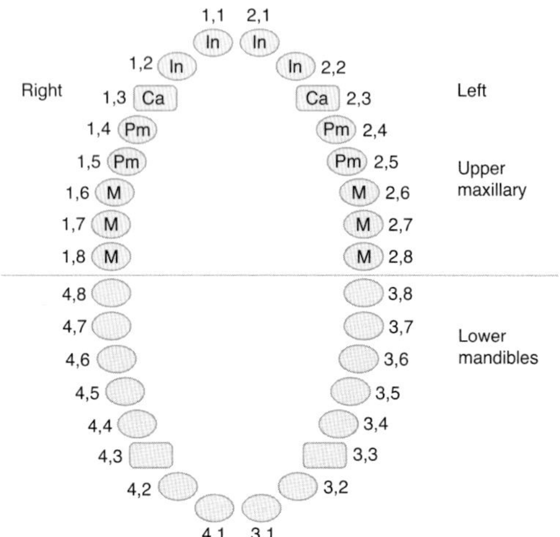

Figure 17.1 Normal adult teeth. In = incisor, Ca = canine, Pm = premolar, M = molar. This is the FDI-World Dental Federation numbering system. Many different systems exist.

Abscess

- Swelling at tooth apex, tender +/– mobile mass, lymph nodes, decrease mouth opening
- Investigations: Orthopantomogram (OPG) shows apical lucency, can also use US or CT if concerned of spreading infection
- Management: Warm saline rinse, analgesia. AB with PO amoxicillin. Dentist for follow-up and drainage
  - Untreated abscess can spread to submandibular infection!

Alveolar osteitis/dry socket

- Risk: Smoker, female, poor hygiene, HRT, trauma
- History/examination: Severe pain radiating to ear, foul odour, trismus, afebrile, white necrotic bone in socket
- Management: Irrigate with warm saline, remove debris, zinc oxide dressing and analgesia. Need dental follow-up. PO metronidazole if severe

Tooth fracture

- Examination: Ellis classification
  - Ellis I: Enamel only
  - Ellis II: Enamel + dentine; pain, sensitive, yellow exposed
  - Ellis III: Enamel, dentine and pulp; pain, pinkish, red
- Management
  - Ellis I: Smooth with emery board
  - Ellis II and III: Cover dentine with calcium hydroxide paste. More difficult to do in Ellis III as blood makes paste not stick
  - See dentist

Avulsed teeth

- History: Ask mechanism, time of injury, dental history
- Examination: Bite, assess TMJ, sensation, mucosal injury, ensure all teeth accounted for especially in children
- In children, check if the teeth are primary (small, white, bulbous, smooth) or secondary (larger, creamier, jagged)
- Investigations: OPG, CXR
- Pre-hospital: Store teeth in milk or saline, pack socket with gauze
- Management
  - Clean the tooth with sterile saline or Hank's solution, don't scrub
  - To prepare socket remove clot, gentle saline rinse
  - Reimplant with firm pressure then patient bite gauze, splint (do not reimplant milk teeth)
- Dental follow-up
- With subluxated teeth, reposition, splint, dental follow-up

Throat

Pharyngitis/tonsillitis

- Most viral, self-limiting, symptomatic treatment
- Forms that need identifying/treatment: EBV (fever, exudative pharyngitis, nodes, splenomegaly; can test EBV serology), influenza (can consider use antivirals if very early; e.g. Tamiflu), HIV primary infection (early recognition important), strep

Group A βhaemolytic strep (GAS)

- Complications: Abscess, rheumatic fever, poststreptococcal glomerulonephritis (PSGN), AOM

- Can use Centor Score or the PAIN Fever score: 1 point each
  - **P**urulence, **A**ttended doctor within 3 days, **I**nflammation of tonsils, **N**o cough, **F**ever in the last day
  - These factors make GAS more likely on rapid antigen testing (RAT) of throat culture
  - Score 0 or 1 = no AB; 2 or 3 = delay AB, > 3 = give AB
- Management
  - AB if PAIN fever score > 2 or 3, patient 2–25 years in at-risk area, scarlet fever (look for rash), systemically unwell, abscess, positive RAT, severe inflammation
  - AB: Phenoxymethylpenicillin 10 mg/kg (500 mg) BD 10/7, alternatives amoxicillin with clavulanate 22 mg/kg (875 mg max.), roxithromycin 4 mg/kg BD to max. 300 mg/day if allergy
  - Steroids if difficult swallowing: Dexamethasone 4 mg (up to 10 mg) PO/IV
  - Admit if toxic, poor intake, suspect airway obstruction, immunosuppressed, severe pain

Fungal/thrush

- White cheesy exudate. Treat with nystatin PO suspension

Peritonsillar abscess

- History: Same as with pharyngitis but higher fevers, longer history, more severe pain, dysphagia. Severe symptoms: Trismus, drooling, airway obstruction
- Examination: Unilateral oedema palate, uvula deviation away, fluctuance, superior/medial displaced tonsil (see Fig. 17.2). Tender cervical nodes. Can be bilateral but rare

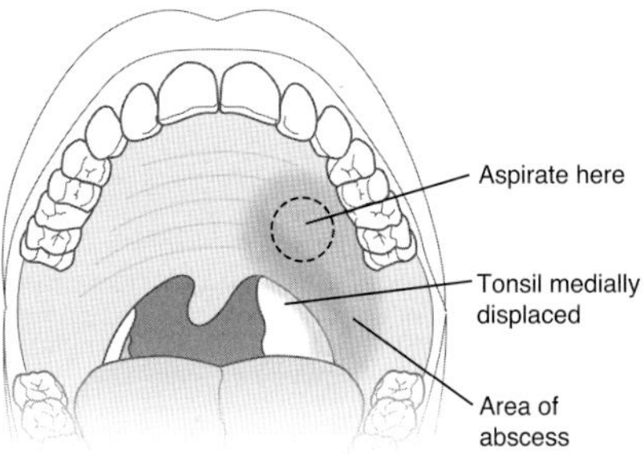

Figure 17.2 What to look for on examination and where to aspirate

- Risk ↑: Previous abscess, chronic tonsillitis, multiple trials PO AB
- Management
  - Drainage by aspiration: Anaesthetic spray (e.g. Co-Phenylcaine) +/– 1–2 mL lignocaine with adrenaline injected into mucosa of anterior tonsillar pillar with 25 G needle. 23 G needle to aspirate just lateral to the displaced tonsil but < 1 cm so as not to hit internal carotid artery
  - Discuss with ENT if aspiration fails
- Post drainage: High dose penicillin or clindamycin 10/7 with ENT follow-up within 24 hours
- Complications: Airway obstruction, aspiration, cavity sinus thrombosis, epiglottitis, sepsis, endocarditis, mediastinitis

Stridor—differential diagnosis

- Epiglottitis, laryngotracheobronchitis (croup), bacterial tracheitis, angio-oedema, inhaled FB, airway trauma, neck infection, laryngeal spasm, vocal cord paralysis, subglottic stenosis

Epiglottitis

- Traditionally caused by haemophilus influenzae type b (Hib). Others: Strep, staph, virus, fungi, ↓↓ cases due to vaccination, now mostly older 40–50 years old
- Can progress to rapid airway obstruction
- History: ↑ dysphagia, SOB especially supine, fever, symptoms progressing over 1–2 days (often < 1 day)
- Examination: Cervical nodes, drooling, pain on palpation of larynx and upper trachea, elevated HR, inspiratory stridor, no or little cough, thick secretions, patient sits themselves up, forward, panting
  - DON'T EXAMINE INSIDE MOUTH UNLESS READY TO INTUBATE
  - Strawberry epiglottis
- Investigations
  - X-ray lateral airways: Thumbprint sign (see Fig. 17.3), narrow airway, hypopharynx extended, C-spine reverse lordosis, thick aryepiglottic folds
  - CT diagnostic but dangerous and most patients can't lie flat
  - Direct vision is definitive. Use fibreoptic with ENT in the room and full preparation for very difficult airway
- Management
  - Never leave patient alone, have them sit up
  - Humidified O_2, heliox if available and obstruction imminent

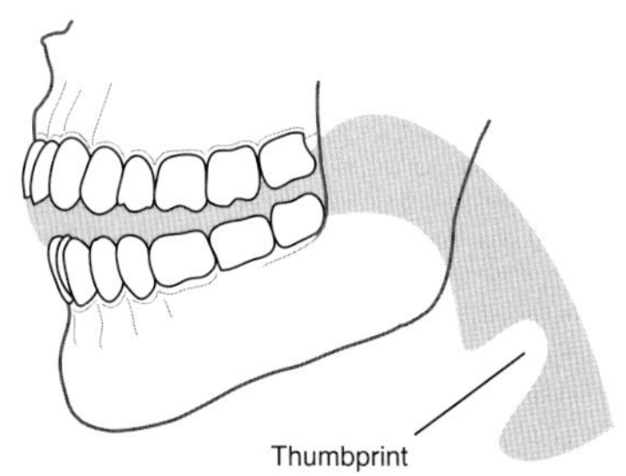

Figure 17.3 Thumbprint sign on a lateral airways x-ray

- IVC with IV fluids, keep well hydrated
- IVAB ceftriaxone 50 mg/kg (2 g)
- URGENT ENT
- Patient should be in resuscitation room, difficult airway trolley by their bed
- Contact tracing: Rifampicin PO to contacts

Retropharyngeal abscess

- Space extends from base of skull to tracheal bifurcation; 2 lymph node chains run through this space
- Mostly children from lymph node pus or FB with perforation
- In adults results from direct extension; e.g. Ludwig's angina
- Complications: Mediastinitis, airway obstruction, carotid artery compression, spinal abscess, cervical OM, jugular venous thrombosis
- History: Insidious onset, mild URTI, dysphagia, SOB, dysphonia, neck pain, decreased ROM neck, decreased intake. If pleuritic chest pain suggest mediastinitis!
- Examination: Fever, C-spine ↓ ROM, cervical nodes, muffled/hoarse voice, drooling; can develop unilateral torticollis, trismus, respiratory distress
    - If can't protrude tongue consider airway obstruction imminent!
- Investigation
    - Lateral airways x-ray: Increased soft tissue shadow, look for FB, gas fluid level, reverse lordosis gas in tissue = perforation or gas forming organism
    - CT neck + contrast (if can lie flat, must be doc accompanied)

- Management
    - URGENT ENT, need operation/incision and drainage
    - IV fluids, IVAB amoxicillin with clavulanate or clindamycin

Mucormycosis/cerebro-rhino orbital phycomycosis

- Invasive fungal infection, high mortality
- Risk groups: Immune suppressed, DM, patients on desferrioxamine
- Assess: Orbital/face pain, fever, periorbital/orbital cellulitis, proptosis, nasal discharge, **black eschar seen on palate**
- Complications: Cavernous sinus thrombosis, intracerebral abscess, central retinal artery occlusion, airway obstruction
- Management: URGENT ENT. Amphotericin B IV and intranasal. Aggressive operation. Cease immune suppressive therapy if taking

Post-tonsillectomy bleed

- ENT emergency: Can be fatal
- URGENT ENT support, get them en route
- Keep patient upright, NBM
- IVC, FBC, cross-match, coagulants (if on thinners), IV fluids
- Quickly get prepared before looking: Move patient to resuscitation room, ensure good lighting, ready equipment (suction, gauze, forceps) and meds (adrenaline for injection, adrenaline-soaked gauze, silver nitrate sticks), difficult airway trolley
- 1 g tranexamic acid gargle or neb, hydrogen peroxide gargle
- Direct pressure with adrenaline-soaked gauze
- If can visualise bleed, use 1% lidocaine (lignocaine) and adrenaline then silver nitrate stick
- Can use nebulised adrenaline 5 mL of 1 in 1000
- Be prepared for difficult intubation
- Be prepared for resuscitation including blood products
- Even if small bleed keep patient and get ENT review
- IVAB: High dose benzyl penicillin

CHAPTER 18

Paediatrics

Resus—advanced life support

- Check for **D**anger, **R**esponse, **S**end for help
- **A**irway: Open (position-tilt, thrust, lift), suction, Guedel, NPA
- **B**reathing: If spontaneous breaths supply oxygen with face mask
- **C**irculation: Assess for signs of circulation/signs of life
  - If signs of life are absent use the flow diagram in Fig. 18.1
- Preparing for incoming paeds resus

  A: Uncuffed tube size = Age/4 + 4 (cuffed = age/4 + 3.5), tube length = age/2 + 12

  B: Oxygen ready

  C: Adrenaline = 10 microgram (0.01 mg) /kg = (0.01 mL/kg of 1 in 1000 for anaphylaxis OR 0.1 mL/kg 1 : 10000 for arrest)

  D: Defibrillation dose = 4 J/kg

  E: Extras—analgesia, antibiotics, antiseizure 0.15 mg/kg midazolam IV/IM double for buccal

  F: Fluids = 20 mL/kg normal saline

  G: Glucose = 2 mL/kg of 10% glucose

  S: Size. Approx. weight = 3 kg at birth, 6 kg at 6 months, 10 kg at 12 months, > 12 months approx. weight = 2 × (age +4)
- Other important drugs for resuscitation in children
  - Calcium = 0.5 mL/kg 10% calcium gluconate (preferred if peripheral IV)
    - o 0.1–0.2 mL/kg of 10% CaCl (BEWARE EXTRAVASATION)
  - Magnesium = 25–50 mg/kg (0.1–0.2 mmol/kg)
  - Lidocaine (lignocaine) = 1 mg/kg
  - $NaHCO_3^-$ = 1 mmol/kg (= 1 mL/kg 8.4%)
  - Amiodarone = 5 mg/kg
- Urgent arrhythmias in children
  - **If bradycardic**
    - o HR < 60, with poor perfusion = severe compromise. Start CPR and adrenaline 10 microgram/kg

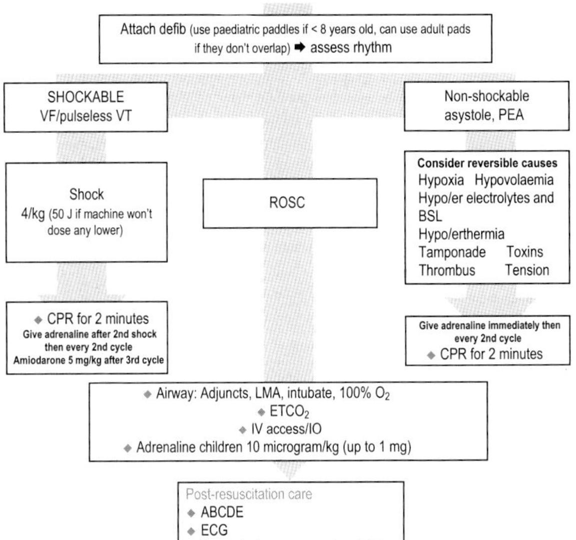

Figure 18.1 Flow diagram for paediatric advanced life support

- ADD atropine 20 microgram/kg
- Consider transthoracic pacing
- Identify and treat cause
- ABCs, maintain airway, give oxygen, monitor, IO/IV access, ECG
- If arrest go to arrest algorithm

- **Tachycardic**
  - ECG or monitor to evaluate QRS
  - If narrow QRS and likely SVT: If child stable can try ice on face (max. 30 seconds), vagal manoeuvres, adenosine 0.1 mg/kg IV in large vein (max. 6 mg). If no response repeat at dose 0.15 mg/kg (max. 12 mg). If no response

repeat at dose 0.3 mg/kg (max. 18 mg). If no response to above or child appears shocked at any stage cardiovert 1–2 J/kg. If stable discuss with cardiologist first. Usually enough time to give analgesia (e.g. fentanyl)

    - Remember adenosine neat, tiny volumes in children—need large flush to get to heart
  - If narrow QRS and likely sinus: Identify and treat cause
  - Wide QRS = possible VT: Cardiovert 1–2 J/kg; if stable consider amiodarone 5 mg/kg IV over 20 minutes to 1 hour
  - Identify and treat cause
    - ABCs, maintain airway, give oxygen, monitor, IO/IV access, ECG

Airway and breathing

- Acute upper airway obstruction
  - Differential diagnosis of stridor (see p. 315)
  - Airway foreign body
    - Usually 1–3 years old
    - Suspect with sudden onset cough, choking
    - Many present > 24 hours, choking episode may not be witnessed
    - BLS: Alternate 5 back blows and 5 chest thrusts, no Heimlich. Start CPR if lose consciousness.
    - Direct visualisation, laryngoscopy and removal of foreign bodies (no blind sweep)
- Bag valve mask
  - 3 sizes of Laerdal bags
    - Neonate: 200 mL bag (only < 1 month)
    - Up to 2 years: 500 mL bag
    - Over 2 years to adult: 2 L bag
- ETT sizes (Table 18.1)
- LMA sizes (Table 18.2)
- High flow humidified nasal prongs (know local protocol)
  - Child up to 10 kg, goal rate is 1–2 L/kg/min
  - Child > 10 kg, goal rate is 1 L/kg/min (max. 50 L)
  - Start at 6 L/min of 50% oxygen
  - Never use 100% FiO_2, max. 85%

Table 18.1 ETT sizes

Age	Estimated weight	Blade	Tube size	Tube length at lips
Newborn	3 kg	0	3.0	8 cm
2 month	5 kg	1	3.5	9 cm
6 month	6 kg	1	4.0	10 cm
≥ 1 year	2 × (Age+4)	≥ 2	Age/4+4 uncuff Age/4 + 3.5 cuff Generally choose cuffed	Age/2 + 12

Table 18.2 LMA sizes (kg guide written on LMA)

Age	Approximate weight	Size
0–2 months	< 5 kg	1
2 months–1 year	5–10 kg	1.5
1–6 years	10–20 kg	2
6–11 years	20–30 kg	2.5
11 years – adult	30–50 kg	3

Neonatal resuscitation

- Neonatal resuscitation guidelines are shown in Fig. 18.2
- APGAR score (Table 18.3)
- Neopuff T-piece
  - Setup
    - o Make sure gas supply connected/on
    - o With test lung in line—check gas flows
    - o Starting flow rate 8–10 L/min
    - o Max. pressure relief valve set to 50 cmH_2O (under flap)
    - o PIP to 20–25 cmH_2O (dial—located on machine)
    - o Set PEEP 5–8 cmH_2O (use PEEP cap—occlusion valve twists on T-piece)
  - Use
    - o Mask held over mouth and nose, valve not occluded = PEEP
    - o Occlude hole to see inflation = PIP
    - o Occlude 0.5–1 sec, release
    - o Can deliver positive pressure via mask or ETT
    - o Once set, PEEP and PIP only depend on mask seal, gas flow
    - o Warning: Changing flow rate will change PEEP and PIP

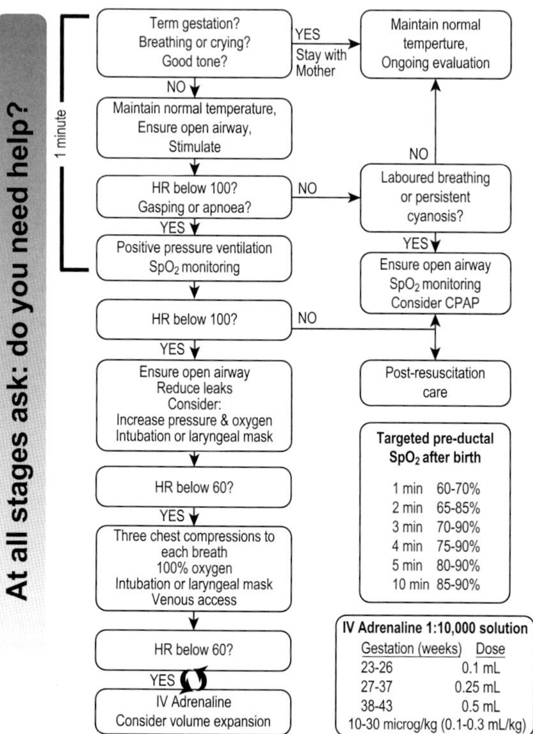

Targeted pre-ductal SpO_2 after birth

1 min	60-70%
2 min	65-85%
3 min	70-90%
4 min	75-90%
5 min	80-90%
10 min	85-90%

IV Adrenaline 1:10,000 solution

Gestation (weeks)	Dose
23-26	0.1 mL
27-37	0.25 mL
38-43	0.5 mL
10-30 microg/kg (0.1-0.3 mL/kg)	

Figure 18.2 Neonatal resuscitation guidelines
Source: Australian Resuscitation Council.

Intraosseous access

- Indications
  - In life-threatening situation and can't get IV access within 60 seconds
  - Can't get IV access in an urgent situation; e.g. trauma/burns/shock

Table 18.3 APGAR score

	Score 0	Score 1	Score 2
Colour	Blue, pale	Acrocyanosis	All pink
Pulse	Absent	< 100	> 100
Irritability	No response	Slight cry	Vigorous cry
Tone	Limp	Some flex	Vigorous movement
Respiration	Absent	Irregular, slow, weak	Strong breath, cry

- Contraindications
  - Bone fracture same limb
  - Prior attempt: Use alternative site
  - Overlying infection
  - Osteogenesis imperfecta, osteopetrosis
- Sites
  - Proximal tibia: 2 fingers below patella, ~1 cm medial to tibial tuberosity (adult)
  - Proximal humerus: 1 cm above surgical neck (greater tubercle)
  - Distal tibia: 3 cm above medial malleolus
  - Femoral: Anterior, lateral 3 cm above lateral condyle
  - Iliac crest
- Needles (for EZ-IO)
  - 45 mm, yellow: Use for humerus, use for obese
  - 25 mm, blue: > 40 kg patient
  - 15 mm, pink: 3–40 kg
- Insertion
  - Hold handle of device
  - BEFORE using drill insert perpendicular to bone until touches periosteum, make sure at least one black line can be visualised above skin for EZ-IO, squeeze the trigger and apply gentle pressure
  - Stop when sudden loss of resistance
  - Stabilise hub and remove driver, remove stylet
  - Aspirate blood marrow (can't always aspirate)
  - Secure site
  - If awake patient, consider flush with lidocaine (lignocaine) (2% lignocaine 0.5 mg/kg; note 2% = 20 mg/mL [max. 2 mL])

  - Connect primed tubing
  - Cannot flow under gravity, needs pump or manual pressure
  - Beware: Phenytoin will crystallise if already given glucose into marrow
- Complications
  - Failure (many will fail after 30 minutes use; prolonged resuscitations often need second insertion)
  - Extravasation
  - Osteomyelitis
  - Skin necrosis
  - Fracture
  - Compartment syndrome (keep checking limb)
  - Necrosis of growth plate
  - Fat, bone embolism: Not clinically significant
- Removal: Within 24 hours or if extravasation or there is swelling
  - Disconnect tubing
  - Connect 10 mL syringe
  - Rotate and pull out
  - Dressing

Apparent life-threatening event (ALTE)/brief, resolved, unexplained event (BRUE)

- Episode frightening to observer characterised by apnoea, colour change, muscle tone change, choking or gagging. Child less than 1 year old
- > 95% benign, physiological cause. No proven association with sudden unexpected death in infancy (SUDI)
- Exclude potentially serious causes (i.e. diagnosis NOT a BRUE)
  - NAI
  - Infection: Sepsis, pertussis, lower respiratory tract infection (LRTI), meningitis
  - Airway obstruction: Congenital, infection, decreased tone
  - Surgical abdomen: Intussusception, torsion
  - Metabolic: Hypoglycaemia, hypocalcaemia, hypokalaemia, inborn error of metabolism

  - Toxins, drugs, withdrawal
  - Cardiac: Arrhythmia, prolonged QT, congenital
  - Neurological: Closed head injury, seizure, infection
- History
  - Event: LOC, seizure, tone, colour
  - Circumstances: Feeding, vomiting, sleeping prone, environment
  - Recent illness
  - Previous history: Comorbidities, respiratory problems etc.
  - Family history: Sudden death
  - Interventions: expired air resuscitation (EAR), CPR by trained provider
- Examination
  - Vitals
  - Cardio, respiratory
  - Neurological
  - Skin
  - Abdomen
  - Fundoscopy (if suspect NAI)
- High-risk features
  - Age < 28 days (some flow charts say 60 days)
  - Premature < 32 weeks
  - Previous history, comorbidities
  - Unwell looking child
  - Recurrent
  - Severe or prolonged symptoms (> 1 minute)
  - Family history
  - CPR by trained provider
  - Concerning history or examination
- Investigations
  - Usually none if no concerns and examination normal
  - Consider pertussis testing, ECG, monitor sats in ED for short period
  - If specific concerns that this is not a BRUE, might consider: FBC, EUC, glucose, NPA, metabolic screen, septic screen, NAI investigation, CTB, EEG, Holter, urine tox

- Management
  - Don't need to admit term well baby with minor event AND normal Hx/Ex with no high-risk features
  - Shared decision-making
  - Good to advise CPR, basic first aid training to anyone with children
  - Education on BRUE

Fluids

- Bolus fluids for hypovolaemia: use normal saline
  - 10–20 mL/kg: Can repeat if required
  - Don't include bolus fluids in subsequent calculations: Do for burns
  - Be very cautious with fluids in DKA
- Maintenance
  - 4 mL/kg for the first 10 kg
  - 2 mL/kg for the second 10 kg
  - 1 mL/kg for every kg over 20 kg
  - Normal saline +5% glucose
  - Use ⅔ maintenance if unwell but not dehydrated, also CNS or respiratory illness
- Deficit: Add to maintenance
  - % deficit × weight × 10
  - Moderate dehydration = 5% deficit. Don't replace more than 5% per 24 hours
  - Deficit to be divided over a given time period (hours to 1–2 days) when added to maintenance
  - Can rapidly replace deficit in gastroenteritis but needs to be slower in DKA, meningitis. Very slow and cautious in hypernatraemia
- Ongoing losses: Add to maintenance and deficit
  - Measure losses and add (often q4hourly)
- Neonates: Use 10% glucose (check local protocols for NaCl content)
- Gastroenteritis rehydration via NG fluids (see Gastroenteritis, p. 338)

Asthma

- Risk factors for severe asthma
  - Previous severe: ICU admissions, intubations
  - Poor compliance

- Poorly controlled asthma: Interval symptoms, multiple ED visits in the last year, no GP
- Sudden attack
- Current steroid use
- Multiple preventers
- Sensitive to NSAIDs

- Assess severity
  - Wheeze is a poor indicator of severity
  - See Table 18.4
- Investigations
  - Not usually required
  - Consider in severe or critical (comorbidity or complication)
  - CXR: Look for pneumothorax, consolidation
  - ABG not required and distressing. Can make child worse
  - Consider bloods if needing IV therapy or if jittery/toxic—check POTASSIUM (may be low, need replacing)
  - FBC, EUC, CRP, VBG
- Management
  - For severe, critical: Get senior help as soon as possible
  - Lung delivery better with MDI + spacer than nebuliser, unless need oxygen

Table 18.4 Assessing severity of an acute asthma attack

Feature	Mild	Moderate	Severe	Critical
Sats	> 94%	90–94%	< 90%	< 90% central cyanosis
HR	Normal	Elevated	Elevated Pulsus paradoxus	Very elevated or bradycardic Pulsus paradoxus
Speech	Normal	Some limitation	Marked limitation	Unable to talk
Mental state	Normal	Normal	Agitated, distressed	Confused, drowsy
Work of breathing (WOB)	Subtle or no increased WOB	Some increased WOB Accessory muscle use Recession	Moderate to marked increased WOB	Max. WOB. Silent chest
Other				Exhaustion

- *General dosing*
  - Salbutamol 1 dose = 6 puffs if < 6 years, 12 puffs > 6 years old
  - Ipratropium bromide 1 dose = 4 puffs < 6 years, 8 puffs > 6 years old
- *Mild*
  - Salbutamol + spacer 1 dose. Review in 20 minutes. If good response consider discharge (see below), or if poor response treat as moderate
- *Moderate*
  - Salbutamol + spacer 1 dose every 20 minutes × 3 doses
  - Prednisone 1 mg/kg PO daily for 3/7 (first dose can be doubled)
  - Oxygen if sats < 92%
  - Review after 20 minutes and after 3 doses complete
- *Severe*
  - Oxygen to keep sats > 92%
  - Salbutamol + spacer 1 dose every 20 minutes, with ongoing review. If improves, decrease frequency. If worsens, treat as critical
  - Ipratropium bromide 1 dose every 20 minutes for 3 doses
  - $MgSO_4$ 50 mg/kg (0.2 mmol/kg) over 20 minutes. Can repeat bolus if needed or can give 30 mg/kg/hr infusion but beware Mg toxicity
  - Prednisone 1 mg/kg PO daily for 3/7 (first dose can be doubled)

    OR
  - Methylprednisolone 1 mg/kg IV (first dose can be doubled)

    OR
  - Hydrocortisone 4 mg/kg IV (first dose can be doubled)
- Can use dexamethasone PO (less volume than PO prednisone)
- Aminophylline if deteriorating 5–10 mg/kg IV over 1 hour (max. 500 mg) loading. Can follow with infusion 0.5–1 mg/kg/hr
- Critical
  - Continuous nebulised salbutamol with oxygen
  - Ipratropium bromide every 20 minutes for 3 doses
  - $MgSO_4$ as above

- IV salbutamol infusion 1 microgram/kg/min up to 5 microgram/kg/min (max. dose for 1 hour only)
- Adrenaline infusion start dose 0.05 microgram/kg/min
- Aminophylline as above
- Consider BiPAP, CPAP, intubation
- Active external decompression of chest can overcome trapping
- May need inotropy/fluid load when adding positive pressure ventilation (PPV) as reduce vascular resistance
- Beware arrest when PPV!

- Criteria for discharge
  - Written action plan
  - Written management plan with details of weaning salbutamol doses, prednisone if needed, preventers and follow-up
  - Fact sheet provided including when to return to ED
  - Parent education, observed given treatment (if first time)
  - Adequate PO intake
  - Adequate oxygenation
  - Salbutamol not needed more frequently than 3 hourly
  - Consider preventer when > 3 courses of prednisone in one year.

Bronchiolitis

- General
  - Viral LRTI
  - Usually children less than 12 months old
  - Peaks at day 3–5
  - Clinical diagnosis
- History
  - Begins with URTI symptoms
  - Followed by respiratory distress and fever
  - Symptoms and signs: Cough, increased RR, increased work of breathing (chest wall retractions, nasal flaring, etc.), widespread crackles or wheeze
- Risk factors for severe illness
  - Indigenous background, immunodeficiency, age less than 10 weeks, chronic lung disease, congestive congenital heart

Table 18.5 Assessing severity of bronchiolitis

	Mild	Moderate	Severe
Behaviour	Normal	Intermittent irritability	Increasing irritability or lethargy or fatigue
RR	Normal or mild increase	Increased RR	Marked increased RR or decreased RR
Accessory muscles	Nil to mild accessory muscle use	Moderate retractions, nasal flaring	Marked retractions and nasal flaring
Oxygen	Sats > 92% room air	Sats 90–92% room air	Sats < 90% room air. Oxygen may not correct
Apnoea	None	May have brief apnoeas	Frequent or prolonged apnoeas possible
Feeding	Normal	Difficulty feeding, reduced feeds	Reluctant or unable to feed

disease, chronic neurological condition, premature baby, exposure to smoking, failure to thrive

- ■ Other red flags for deterioration: feeding < 50%, looks unwell day 1–2, oxygen requirement

- Assess severity (see Table 18.5)
- Investigations
  - ■ Not needed unless diagnosis uncertain or sicker than expected; e.g.:
    - o CXR may be used if concerned about alternative diagnosis such as pneumothorax, pneumonia, cardiac failure
    - o Blood tests may be used if concerned about infections or electrolyte imbalances if child not feeding
    - o NPA may be used for patient cohorting or suspected influenza in infant (would consider antiviral treatment < 6 month)
- Management
  - ■ General: Supportive, ensure fluid intake, minimal handling
  - ■ Generally do NOT need: Corticosteroids, bronchodilators, antibiotics
  - ■ Mild
    - o Likely discharge, ensure good follow-up
    - o Observe in ED pre-discharge. Document vitals
    - o Nasal saline AC feed and on waking (babies are obligate nose breathers)

- Moderate
  - Likely admission
  - Observation (does not need to be continuous)
  - Nasal saline AC feed and on waking
  - Nasal suction to help with feeding and respiratory distress
  - Oxygen to keep sats > 90%
    - Begin with nasal prongs, increase to heated humidified high-flow nasal cannula (HFNC) if fails; 1–2 L/kg
  - If feeds inadequate give NG hydration at ⅔ maintenance
  - NG is preferred to IV. If using IV give ⅔ maintenance
- Severe
  - Admission. Consider need to transfer to paediatric intensive care unit (PICU) if available
  - Continuous observation
  - Oxygen to keep sats > 90%
    - HFNC oxygen 1–2 L/kg or CPAP
  - Will need escalation, ICU admission if does not improve
  - NG hydration at ⅔ maintenance
  - NG is preferred to IV. If using IV give ⅔ maintenance

- Discharge
  - Once maintaining adequate oxygenation without support
  - Once maintaining adequate PO intake
  - Provide parent education
  - Consider phase of illness, geographical and social factors

Croup—laryngotracheobronchitis

- General
  - Viral inflammation upper airway
  - Worse at night
  - Typical age between 6 months and 3 years of age
  - Peaks day 2–3
- History
  - Harsh barking cough, inspiratory stridor
  - Increased work of breathing
  - Often febrile, miserable

Table 18.6 Assessing severity of croup

	Mild	Moderate	Severe
Behaviour	Normal	Intermittent irritability	Increasing irritability or lethargy
RR	Normal	Increased RR	Marked increased RR or decreased RR
Accessory muscles	None or minimal	Tracheal tug, moderate retractions, nasal flaring	Marked retractions, tracheal tug and nasal flaring
Oxygen	None required	None required	Hypoxia is a late sign
Stridor	Barking cough. Stridor only when active or upset	Some stridor at rest	Stridor at rest

  - Otherwise well looking
  - Consider differential diagnosis (see list of differentials of stridor on p. 333) especially if less than 6 months old or greater than 6 years old
- Risk factors for severe illness
  - Prior severe croup, narrow airway (Down Syndrome, subglottic stenosis)
- Assess severity (see Table 18.6)
- Investigations
  - Not needed unless diagnosis uncertain
  - CXR, blood tests, NPA etc. not usually needed and may distress child
- Management
  - General: DON'T DISTRESS CHILD. Minimal handling. Nurse with parents
  - Mild–moderate
    - Dexamethasone 0.15 mg/kg PO (usually steroid of choice) OR
    - Prednisolone 1 mg/kg PO with 2nd dose next morning
    - Discharge once stridor-free at rest
  - Severe
    - 0.5 mL/kg of 1 : 1000 (max. 5 mg/5 mL) adrenaline nebulised AND
    - Dexamethasone IV/IM/PO 0.6 mg/kg (12 mg max.)
    - If no improvement repeat adrenaline

  - Treatment failure
    - o GET URGENT HELP: Senior clinician, anaesthetics
    - o Consider an alternative diagnosis
    - o Give oxygen with non-rebreather
    - o Urgent gaseous induction
- Discharge—if no high-risk features or other concerns
  - Observe minimum 4 hours post adrenaline and ½ hour post steroids
  - Should be stridor-free at rest
  - Provide parent education
  - Consider phase of illness, geographical and social factors
  - Advise to return if stridor at rest

Stridor/acute upper airway obstruction—differential diagnosis

- Congenital: Preexisting stridor, baby < 6 months
- Haemangioma (look for skin haemangiomas especially in midline): Vascular ring, subglottic stenosis
- Laryngomalacia: Manifests shortly after birth, worse with agitation and post feed, improves with neck extension and being prone
- Croup: Harsh barking cough, febrile, miserable, otherwise well
- Epiglottitis: No cough, low-pitch expiratory stridor, drooling, high fever, neck hyperextension, dysphagia, refusing to speak and/or drink, unimmunised
- Retropharyngeal or peritonsillar abscess: High fever, drooling, hyperextension of neck, torticollis, trismus
- Bacterial tracheitis: Toxic appearance, very tender trachea especially larynx
- Inhaled foreign body: Sudden onset, otherwise well, cough or choking episode, apnoea
- Anaphylaxis: Swelling of face, wheeze, rash (erythema, urticarial), other systems (e.g. vomiting, abdominal pain)
- Preexisting stridor: Congenital abnormality, subglottic stenosis. Baby < 6 months

Fevers

- General
  - Consider fever with temperature > 38
  - Forehead strips and ear thermometer not always reliable

  - Degree of fever, rapidity of onset, its response to antipyretics and febrile convulsions are not good predictors of severity of illness
  - Hypothermia especially in babies also can be a sign of serious illness/sepsis
- Assessment
  - History
    - Localising symptoms
    - Travel
    - Sick contacts
    - Immunisations up to date (full course is age dependent!)
    - Fluid balance: Input versus output
    - Previous history
  - Examination
    - General—behaviour and appearance: Best indicator of severity of illness
    - Signs of an unwell child: Lethargic, poor interaction, inconsolable, tachycardia, tachypnoea, cyanosis, poor peripheral perfusion
    - Localising signs: ENT, meningism, work of breathing, abdominal signs, skin (rashes, cellulitis), joints (remember spine)
- Investigations
  - Under 1 month old corrected age: Full septic workup including LP and empirical antibiotics per local protocols, always consider adding aciclovir if CSF abnormal.
  - 1–3 months old age corrected: If obvious focus Ix/Mx as per focus
    - +/– CXR if respiratory signs and symptoms
    - +/– LP; remember small babies don't get classic signs of meningitis, may just be lethargic
    - Can discharge for review within 12 hours if all tests normal, well child, previously healthy child
    - Admit if unwell or abnormal findings
    - Know local protocols
  - > 3 months and clear focus
    - Treat focus as appropriate
    - Admission if looking unwell

  - > 3 months no focus
    - Well child: Consider urine, especially if < 12 months old or fevers for > 48 hours. Discharge with symptomatic treatment. Review within 24 hours
    - Unwell child: FBC, blood culture, urine culture, +/– CXR +/– LP, admit and observe +/– IVAB
  - If child has impaired level of consciousness, focal neuro signs or are unstable haemodynamically, defer LP and treat for meningitis/encephalitis
- Management
  - If child looks unwell regardless of other findings investigate and admit
  - If child is unimmunised, needs investigations and likely admit
  - All children under 1 month need admission, investigation, treatment
  - Antibiotics: Should target source, should always check your local guidelines. Recommendations change constantly!
  - Empiric treatment of sepsis stat IV doses
    - < 2 months
      - Cover: GBS, *E. coli*, listeriosis
      - Benzylpenicillin 60 mg/kg IV/IM or amoxicillin IV/IM
      - + cefotaxime 50 mg/kg IV/IM (avoid ceftriaxone)
      - +/– flucloxacillin 50 mg/kg IV if suspect staph (e.g. umbilical infection)
    - < 2 months and abdominal source
      - Ampicillin 50 mg/kg IV/IM
      - + gentamicin 7.5 mg/kg IV/IM
      - + metronidazole 15 mg/kg IV
    - > 2 months:
      - Cover: *S. pneumoniae*, *N. meningitidis*, *Staphylococcus aureus*, GAS, *E. coli*
      - Flucloxacillin 50 mg/kg
      - + ceftriaxone or cefotaxime 50 mg/kg IV/IM
      - Piperacillin/tazobactam 100 mg/kg (piperacillin) if neutropenic
    - Consider aciclovir if suspect encephalitis 20 mg/kg

- Discharge
  - 1–3 months old
    - If well
    - All investigations normal
    - Follow-up within 12 hours
  - > 3 months old
    - Well child
    - Follow-up arranged
  - Parental information provided
  - Always consider social and geographical elements

Lumbar puncture

- Indications
  - Suspected meningitis or encephalitis
  - Suspected SAH with normal CT (see Subarachnoid haemorrhage, p. 170)
- Contraindications
  - Don't LP a child that is so sick you are going to give antibiotics anyway
  - Give treatment (dexamethasone, antibiotics) and delay LP if:
    - Coma
    - Raised ICP (drowsy, diplopia, abnormal pupils, motor posturing, papillo-oedema)
    - Cardiovascular or respiratory compromise
    - Focal neurological seizure, recent seizure, focal signs
    - Coagulopathic, decreased platelets
    - Local infection at LP site
    - Fever + purpura with suspected meningococcal
    - Consider deferred LP and treat if sacral dimple (suspected tethered cord)
- Sedation/analgesia
  - AnGel or EMLA at site
  - Lidocaine (lignocaine)
  - Oral sucrose for < 3 months
  - Nitrous oxide for > 6 months (see Procedural sedation, p. 49)

- Equipment
  - Spinal needles
    - o Use needles with stylet, blunt/non-cutting needles in older children
    - o Use 22 or 25 gauge (25 G will be really slow)
    - o Size/length: < 2 year old 3 cm, 2–5 years old 4 cm, 5–12 years old 5 cm, > 12 year old 6 cm
    - o Insertion distance = 0.03 × height (cm) of child
  - Trained assistant: Very important (must be curved enough to part the spinous processes), *BEWARE airway obstruction*
  - Sterile gloves, drapes, tray, CSF tubes, mask
  - Skin prep
  - LA
- Procedure
  - Patient on side or sitting, spine at max. flexion. Don't flex neck too much
  - Ensure plane of back perpendicular to bed
  - L3–L4 = approx. level of iliac crest
  - Note: Spinal cord finishes at L3 at birth and L1–L2 by adulthood so go level just below iliac crest in infants, can go one above in older children
  - Aseptic technique, wash hands, drape, glove, mask
  - Prep skin, allow to dry, prepare tray and remove lids of CSF tubes
  - Use LA, 1% lidocaine (lignocaine) 25 G, subcutaneous
  - Use needle, bevel towards ceiling (if patient on side) or towards side (if patient sitting)
  - Pierce the skin then wait for child to stop wriggling
  - Advance needle aiming for umbilicus
  - Always reference the plane of the back rather than the bed as children wiggle
  - If hit bone, usually need to angle a bit more rostrally
  - Stop when there is a fall in resistance. Remove stylet
  - If no CSF replace stylet and advance slightly further
  - Can choose not to replace the stylet and just advance (increased success rate)
  - Collect CSF 5–10 drops per tube

- Replace stylet (reduces risk of headache), remove needle
- Apply pressure briefly, apply Band-Aid
- Send to lab: MCS, protein and glucose +/– xanthochromia
- Consider viral PCR (enterovirus, HSV etc.)
- No need for bed rest

- Complications
  - Failure to get sample or blood stained
  - Headache (5–15%)
  - Transient or persistent paraesthesia (rare if insertion point L4 IS)
  - Respiratory compromise or arrest from positioning
  - Spinal haematoma
  - Spinal abscess
  - Tonsillar herniation

Gastroenteritis

- Assessment
  - Usual symptoms: Diarrhoea +/– vomiting, +/– crampy abdominal pain, +/– fever
  - Must have diarrhoea at some stage to diagnose gastroenteritis
  - Always consider differential diagnosis
    - Appendicitis, torsion, other surgical abdomen
    - UTI, other infections (pneumonia, bacteraemia, sepsis)
  - Red flags: Consider other diagnosis if any of the following (may still be gastroenteritis)
    - Severe abdominal pain, abdominal signs
    - Isolated vomiting
    - Persisting diarrhoea (> 10 days)
    - Blood in stool
    - Bilious vomit (true green)
    - Very unwell looking child
  - Be cautious in children with comorbidities
    - Short gut syndrome, ileostomy
    - Heart disease, renal disease or transplant
    - Children needing fortified feeds
    - Chronic disease

    - Poor growth
    - Very young children (< 6 months)
    - Recent use of hypertonic fluids
    - Morning vomits
  - Be cautious with the patient that re-presents to ED after discharge. Consider treatment failure needing admission, also need to have an increased index of suspicion for alternative diagnosis
  - Consider complications of gastroenteritis: It may have started as gastroenteritis but evolved
    - HUS
    - Intussusception
  - Assess degree of dehydration
- Investigations
  - Usually none required
  - Consider stool culture if: Ongoing diarrhoea (> 7 days), recent travel, suspected septic child, blood or mucus in stool, immunocompromised child
  - Bloods (EUC, glucose, VBG) if: Severe dehydration, renal disease, diuretic use, altered level of consciousness, potential hypernatraemia (skin doughy), home therapies with excess hypertonic (fluids with salt added) or hypotonic fluids (plain water), prolonged or severe losses, ileostomy
- Management
  - Ondansetron (only give once, not for < 6 kg or < 6 months)
  - Dose: 0.15 mg/kg up to 4 mg
    - Can use the following guide for dose as per weight range
      - 6–15 kg: 1–2 mg
      - 15–30 kg: 4 mg
      - > 30 kg: 8 mg
  - Oral rehydration
    - Oral rehydration solution; e.g. Gastrolyte, Hydralyte
    - Continue breastfeeding
    - Stop feed fortifications
    - Early feeding. Normal diet once rehydrated
    - If diarrhoea worsens with formula consider 2 weeks on lactose-free formula
    - Trial of oral fluids in ED: Small frequent amounts. Aim for 10–20 mL/kg over 1 hour

- Nasogastric rehydration
  - Most children with moderate dehydration, otherwise well
  - NGT fluids preferred over IV
  - Can rapidly rehydrate with oral rehydrating solution in a normally well child with no medical issues that is > 6 months of age and does not have significant abdominal pain
  - 10 mL/kg/hr for 4 hours
  - Gastrolyte preferred for NGT as better electrolytes, don't need to taste
- IV fluids
  - Use in severe dehydration, children with IVC already, if NGT fluids fail, specific comorbidities (e.g. short gut)
  - Bolus normal saline 20 mL/kg if shocked. Can repeat.
  - Don't just bolus to 'get things going'
  - See section on fluids (p. 326)
- Monitor for rehydration
  - Look for weight change, signs of fluid overload (puffy face and extremities, more common with IV fluids compared to NG)
  - Signs of dehydration
  - Ongoing losses
- Discharge home
  - Tolerating PO fluids
  - No significant red flags, ongoing losses
  - Parent fact sheet and education
  - Parents able to obtain follow-up or seek medical attention again if required

Infectious diseases

***Note on immunisations**: Always check immunisation status. Immunisations 'up to date' does not necessarily mean fully immune so check schedule; e.g. a 9 month old will not have had measles vaccine yet.*

Meningococcal sepsis

- Peak incidence 0–4 and 15–25 years; immunisation is changing profile
- Assessment
  - Early symptoms: Leg pain, cool peripheries, viral-looking blanching rash

- Fever, increased RR, vomiting, decreased feeding, muscle pain, abdominal pain, drowsy, non-blanching rash—petechiae/purpura, +/– meningisms
- Patients can initially look well but can deteriorate quickly
- BEWARE patients partially treated with oral antibiotics as symptoms may be much milder and longer duration; ALWAYS ask about antibiotic use

- Investigations
  - Blood culture, FBC, CRP, VBG, EUC, meningococcal PCR
  - NPA
  - +/– CSF
- Management
  - PPE: Mask for yourself, staff and family
  - Pre-hospital: Benzylpenicillin, ceftriaxone
  - IV/IM ceftriaxone or cefotaxime 50 mg/kg (up to 2 g)
  - IV dexamethasone 0.15 mg/kg max. 10 mg
  - Fluid resuscitation
  - ICU
  - Report: Public Health to contact trace. Chemoprophylaxis to contacts rifampicin, ciprofloxacin

Meningitis

- 90% of patients < 5 years old
- Usually haematogenous spread: URTI, sinus, AOM etc.
- Note: Not all meningococcal disease is meningitis and not all meningitis is meningococcal. Think other bacteria. Think viral
- Assessment
  - Infants: Non-specific, fever, irritable, lethargy, poor feeding, vomiting and diarrhoea
  - Headache, photophobia in older children
  - Seizures
  - BEWARE partial treatment with antibiotics, may alter presentation
- Examination
  - Full fontanelle
  - Look for photophobia and pain with eye movements
  - Neck stiffness: Unreliable

  - Purpuric rash = meningococcal
  - Kernig's sign: Hip flexion with extended knee causes pain in back and legs
  - CSF shunts, cranial abnormalities
  - Altered level of consciousness, focal neurological findings: Encephalitis
- Investigations
  - LP (see Lumbar puncture, p. 336)
  - FBC, EUC, glucose, blood culture, CRP, pro-calcitonin
- Management
  - Don't delay antibiotics
  - < 3 months old: Cefotaxime 50 mg/kg and benzylpenicillin 60 mg/kg IV/IM, consider adding aciclovir 10 mg/kg 8-hourly
  - > 3 months old ceftriaxone 50 mg/kg and dexamethasone 0.15 mg/kg max. 10 mg, 15 minutes prior to or up to 1 hour post first dose antibiotics (evidence that early steroids improve neurological sequelae of bacterial meningitis [i.e. hearing loss] but do not improve mortality)
  - ABC, support, fluid resuscitation
  - Treat seizures immediately
  - Chemoprophylaxis
  - Monitor electrolytes, ICP

Measles

- Highly infectious, airborne, full vaccine series confers excellent immunity (remember schedule: 12 and 18 months)
- Assessment
  - Cough, fever, coryza, conjunctivitis, +/– diarrhoea
  - Rash: Maculopapular head then neck then body, soles and palms (this pattern is universal)
  - Koplik's spots
- Investigations
  - Swab, urine (double bag specimens, don't put in pneumatic tube), PCR, IgM
- Management
  - Isolate (i.e. home quarantine until cleared), respiratory precautions, call Public Health

    - Supportive care, vitamin A (deficiency is a risk factor for severe disease), antibiotics for secondary infection
    - Identify contacts for vaccination with Ig, notify Public Health
- Complications
    - Encephalitis, AOM, pneumonia, pericarditis, myocarditis, nephritis, subacute sclerosing pan encephalitis, hepatitis

Varicella

- Droplet infection
- Itchy rash trunk, face, mucous membranes. Macular then papular then vesicles then crusts ('dewdrops on a rose petal' at peak)
- Disease presentation has been modified by vaccination (milder but still possible)
- Centrifugal spread (torso—outwards)
- Management
    - Supportive, report
    - Keep skin cool, keep nails short, calamine lotion, antihistamines at night, some prefer emollients
    - If < 24 hours from rash onset and well and > 12 years old can give PO aciclovir (but only shortens duration by 1 day)
    - If immunocompromised, pregnant, neonate, secondary complications: Give IV aciclovir +/– varicella zoster immune globulin (VZIG)
    - Antibiotics if secondary infections
- Complications
    - Secondary skin infection (impetigo, cellulitis, invasive streptococcal), encephalitis, pneumonia, AOM, hepatitis, arthritis, Reye syndrome, congenital, zoster

Mumps

- Droplet infection
- Assessment
    - Fever, malaise, parotitis, submandibular glands
    - Parotid gland crosses mandible
- Complications
    - Meningitis, encephalitis, epididymo-orchitis/oophoritis, pancreatitis, arthritis, myocarditis, pneumonia, thyroiditis, deafness
    - Post-pubertal males up to ⅓ unilateral orchitis; 10–20% bilateral (can't do anything about it other than vaccinate!)

Hand-foot-and-mouth disease

- Usually children < 5 years old
- Assessment
  - Mild febrile illness
  - Macular: Papular rash palms/soles, can become papulovesicular. Vesicles and ulcers in mouth
  - Oral symptoms throughout mouth but usually starts at back
- Investigations: Can consider as required—swab/PCR, CSF, echo
- Complications: Encephalopathy, paralysis, heart failure, nail shedding (common)

Scarlet fever

- Group A strep toxin
- Assessment
  - Tonsillitis, fever, headache
  - Rash: Generalised, fine papules, sandpapery, starts torso and axillae—fades, desquamates. Linear petechiae antecubital and axillary skin folds (Pastia's lines)
  - Tongue inflamed, prominent papillae, may have white coat—strawberry tongue (classic strawberry or white strawberry)
- Management: Penicillin IV/beta lactam/macrolide if allergy
- Complications: AOM, sinusitis, rheumatic fever, PSGN

Pertussis

- Droplet infection. Patients infectious just prior to cough and for 21 days if untreated (still infectious 5 days post starting treatment)
- Assessment
  - Initially looks just like classic URTI with rhinorrhoea, so need high index of suspicion in high-risk (young) patients
  - Then 1–2 weeks classic paroxysms of cough; whoop is pathognomonic but small infants may not show whoop as unable to generate enough negative intrathoracic pressure. Generally, cough is non-productive but small infants will appear to choke. Increased cough nocte, vomiting, cyanosis, subconjunctival haemorrhage. Often well between coughing spasms
  - Patients that are vaccinated can still contract disease but generally less severe
  - Contacts with cough (> 70% of household contacts will be infected also). Note: Adults are generally the index case ('cough they just can't shake')
  - Fever uncommon

- Investigations
  - WCC can be > 20,000: Lymphocytes
  - Afebrile baby with increased lymphocytes = pertussis
  - NPA PCR (usually negative after 21 days or 5 days of antibiotics)
- Management
  - Oxygen, NG feeds, admit if < 6 months
  - Azithromycin 10 mg/kg (max. 500 mg) PO daily for 5 days or clarithromycin 7.5 mg/kg (max. 500 mg) PO BD for 7 days
  - Antibiotic prophylaxis in close contact while patient was infectious and one of the following: Child < 6 months old, child with < 3 doses of vaccine, anyone living with a child < 6 months, expectant mothers (last month pregnancy), child attending childcare with babies under 6 months, healthcare or childcare worker that will be caring for children < 6 months
  - Isolation: Only first 3 weeks or 5 days of antibiotics
- Complications
  - Pneumonia, cyanosis, apnoea, death. Babies most at risk

Seizures

- General
  - Most self-limiting, don't need treatment
  - Treat if > 5 minutes or known cause warrants treatment (e.g. meningitis, hypoxic injury, trauma, known difficult-to-treat seizure disorder such as Dravet syndrome)
- Assessment
  - Assess and manage at the same time: ABC
  - Don't ever forget glucose!
  - History: Fevers, focal features, symptoms preceding seizure, previous seizures, past medical history, any medications, antiseizure meds (missed doses)
  - Look for causes: Hypoglycaemia, electrolyte disturbance, overdose, infections (encephalitis/meningitis), trauma, CVA, ICH, cardiac (check ECG, signs myocarditis)
- Management
  - Supportive care, ABC, oxygen, monitor, IVC/IO if needed
  - Ongoing seizure > 5 minutes or unknown duration

- Terminate seizure and prevent recurrence
  - Medications sequence (doses to follow)
    - Benzos

    Ongoing seizure 5 minutes
    - Benzos repeated

    Ongoing seizure 5 minutes
    - IV phenytoin OR levetiracetam (don't use phenytoin in Dravet syndrome or babies < 1 month old); IV phenobarbitone < 1 month old; consider pyridoxine in young infant if seizures refractory

    Ongoing
    - IV phenytoin OR levetiracetam (give the medication that you didn't give in step 3)
    - RSI with thiopentone or propofol
- NOTE: Don't wait around between steps; be drawing up ready if seizure has not terminated. The longer the seizure goes the harder it gets to stop it!
- Medication doses
  - Midazolam IV/IO/IM 0.1 mg/kg (max. 10 mg) buccal or intranasal 0.3 mg/kg (max. 10 mg)
  - Diazepam IV/IO 0.3 mg/kg (max. 10 mg), DO NOT GIVE IM, PR 0.5 mg/kg (max. 10 mg)
  - Phenytoin 20 mg/kg IV/IO over 20 minutes (max. 50 mg/min, monitored)
  - Levetiracetam 40 mg/kg IV/IO (max. 3 g) over 5 minutes
  - Phenobarbitone 20 mg/kg IV (max. 1 g, monitored)
  - Midazolam infusion IV/IO 1 microgram/kg/min
  - Propofol IV/IO 2.5 mg/kg stat then 1–3 mg/kg/hr
  - Thiopentone IV/IO 2–5 mg/kg slowly stat then 1–4 mg/kg/hr
  - Pyridoxine 100 mg slow IV
- Identify and treat complications: Glucose, VBG, electrolytes, Ca
- When seizure terminated: Place child in recovery position, monitor and maintain airway

Neonatal seizures

- Causes: Hypoxic ischaemic encephalopathy (most common), ICH, CNS infection, metabolic, VCA, withdrawal/NAS, congenital, IEOM (inborn errors of metabolism), familial, NAI
- Often seizures are subtle (think mouthing, blinking, cycling)

- Investigations
  - Metabolic screen (urine, BSL, EUC, CMP, VBG, ammonia on ice)
  - Infective screen (FBC, blood culture, CSF)
  - EEG
  - Structural screen (US, MRI)
  - Seek newborn screen result
- Management
  - Phenobarbitone 20 mg/kg IVI (watch for respiratory depression)
  - If continuous further 5 mg/kg phenobarbitone IVI
  - If continuous phenytoin 20 mg/kg IVI
  - Pyridoxine 100 mg slow IV if < 2 years
  - Consider midazolam, clonazepam 100 microgram/kg IV, lidocaine (lignocaine) 2 mg/kg IV
  - Treat identified causes

Febrile seizures

- Definition
  - 6 months to 6 years old
  - No underlying neurological abnormality
  - No afebrile seizure
  - No CNS infection
  - Acute febrile illness (may not necessarily need fever at time of seizure)
- Classification
  - Simple: Tonic-clonic generalised, self-limited < 15 minutes, doesn't recur this illness, no focal features, complete recovery in < 1 hour
  - Complex: > 15 minutes, focal features, recur same illness, incomplete recovery < in 1 hour
  - Febrile status: > 30 minutes
- Assessment and management
  - Cease the seizure (see above medications and sequence)
  - Exclude other causes
  - Consider LP if < 6 months old, 6–12 months old and unimmunised, already on PO AB, clinically unwell, no focus, recurrent seizures in 24 hours, incomplete recovery between seizures

- Discharge
    - Neurologically normal
    - Simple febrile seizure (see above)
    - Serious bacterial infection excluded, preferably patients have an identified focus of infection
    - Parent education written and verbal with follow-up

Limping

- General
    - Always consider meningococcal, leukaemia, trauma, NAI
- Causes to consider by age
    - Any age: Trauma, infection, tumour, serum sickness, nodes
    - Toddler: Transient synovitis, juvenile arthritis, ALL, haemophilia, NAI, toddler fracture, HSP, neuromuscular disease, rickets, development dysplasia
    - 4–10 years: Transient synovitis, juvenile arthritis, ALL, haemophilia, HSP, Perthes' disease, rheumatic fever
    - Adolescent 10–15 years: Slipped upper femoral epiphysis (SUFE), overuse syndromes, tumour, osteochondritis dissecans, complex regional pain syndrome (CRPS), chondromalacia
- History
    - Duration, number of joints involved, severity
    - Systemic features, fever, viral illness/coryza, pallor, weight loss
    - Trauma (note: *most* children do have some history of trauma!)
    - Medications
    - Previous history
    - NAI
- Investigations
    - WCC, ESR, CRP, CK, blood culture, x-ray
    - Consider US, bone scan, MRI
    - Consider joint aspirate, usually done by orthopaedics; if possible, aspirate before antibiotics

Orthopaedics

Osteomyelitis (OM)/septic arthritis (SA)

- At-risk patients: Neonates, male, sickle cell anaemia, open fractures, chronic ulcer

- Children versus adults
  - Usually: Long bone (hips and knees), haematogenous spread and no underlying cause
  - Most *S. aureus* (others: Hib, GAS, *Enterobacter*, *Kingella* spp.)
- OM features
  - Subacute limp, refuse to walk
  - Local pain and tenderness
  - Pain on movement, pain with hip rotation
  - Soft tissue redness/swelling may be absent or hidden
  - +/– fever
- SA features
  - More acute onset
  - Pain on movement and at rest
  - Limited ROM, loss of movement
  - Soft tissue redness/swelling often present
  - Fever, can be unwell
- Investigations
  - FBC, CRP, ESR (sensitive not specific), blood culture
  - X-ray (often normal)
  - MRI, US, bone scan, CT
  - Aspirate
  - Kocher study: Increased risk SA if
    - Non-weight bear
    - WCC > 12
    - ESR > 40
    - Fever > 38.5
- Management
  - Consult orthopaedics urgently if possible septic arthritis—often do not want antibiotics prior to sample/washout
  - Flucloxacillin 50 mg/kg IV

Knee pain

- Acute synovitis
  - Typically teenage girls. Pain over 24 hours, looks well
  - Minimal swelling, pain and crepitus patellofemoral

- Chondromalacia patella: Softening cartilage
  - Girls > boys, often with increased activity
  - Crepitus. Pain with patella palpation
  - MRI
- Osteochondritis dissecans: Pathologic lesion of articular cartilage
  - Boys aged 10–15 years
  - Intermittent swelling and locking
  - Order intercondylar x-ray
- Osgood-Schlatter disease: Traction apophysitis tibial tubercle
  - Boys > girls. Growth spurt (girls 8–12 years of age, boys 12–15 years)
  - Tibial tuberosity pain and tenderness
  - Pain on resisted knee extension
  - X-ray +/– MRI
- Refer to orthopaedics for considerations of operative and non-operative management

Hip pain

- Septic arthritis
- Perthes' disease
  - Avascular necrosis femoral head
  - Age 5–10 years, usually male > female
  - 20% bilateral
  - Well child, intermittent limp, hip/knee pain, insidious onset
  - Decreased ROM, unequal leg length, pain with or loss of internal rotation
  - X-ray: Flattening and increased density of femoral head, sclerosis, epiphyseal OP, decreased joint space. Late signs = femoral head fragmentation, subchondral fracture
  - Management: Osteotomy, brace
- Slipped femoral epiphysis (upper—SUFE, capital—SCFE)
  - Age 10–15 years, males > females
  - Risks: Obese, hypothyroid, hypopituitary, hyperparathyroid
  - X-ray—frog leg lateral: Klein's line passes above instead of through the femoral epiphysis, widened physis
  - Management: Traction, operative
  - Complications: 50% bilateral, 15% avascular necrosis

- Transient synovitis (70% of hip pain in children)
    - Age 3–10 years most common, male > female
    - Hip/knee pain (hip refers to knee), usually unilateral, can walk
    - History: Nocte cry, limp, 50% recent URTI, recent trauma
    - Exam: Well, no fever, mild decreased ROM, pain and tenderness active +/– passive movement
    - Log roll test: Involuntary muscle guarding
    - Investigations: Effusion on US, x-ray normal, WCC/ESR slightly elevated or normal
    - Management: Exclude septic arthritis, analgesia, anti-inflammatories, should resolve 1 week, 10% recur

Surgical abdomen

Pyloric stenosis

- Age group usually 2–6 weeks, males > females, firstborn, family Hx
- History: Vomiting (may be projectile) soon after feed, milk, non-bilious can be blood stained, decreased stools, hungry infant, dehydration, failure to thrive
- Examination: Usually well-looking infant (unless presenting late), signs of dehydration, distended abdomen, visible peristalsis, olive (rare to find = mass epigastric/RUQ)
- Investigations
    - Decreased Na, K
    - Hypochloraemic metabolic alkalosis, paradoxic aciduria
    - Abdomen x-ray: Distended stomach
    - US: Bullseye/doughnut sign, pyloric muscle thickness > 3 mm
- Differential diagnosis: Achalasia, hiatus hernia, GORD, overfeeding, adrenal insufficiency, inborn errors of metabolism, infection
- Management: Needs surgical correction (myomectomy), usually delayed to correct fluid and electrolytes
    - Correct fluid balance, bolus if required
    - Electrolytes especially bicarbonate and potassium
    - Cease feeds
    - NGT if profuse vomiting

Intussusception

- Age 3 months to 3 years, usually < 1 year of age
- Causes: Idiopathic, Meckel's diverticulum, polyp, HSP, HUS, CF, lymphoma, gastroenteritis especially adenovirus (all cause lead point)

- History
  - Intermittent severe, colicky abdominal pain. Child may draw legs up; child may look pale. Rarely may not have pain episodes
  - Episodes of pain often 2–3 hours
  - Pallor and lethargy between episodes as worsens
  - Often vomiting (bile stained is a late sign)
  - Blood or mucus in stool, 'red currant jelly' is a late sign
  - Can have diarrhoea
  - Can have preceding viral illness
  - Can be associated with bradycardia
- Examination
  - Pallor, lethargy. Child may look well between episodes
  - Abdominal mass usually RUQ (if classic ileo-caecal)
  - Stool with blood
  - Signs of shock: Late sign
- Investigations
  - X-ray abdomen: Can be normal. Target sign usually RUQ, crescent sign LUQ, absent gas RUQ, obstructive pattern
  - US (investigation of choice): Pseudokidney, target sign
  - Air enema (investigation of choice if highly clinically likely), diagnostic and therapeutic
  - Bloods: G&H, FBC, EUC, glucose, VBG
- Management
  - Resuscitation
  - Analgesia
  - NBM
  - NGT if bowel obstruction
  - Air enema if able
  - Urgent operation if shock or perforation

Bilious vomiting

- True bilious vomit = obstruction: Get urgent surgical consult
- Causes
  - Intestinal atresia: Usually diagnosed intrauterine or 1st day life
  - Anorectal anomaly: Usually diagnosed day 1–2 of life
  - Meconium ileus: Rare without CF
  - Hirschsprung's disease: Abnormal enteric nervous system—fail to pass meconium within 48 hours. Usually bilious vomiting day

1–2 but can present later (up to 2 years), even into adulthood if very short segment affected

  - Inflammatory: Complicated appendicitis, Meckel's diverticulum, IBD; i.e. inflammatory mass causing obstruction
  - Malrotation and volvulus: Can cause bowel obstruction, ischaemia. Presents usually 1st month of life. Can be any age to adult
  - Meckel's diverticulum: Can cause bowel obstruction, intussusception, volvulus, internal hernia, inflammatory mass (usually Meckel's just causes large volume painless rectal bleed)
  - Other surgical causes: Irreducible inguinal hernia, intussusception, adhesions (rare), pyloric stenosis
  - Non-surgical causes: Severe gastroenteritis, sepsis, hypothyroid cyclic vomiting (need to rule out surgical causes first)
- Investigations
  - Bloods: Often normal or signs of dehydration, increased WCC in ischaemia, lactate
  - Glucose
  - UA
  - Erect x-ray (usually supine in babies): Free air, fluid levels
  - US
- Management
  - Resuscitation. Fluids, electrolytes. Keep warm
  - Analgesia
  - Urgent surgical review (don't delay for US)
  - NBM
  - NGT
- Complications depend on cause
  - Ischaemia
  - Perforation
  - Sepsis
  - Short bowel syndrome

Malignancy

Leukaemia

- Mostly ALL
- Symptoms: Malaise, fever, bone pain, limp, weight loss, petechia
- WCC > 20 or < 4, thrombocytopenia, anaemia, pancytopenia
  - High index of suspicion if find ≥ 2 cell lines abnormal FBC

- Burkitt's lymphoma: Rapidly enlarging lymph node tumour in chest/abdomen; i.e. abdominal pain/difficulty breathing, +/– fevers, 5–10 years of age, risk of tumour lysis at presentation

CNS malignancies

- Delayed diagnosis and presentation
- Children usually posterior fossa, present when ICP elevated
- Headaches, vomiting, behavioural issues, abnormal gait, vision issues, sunset eyes, squint, growth delay, seizures

Nephroblastoma

- Usually incidental renal mass palpable
- 60% < 3 years old

Analgesia and sedation

Analgesia

- See Table 18.7 for common analgesics and how to use them
- Topical analgesia
  - EMLA = lidocaine (lignocaine) + prilocaine (prilocaine can trigger methaemoglobinaemia in < 3 months of age)

Table 18.7 Commonly used analgesics, route and dose

Analgesia	Route	Load	Continued dose	Max. dose
Sucrose*	PO		0.1–0.5 mL	5 mL
Paracetamol	PO/IV PR		15 mg/kg QID 15–20 mg/kg PR	1 g per dose (60 mg/kg/day)
Ibuprofen (not for < 3 months old)	PO		10 mg/kg TDS	400 mg TDS
Oxycodone (half dose < 12 months old)	PO		0.1–0.2 mg/kg 4-hourly	5–10 mg 4-hourly
Morphine (half dose < 12 months old)	IV	0.1–0.2 mg/kg	Titrate	10 mg/dose
Fentanyl (not for < 12 months old)	IN	1.5 microgram/kg	0.5–0.15 microgram/kg	75 microgram or 3 microgram/kg

*Highest efficacy < 6 weeks (some up to 6 months)

  - ALA = tetracaine (amethocaine), lidocaine (lignocaine) and adrenaline
  - Co-Phenylcaine = lidocaine (lignocaine) and phenylephrine
  - Always remember that babies CAN feel pain, physiologic response to pain is unhelpful

Sedation with ketamine

- Actions: Dissociative, analgesia, amnesic, cardiovascular stable
- Contraindications (varies, you must use your local protocol): Age < 12 months, not fasted for 4–6 hours solid, 2 hours liquid (controversies with fasting times), URTI/lung disease, history or prior airway operation or congenital abnormality, head injury with LOC/ altered consciousness/vomiting, glaucoma, acute globe injury, porphyria, thyroid disease, cardiovascular disease, HT, psychosis, procedures that stimulate the posterior pharynx
- Side effects: Vomiting, emergence, hypersalivation, laryngospasm, apnoea, decreased respiration, emesis, agitation, random movement, rash
- Preparation: Need 2 doctors (1 for sedation and 1 for procedure) and nurse, need cardiac monitoring and pulse oximetry. Have written consent. Check baseline observations
- Dose
  - IV 1–1.5 mg/kg (max. 50 mg) over 1–2 minutes (rapid infusion can cause respiratory depression). 0.5 mg/kg (max. 25 mg) extra bolus if needed
  - IM 3–4 mg/kg repeat 2–4 mg/kg onset in 5 minutes
- Adjuncts
  - Atropine for hypersalivation: 0.02 mg/kg max. 0.6 mg
  - Midazolam for emergence: 0.02 mg/kg (age > 5 years)
  - Ondansetron: High risk of vomiting
- Observe patient until back to pre-procedure mental status

Sedation with nitrous oxide

- Action: Analgesic and amnesic
- Contraindications: Head injury with LOC or altered consciousness, chest injury, possible pneumothorax, current asthma, patient uncooperative (usually need to be over 4 years old), otitis media
- Side effects: Nausea, vomiting, headache, sleepiness, sweats
- Preparation: NBM 2 hours prior, need 2 doctors or 1 doctor and 1 nurse trained in nitrous use. Check continuous flow meter, scavenger and check canister. Check mask and seal, continuous O_2 monitoring

- Procedure: Start with 100% oxygen. Adjust nitrous to 30–70% and as needed, administer for 2–3 minutes pre procedure. Post procedure use 100% oxygen for 2–3 minutes
- Observe patient until back to pre-procedure mental status

Unwell neonate

Jaundice

- Maternal risk factors
  - Blood type ABO or rhesus incompatibility
  - Breastfeeding (especially first time)
  - Gestational diabetes
  - Asian, native American
  - Medications: Diazepam, oxytocin
- Patient risk factors
  - Birth trauma
  - Excessive weight loss, infrequent feeds
  - Male, jaundice in siblings
  - Premature
  - Polycythaemia
  - TORCH/infections
  - Meds: Erythromycin, chloramphenicol
- Evaluation
  - Baby less than 24 hours old: Usually pathological causes
    - Sepsis, infection, TORCH
    - Haemorrhage, haemolysis
  - Baby 24 hours to 2 weeks: Likely non-pathological
    - Look for causes depending on severity of jaundice, if child unwell, if risk factors
    - Can plot bilirubin on graph and treat accordingly with e.g. phototherapy as required (bilirubin threshold for phototherapy)
  - Baby > 2 weeks: Need to look for causes
    - Sepsis
    - Metabolic
    - Thyroid

    - o Obstruction
    - o Cardiac
  - Investigations if needed: FBC, reticulocyte count, bilirubin (conjugated and unconjugated), TSH, TORCH, blood culture, Coombs' test, blood group, G6PD level

Cyanosis

- Difficult to detect if anaemic
- Causes
  - Central
    - o Airway: Obstruction
    - o Breathing: Lung disease, CNS disease, respiratory muscle issue, decreased respiratory drive
    - o Circulation: Intra-cardiac shunt right to left, pulmonary HT, intrapulmonary shunt
  - Peripheral
    - o Circulatory shock; e.g. sepsis
    - o CCF; e.g. left-to-right shunt
    - o Environmental (cold)
    - o Acrocyanosis of newborn
    - o Methaemoglobinaemia
- Hyperoxia test
  - Measure saturations on room air, remeasure after 15 minutes of 100% oxygen. If saturations are still low possibly fixed cardiac shunt. If saturations increased lung pathology likely, cyanotic heart disease excluded
  - Examination for suspected cardiac cause
    - o Check BP all 4 limbs
    - o Pre (right arm) and post (left arm, any leg) ductal sats
    - o Femoral pulses
    - o Palpate liver
    - o Murmur
    - o Peripheral oedema
  - Investigations
    - o VBG, EUC, FBC, glucose, blood culture
    - o CXR

- o ECG
- o ECHO

■ Management of duct dependent lesion: Needs specialist help!
- o Prostaglandin E_1 IV infusion: 60 microgram/kg in 50 mL normal saline
- o Therefore 1 mL/hr = 20 ng/kg/min
- o To OPEN a closed duct, will need 50–100 ng/kg/min
- o Give 2.5 mL over 30 minutes then reassess
- o To maintain a duct open use 10–20 ng/kg/min
- o Double dilution protocols facilitate tiny doses

■ **Side effects include apnoea, bradycardia, hypotension, seizure**

The crying baby

- Differential diagnosis to consider
  - ■ Sepsis
  - ■ Surgical cause: Intussusception, anal fissure
  - ■ Feeding difficulty
  - ■ GORD
  - ■ NAI
  - ■ Fracture
  - ■ Constipation
  - ■ Corneal abrasion
  - ■ Hair tourniquet (digits, phallus)
  - ■ Foreign body
  - ■ Otitis media
  - ■ Metabolic causes
  - ■ Normal baby versus parental expectations
- Examination: Alertness, tone, activity, scalp, fontanelle, perfusion, hydration, digits, penis, cornea, skin, perianal, squeeze all limbs
- Admit/observe child at risk or other concerns (even if think 'normal baby' sometimes!)

Metabolic disorders

- Most diagnosed at birth on screening
- Increased risk: Consanguinity, sibling death

- Presentation: Sudden unwellness, precipitated by illness, CNS abnormality, arrhythmia, vomiting, can look like sepsis/acute collapse
- Examination: Not sensitive
- Investigations: EUC, glucose, VBG, lactate, ammonia, pyruvate, LFT, Ca, Mg, urine metabolic—many need to be ON ICE (all okay to be cold)
  - If infant/child presents with BSL < 2.5 do metabolic screen (usually have packs in department which include bloods and urine which need to be taken prior to correction of BSL)
- Management: Get expert help
  - Make child NBM (removes substrate)
    - Correct fluids, run normal saline + 10% glucose
    - Bolus glucose if hypoglycaemic 10% glucose 2 mL/kg IV
    - $NaHCO_3^-$ 1–2 mmol/kg IV may be needed; seek expert advice
    - Carnitine 100 mg/kg/day under specialist advice (give if suspected metabolic issues, minimal adverse effects)
    - Other treatments: Biotin, thiamine, arginine, intralipid

Non-accidental injury (NAI)

- 75% < 12 months old, 60% < 6 months old
- Behaviour: Detached, depressed, poor eye contact, delayed milestones, or overly clingy/immediate attachment to strangers
- Features on presentation
  - Changing history of events, inconsistent
  - Multiple sites, multiple ages of injuries
  - Delayed presentation
- Specific fractures
  - Infants less than 1 year of age: 75% of fractures likely NAI
  - Metaphyseal long bone
  - Chip fracture corner metaphysis
  - Epiphyseal
  - Spiral long bone
  - Scapula
  - Spinous process
  - Sternal

    - Rib
    - Skull
- Injuries
    - Soft tissue (80%)
        - Grab, stab, restraint, object marks, bites
        - Non-bony prominence: Cheek, abdomen, head, upper arm
        - Multiple
    - Burns
        - Pattern
        - Immersion without splash
        - Vivid demarcation
        - Cigarette burn
    - Head
        - Coma
        - Seizure
        - SDH
        - Retinal haemorrhages
    - Abdomen
        - Intramural duodenal haematoma
        - Pancreas
        - Bowel perforation
        - Retroperitoneal haematoma
        - Liver, spleen injury
    - Neglect
        - Hygiene
        - Inadequate shelter/food/clothes/medical care
    - Sexual
    - Emotional
- Investigations
    - Coag
    - CTB
    - Urine
    - FTT workup
    - Skeletal survey (all children < 2 years old, rarely in > 5 years old)
    - Document all interactions, clearly and without emotion

- Management
  - Remember we are mandatory reporters!
  - Consider the CHAIN ER (Child Abuse Inventory in ER) questions. If yes to any consult paediatric or child protection team (know your local referral pattern!)
    - Injury incompatible with history or age
    - History inconsistent
    - Delayed attendance without good explanation
    - Suspicious head to toe examination
    - Unexplained other injuries
    - Inappropriate interaction

CHAPTER 19

ECG—detailed guide

There are many ways to read an electrocardiogram (ECG) (see Fig. 19.1 for the standard ECG waves and intervals). It is important to develop your own sequence of review and do it the same every time. This minimises the chance of errors. Here is my stepwise approach to reading an ECG.

- Look for rate: Ventricular and atrial
  - 300/number of large squares P-P or R-R

    OR
  - 1500/number or small squares P-P or R-R

    OR
  - Number of complexes on rhythm strip × 6
- Look for rhythm
  - Sinus = P followed by QRS every time. P up in I, II, III aVF down in aVR
  - **Tachy** > 100, normal or **brady** < 60
  - P relation to QRS: Is it **regular**, irregular with a **pattern** or **irregular** with no pattern.
    - Increased HR: 1st-degree heart block: **Regular**
    - Sequential increased PR then dropped QRS—Mobitz 1: **Pattern**
    - PR (and PP) constant, intermit dropped QRS—Mobitz II: **Pattern**
  - Complete dissociation P and QRS
    - 3rd-degree heart block, **brady**
    - Idioventricular rhythm **brady** (called accelerated if > 40 bpm)
    - VT (capture and fusion beats, QRS concordance V1–6) **tachy (usually > 200)**, **regular**
  - Intermit cease P wave or long pauses—sick sinus syndrome (SSS): **Irregular**
  - P wave hidden or retrograde (inverted, pre-QRS, short PR) or post QRS—junctional rhythm (sinoatrial node [SAN] conducts slower than atrioventricular node [AVN]): **Regular**

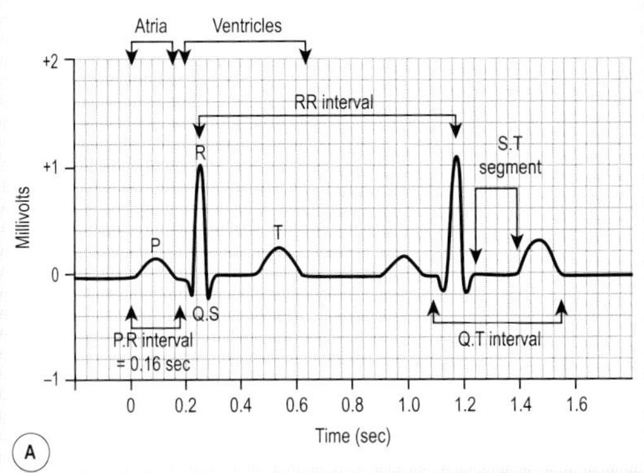

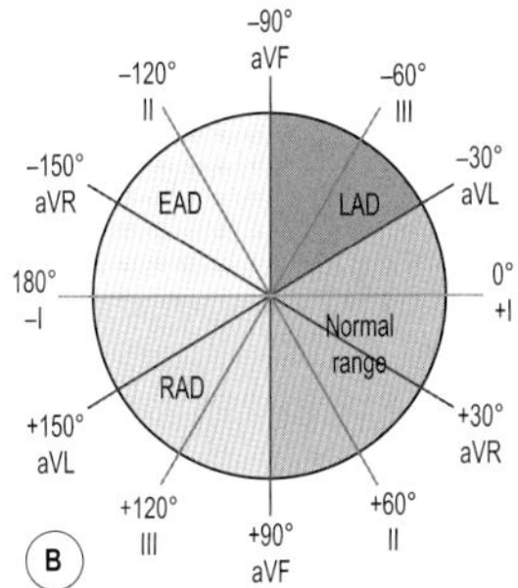

Figure 19.1 The standard ECG. (a) Waves and intervals with timings. (b) Cardiac axis and the ECG.

  - No P waves
    - AF irregular
    - A flutter (flutter waves, usually regular, often rate 150, QRS narrow)
    - SVT (regular, narrow QRS, P buried in T)
    - AF + Pre-excitation/WPW (irregular broad bizarre changing QRS, occasional normal QRS, changing RR interval) **irregular**
- Look at P wave (best lead is usually V1)
  - Occasional abnormal P wave: Atrial ectopic
  - 3 or more different P wave morphology: Multifocal atrial **tachy**
  - Tall, peaked (P pulmonale): RA hypertrophy/right atrial enlargement (RAE)
  - Broad, notched/biphasic in lead II (P mitrale): left atrial hypertrophy/left atrial enlargement
- Look at PR
  - Prolonged = PR > 200 (5 small squares): Heart blocks (see above), hypokalaemia
  - Shortened = PR < 120 (3 small squares): Junctional rhythm, WPW (look for delta wave—upstroke of QRS)
- Look at axis (see Figs 19.1(b) and 19.2)
  - Left axis deviation (LAD): QRS more +ve in I, more –ve in III and with worse LAD also –ve II
  - RAD: QRS more +ve in III, more –ve in I
  - Left anterior fascicular block: LAD, normal QRS AND rS in III, qR or R in I/aVL
  - Left post fascicular block: RAD, normal QRS AND qR in III
- Look at QRS width
  - Wide: > 120 (3 small squares)
  - LBBB: +ve terminal QRS in V6, –ve terminal QRS in V1. Typical (but not always seen) W pattern in V1, M in V6 (WILLIAM)
  - RBBB: +ve terminal QRS in V1, –ve terminal QRS in V6. Typical (but not always seen) M pattern in V1, W in V6 (MORROW)
  - Other causes wide QRS: Hyperkalaemia, drugs (TCA), pacing, WPW, vent escape

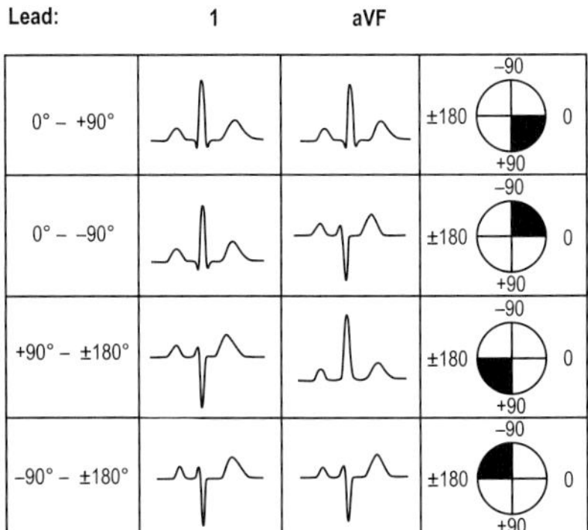

Figure 19.2 Quick method for determining cardiac axis

- Brugada: Incomplete RBBB + coved ST elevation V1, V2 with terminal T inversion; other variants exist
- Sgarbossa criteria: With LBBB, ST elevation/depression is normal but should be opposite direction to terminal QRS and < 6 mm. If ST changes are > 6 mm OR ST changes are in the same direction as the terminal QRS then consider AMI
- Bifascicular block: RBBB + LAFB or RBBB + LPFB
- Trifascicular block: Bifascicular block + 1st-degree heart block OR LBBB + 1st-degree heart block OR alt LBBB with RBBB
- Na channel blocker overdose: Sinus tachy, wide QRS, RAD, terminal R > 3 mm aVR, R/S > 0.7 aVR

- Look at QRS morphology
    - Left ventricular hypertrophy (LVH): S (V1 or V2) + R (V5 or V6) > 35 mm. Any R > 20 (limb lead) > 25 (chest leads), R in V1 + S in III > 25
    - LVH + strain: ST depression with asymmetric T
    - Right ventricular hypertrophy (RVH): R/S ratio > 1 in V1 AND R/S ratio < 1 in V6 AND *RAD*, R in V1 > 6 mm
    - Poor R wave progression: R in V3 < 3 mm, low ejection fraction
    - Q waves: Previous AMI

  - Low voltage: QRS amplitudes in all praecordial leads < 10. Seen in pericardial effusion, pleural effusion, pneumothorax, obesity, emphysema
- Look at ST segment: Compare against baseline TP segment
  - Elevation: Benign early repolarisation (BER) (fishhook), AMI, pericarditis, aneurysm, vasospasm, BBB
  - Coronary vessel occlusion patterns
    - Anterior: ST elevation V1, 2, 3, aVF usually left anterior descending artery
    - Ant/Lat: ST elevation V5, 6 aVL, I depression V1, 2, 3 usually circumflex artery
    - ST elevation aVR > 1 mm, aVR >V1 elevation. Horizontal ST depression especially I, II, V4, 5, 6. Consider left main coronary artery. NEED urgent PCI
    - Inferior: ST elevation III > II, dep I, aVL usually right coronary artery (RCA)
    - Posterior MI: horizontal ST depression V1, 2, 3 with upright T and tall R. Check posterior leads V7 (post axillary line, 5th IC space), 8, 9 (5th IC space 2 cm apart) for ST elevation
    - RV infarction: ST elevated V1 > V2, or V1 with depressed V2. ST elevated V3R–V6R (mirror of chest leads on right side) ***DON'T USE NITRATES***
  - Depression: LVH + strain, digoxin, hypokalaemia, AMI/ ischaemia, reciprocal changes
  - Global ischaemia or ST depressed with elevation in aVR or aVL: Consider left main disease
  - Osborn (J) waves: Upward slurring of ST—severe hypothermia
- Look at T waves
  - Tall: Ischaemia, hyperkalaemia
  - De-winter (J wave depression with tall T) = AMI
  - Inversion: AMI, PE, CNS, LV strain
  - Wellens syndrome: Deep T inversion or biphasic T in V2, 3 or 4 = critical stenosis of proximal left anterior descending. Often pain has resolved so can be missed. Need urgent consult with cardiologist
  - Camel hump T: Biphasic T, U wave, buried P wave
  - T wave balance: T V1 > T V6—cardiac disease (T in V1 usually inv or small)
  - Marriott: T inversion anterior and inferior = consider PE

- Look at QT: Measure in lead II, V5/6. cQT = QT/(square root of RR)
  - Prolonged > 440 men 460 women (2 large squares is 400): drugs, U waves, electrolytes, increased ICP, ACS, hypothermia, hereditary
  - Short QT < 350: Hypercalcaemia, Dig, congenital
- Look for U waves: Seen in hypokalaemia
  - Inverted U waves: Ischaemia
- Other specific diagnosis
  - Idiopathic VT—RV outflow tract VT: LBBB, very rapid, VT
  - Idiopathic VT—LV tachycardia: Mildly broad QRS with RBBB morph, LAD
  - Pericardial effusion: Low voltage leads + tachycardia +/– electrical alternans
  - PE: Tachycardia, S1Q3T3, right axis, incomplete RBBB, T inversion inferior and anteroseptal. Pointy P in V1 (right heart strain). Non-specific ST/T changes
  - Digoxin excess = slow, regular rhythm, swooping ST segments (reverse tick), ST depression, ectopics, slow AF, any AV block, VT, bi-directional VT
  - Hypertrophic obstructive cardiomyopathy (HOCM): High voltage, large QRS, Qs deep and narrow I, aVL, V5, V6
  - Hyperkalaemia: Tall T, wide QRS, loss of P waves, sine wave
- VT versus SVT with aberrancy (BBB or WPW)
  - If in doubt treat as VT: Suspect VT if
    - Absence of BBB morphology
    - Extreme axis deviation
    - QRS complexes very broad: > 160
    - AV dissociation
    - Capture beats: A normal duration QRS
    - Fusion beats—sinus and ventricular beat coincides: Hybrid QRS complex
    - Positive or negative concordance of QRS throughout chest leads. All entirely R or entirely QS. No RS
    - Brugada's sign: Distance from onset of QRS to nadir of S wave is > 100
    - Josephson's sign: Notching near nadir of S wave

        - RSR′ complex with left rabbit ear taller. Most specific finding. Right bundle branch (RBB) usually has right ear taller
        - Patient factors: Age > 35, IHD, structural heart disease, previous MI, CCF, cardiomyopathy, FHx of sudden death
        - Cannon A wave, variable S1, unchanged S2, angina
- SVTs
    - Atrioventricular nodal re-entry tachycardia (AVNRT): Rate 140–280, QRS < 120 unless BBB, QRS alternans, may have ST depression, P waves retrograde or buried
    - Atrioventricular re-entrant tachycardia (AVRT): Pre-excitation, re-entry circuit (delta wave, short PR) (e.g. WPW), rate 200–300, P buried or retrograde, QRS alternans, may have ST depression, QRS < 120 unless BBB
    - Atrial tachycardia: Rate > 100, abnormal P wave morph and axis inverted II, III, aVF, QRS < 120 unless BBB, at least 3 consecutive ectopic P waves
    - Junctional tachycardia: Retrograde P usually inverted II, III, aVF, short PR, may be associated with digoxin toxicity
    - MAT: Irregular, 3 or more different P wave morphologies
    - AF: A flutter
- Rhythm assessment by rate
    - Is it brady?
        - Regular: SR, junctional rhythm, 1st-degree heart block
        - Irregular with a pattern: 2nd-degree heart block
        - Irregular, no pattern: Complete dissociation P and QRS = 3rd-degree heart block, idioventricular rhythm, SSS
    - Is it normal rate?
        - Regular: SR, junctional rhythm, atrial flutter
        - Irregular with a pattern: 1st-degree heart block, 2nd-degree heart block
        - Irregular no pattern: Accelerated idioventricular rhythm (dissociated), AF (no P waves)
    - Is it tachy?
        - Regular: SR, junctional rhythm, atrial flutter, SVT, VT
        - Irregular: AF, AF + WPW, ectopics

Reading a paediatric ECG

(Adapted from Burns, E. 2019. Paediatric ECG interpretation. Life in the Fast Lane (ITFL). 7 Nov. Retrieved from http://lifeinthefastlane.com/ecg-library/paediatric-ecg-interpretation/)

- Why are children different from adults?
  - At birth, the RV is larger and thicker than the LV (from pumping blood through the relatively high-resistance pulmonary circulation)
  - ECG therefore looks like RV hypertrophy in the adult
  - Marked rightward axis, dominant R wave in V1 and T wave inversions in V1–3
  - Conduction intervals (PR interval, QRS duration) are shorter than adults due to the smaller cardiac size
  - Heart rates are much faster in neonates and infants, decreasing as the child grows older
- Placement of leads: Children under 5—RV extends to right side of sternum. Need an extra lead; right-sided V4
  - New lead = V4R: 5th intercostal space, right midclavicular line
  - V1: 4th intercostal space, right sternal border
  - V2: 4th intercostal space, left sternal border
  - V3: Midway between V2 and the normal V4 (5th IC space, left midclavicular line)
  - V4R: 5th intercostal space, right midclavicular line
  - V5: Anterior axillary line, same horizontal plane as V4
  - V6: Midaxillary line, same horizontal line as V4
- Assess rate
  - 300/number of large squares between R-R and/or P-P

    OR
  - 1500/number of small squares R-R and/or P-P
  - Number of complexes in the rhythm strip × 6
  - Normal rate varies with age
- Assess rhythm
  - P before every QRS
  - Normal P wave axis: P upright in I and aVF
  - Tachy or brady: Depending on age
  - Dysrhythmias as in adults: Look at P wave in relation to QRS

    - 90% of paediatric dysrhythmias are SVT
    - 90% of these are re-entrant
- Look at P wave
    - Normal P wave is < 3 mm high and < 90 sec duration children, 70 sec in infants
    - Tall, peaked (> 3 mm): RA hypertrophy/RAE
    - Broad, wide (> 90 children, 70 infants): Left atrial hypertrophy/ left atrial enlargement
    - Combination tall and wide: Combined atrial hypertrophy
- Look at PR: Varies with age and HR
    - Younger children have shorter PRs
    - PR will decrease with HR
    - Normal PR at a normal HR
        - 0–1 months: 100 (upper limit 120)
        - 6–12 months: 110 (upper limit 140)
        - 3–8 years: 140 (upper limit 160)
        - 12–16 years: 150 (upper limit 180)
    - Prolonged: Myocarditis, myocardial dysfunction, CHD, hyperkalaemia, digoxin toxicity
    - Shortened = pre-excitation: WPW, glycogen storage disease
    - Variable: Wenckebach heart block, wandering atrial pacemaker
- Look at axis: Normal axis varies with age
    - Calculate axis (see Figs 19.1(b) and 19.2)
    - Normal axis
        - 1 week to 1 month: +110 (range +30 to +180)
        - 1 month to 3 months: +70 (range +10 to +125)
        - 3 months to 3 years: +60 (range +10 to +110)
        - Over 3 years: + 60 (range +20 to +120)
        - Adult: +50 (range –30 to +105)
- Look at QRS width: Varies with age
    - Normal QRS
        - 0–1 year: 50 (upper limit 70)
        - 1–3 years: 60 (upper limit 70)

        - 3–8 years: 70 (upper limit 80)
        - 8–12 years: 70 (upper limit 90)
        - 12–16 years: 70 (upper limit 100)
    - Prolonged: BBB, pre-excitation, intra-ventricular blocks, ventricular arrhythmia
- Look at QRS amplitude: Varies with age and lead
    - High amplitude: Ventricular hypertrophy, ventricular conduction disturbance (BBB, WPW)
    - Low amplitude: Pericarditis, myocarditis, hypothyroidism, normal newborns, obesity, effusion, pleural effusion, pneumothorax
    - Ventricular hypertrophy will change one or more of the following: QRS axis, QRS voltage, R/S ratio, T axis
    - Ventricular hypertrophy
        - LVH: LAD for age, tall R V5 V6, deep S V4R, V1, decreased R/S V1–2, Q in V5 V6
        - LVH + strain: Inverted T I and aVL
        - RVH: RAD for age, tall R V4R, V1, deep S V5, V6, R/S ratio increased V1–2, R/S ratio < 1 V6
        - Upright T waves in V1 V4R in children 3 days to 6 years alone: RVH
        - qR in V1: Specific for RVH
        - Biventricular hypertrophy
            - Positive criteria for RVH and LVH
            - Large equiphasic QRS complexes on 2 or more limb leads and V2–V5
- Q waves
    - Normal if narrow (< 30) and in left praecordial leads and aVF and no deeper than 5 mm, 8 mm in III in children < 3
    - Abnormal if in right praecordial leads (e.g. V1), absent in left praecordial leads, abnormally deep (vent hypertrophy), abnormally wide and deep (MI, fibrosis)
- Look at ST segment: In relation to TP segment
    - Normal changes
        - Limb lead ST depression or elevation up to 1 mm
        - J point depression/upsloping ST depression
        - Early repolarisation in adolescents

    - Abnormal
        - Downward slope of ST followed by biphasic inverted T
        - Sustained horizontal ST depression > 80
        - Occur in pericarditis, MI, severe ventricular hypertrophy, digoxin effect
- Look at T waves: Configuration changes over time
    - Normal
        - 0–1 week: T waves upright praecordial
        - After 1 week: T waves inverted V1–3 = juvenile T wave pattern
        - After approx. 8 years T waves become upright V1–3
        - T wave pattern can persist into young adulthood = persistent juvenile T wave pattern
    - Tall peaked T waves: Hyperkalaemia, LVH (vol. overload), BER
    - Flat T waves = normal newborn, hypothyroid, hypokalaemia, digoxin, pericarditis, myocarditis, MI
    - Large deep inverted T waves: Raised ICP; e.g. bleed, tumour
- Look at QT: Measure in lead II, V5/6. cQT = QT/(square root of RR)
    - Normal QT: Is longer in babies
    - Infants less than 6 months: < 490
    - Children older than 6 months: < 440
    - Prolonged: Drugs, head injury, electrolytes—hypocalcaemia, myocarditis, hereditary—long QT syndrome
    - Short QT: Hypercalcaemia, digoxin, congenital short QT
- Look for U waves: Seen in hypokalaemia. Normal in sinus bradycardia
- Specific diagnosis
    - Pericarditis
        - Widespread concave ST elevation and PR depression. Normalises 1–3 weeks
        - T wave inversion from 2–4 weeks post onset
    - Myocarditis
        - AV conduction disturbances from prolonged PR to dissociation
        - Low QRS voltage

- Decreased T waves
- QT prolonged
- Tachyarrhythmia
- Infarction pattern: Deep Q and poor R wave prog

- MI: In children with anomalous coronary artery/post cardiac OT/thrombophilia
  - ST elevation contiguous leads with reciprocal depression
  - Horizontal ST depression
- Hypo/hypercalcaemia
  - Hypocalcaemia: Prolong ST and QT
  - Hypercalcaemia: Short ST and QT
- Hypo/hyperkalaemia
  - Hypokalaemia: U waves, flat/biphasic T, ST depression progressing to PR prolonged, sinoatrial block
  - Hyperkalaemia: Tall T, prolongs QRS, prolonged PR, P disappears, wide bizarre QRS, asystole
- WPW
  - Short PR, wide QRS, slurred upstroke: Delta wave to QRS
- SVT: 90% of paeds dysrhythmias are SVT, 90% re-entrant; > 95% of wide complex tachycardias in paeds are SVT with aberrancy
  - Rapid, regular, narrow QRS
  - P wave usually invisible but may precede or follow QRS
  - Re-entrant: Requires bypass pathway; e.g. WPW. Adenosine works well
  - Automatic SVT: Abnormal or accelerated normal automaticity; e.g. sinus tachy, atrial tachy, junctional ectopic tachy (usually post operation and difficult to treat)
  - ¼ will have CHD, ¼ will have WPW, ½ normal
  - Consider fever or drugs as cause
  - Management
    - Vagal manoeuvres, ice + water in a bag on face for 10 seconds
    - Adenosine 0.1 mg/kg (max. 6 mg) IV into large vein. If no response repeat at dose 0.15 mg/kg (max. 12 mg), if no response repeat at dose 0.3 mg/kg (max. 18 mg)

      - Cardioversion usually 1–2 J/kg (if in shock, be wary if conscious as anaesthesia may cause rapid deterioration)
    - DO NOT GIVE VERAPAMIL OR BETA-BLOCKER
  - Broad complex tachycardia
    - VT is extremely rare. Usually Hx of CHD
    - Torsades occurs with long QT syndrome and some drugs
    - VF extremely rare. Usually associated with CHD. DC shock 4 J/kg
- Abnormal in adults but normal in child's ECG
  - HR > 100 bpm
  - Rightward QRS axis > +90°
  - T wave inversions in V1–3 ('juvenile T wave pattern')
  - Dominant R wave in V1
  - RSR′ pattern in V1
  - Marked sinus arrhythmia
  - Short PR interval (< 120 ms) and QRS duration (< 80 ms)
  - Slightly peaked P waves (< 3 mm in height is normal if ≤ 6 months)
  - Slightly long QTc (≤ 490 ms in infants ≤ 6 months)
  - Q waves in the inferior and left praecordial leads.

CHAPTER 20

ABG—detailed guide

There are lots of methods for assessing an arterial blood gas (ABG). Here is my stepwise approach to reading an ABG. Remember that you actually cannot interpret an ABG without the clinical context. Two ABGs can be identical but have two very different interpretations in two different patients.

- Check all values—identify what is normal and abnormal. ***Every time someone hands you a blood gas slip: Circle every abnormal value, tick every normal value otherwise one day you will overlook an important abnormal value!***
  - pH: 7.35–7.44 arterial
  - pO_2: 80–100 mmHg arterial gas
  - pCO_2: 35–45 mmHg arterial
  - HCO_3^-: 21–28 mmol/L
  - $-1 <$ base excess < 1
  - O_2 sats: 95–100% (arterial gas)
  - Lactate: < 2 mmol/L
  - Na: corrected Na = Na + (glucose – 5)/3: 136–146 mmol/L
  - K: 3.7–4.7 mmol/L
  - Cl: 95–110 mmol/L
  - Cr: 45–90 micromol/L
  - Glucose: 3.5–5.4 mmol/L
  - Hb: 120–150 g/L
  - Ca ionised: 1.15–1.3 mmol/L
  - Others: e.g. COHb
- How is ventilation going?
  - Normal pCO_2 35–45 mmHg
  - Hypoventilation/retaining CO_2: ↑ $pCO_2 > 45$
  - Hyperventilation: ↓ $pCO_2 < 35$
- How is oxygenation going (arterial gas)?
  - Normal pO_2: 80–100 mmHg
  - O_2 sats: 95–200%
  - Do sats correlate with monitor reading? (confirming arterial or venous sample)

- Acid–base: Remember the Henderson–Hasselbalch equation

$$H_2CO_3 = HCO_3^- + H^+ = CO_2 + H_2O$$

$$pH = pK + \log (HCO_3^- / H_2CO_3)$$

Therefore, if you add CO_2 then you make acid

$$H_2CO_3 = HCO_3^- + H^+ \rightarrow CO_2 + H_2O$$

If you take CO_2 away, you use acid

$$H_2CO_3 = HCO_3^- + H^+ \rightarrow CO_2 + H_2O$$

↘ lungs

- Acid–base: Look at pH, is it normal, ↑ or ↓
  - Acidosis = ↓ pH < 7.35; look at pCO_2, HCO_3 and BE, lactate
    - Primary respiratory acidosis
      - If ↑ $pCO_2 > 45$ = primary respiratory acidosis
      - If ↑ $HCO_3^- > 28$ = compensation
    - Primary metabolic acidosis
      - If ↓ BE < –1 = primary metabolic acidosis
      - If ↓ $pCO_2 < 45$ = compensation
    - Lactate: Is ↑ lactate contributing to acidosis?
  - Alkalosis = ↑ pH > 7.45; look at pCO_2, HCO_3 and BE
    - Primary respiratory alkalosis
      - If ↓ $pCO_2 < 35$ = primary respiratory alkalosis
      - If ↓ $HCO_3^- < 21$ = compensation
    - Primary metabolic alkalosis
      - If ↑ BE > 1 = primary metabolic alkalosis
      - If ↑ $pCO_2 > 45$ = compensation
  - Normal = pH 7.35–7.45. There still may be acidosis or alkalosis; look at pCO_2, HCO_3, BE, lactate
    - Consider complete compensation
    - Chronic respiratory alkalosis is the only derangement that pH completely compensates
    - Consider mixed acid–base

- Mixed acid–base disorder
  - Respiratory acidosis
    - Acute respiratory acidosis
      - Expected $HCO_3^- = 24 + (pCO_2 - 40)/10$
      - HCO_3 should increase by $\Delta\ pCO_2/10$
    - Chronic respiratory acidosis
      - Expected $HCO_3^- = 24 + ([pCO_2 - 40])/10) \times 4$
      - HCO_3 should increase by $\Delta\ pCO_2/10 \times 4$
  - Metabolic acidosis
    - Expected $pCO_2 = 1.5 \times HCO_3^- + 8$ (+/–5)
    - If pCO_2 is higher than expected, there is also respiratory acidosis
    - If pCO_2 is lower than expected, there is also respiratory alkalosis
  - Respiratory alkalosis
    - Acute respiratory alkalosis
      - Expected $HCO_3^- = 24 - ([40 - pCO_2]/10 \times 2)$
      - HCO_3 should decrease by $\Delta\ pCO_2/10 \times 2$
    - Chronic respiratory alkalosis
      - Expected $HCO_3^- = 24 - ([40 - pCO_2]/10 \times 5)$
      - HCO_3 should decrease by $\Delta\ pCO_2/10 \times 5$
  - Metabolic alkalosis
    - Expected $pCO_2 = 0.7 \times HCO_3^- + 20$ (+/–5)
    - Higher than expected = there is also respiratory acidosis
    - Lower than expected = there is also respiratory alkalosis
- Anion gap
  - $AG = Na^+ - HCO_3^- - Cl^-$
  - DON'T USE CORRECTED Na
  - Normal 8–16
  - Change in (delta) AG should = change in (delta) HCO_3
    - Delta ratio = increase in AG/decrease in HCO_3^- = $(AG - 12)/(24 - HCO_3^-)$
    - If ratio < 0.4 NAGMA
    - If ratio 0.4–0.8 consider HAGMA + NAGMA
    - If ratio 0.8–2 uncomplicated HAGMA

    - If ratio > 2 MA + metabolic alkalosis or chronic comp resp acidosis

- Osmolar gap
  - Calculated osmolarity = (2 × [Na+]) + (glucose) + (urea)
  - Osmolar gap = Osmolality (measured) – Osmolarity
  - Normal = < 10
  - Causes of elevated osmolar gap: Mannitol, methanol, maltose, ethylene glycol, propylene glycol, glycine, sorbitol
- Ur:Cr ratio
  - 100 = normal, > 100 = prerenal, 50–100 = postrenal, acute kidney, < 50 = intrarenal, chronic disease
  - Causes of high ratio: Sepsis, upper gastrointestinal tract (GIT) bleed (ratio < 200, 90% sensitivity), decreased RBF (CCF, renal artery stenosis, dehydration), steroids, tetracyclines
  - Causes of decreased ratio: Hepatic failure, pregnancy, trimethoprim, muscle trauma
  - Interference: Jaffe reaction, vitamin C, trimethoprim, cephalosporins, cimetidine, ketoacids, bilirubin, dobutamine, nitromethane
- Calculate A–a gradient
  - A–a gradient = PiO_2 – (pCO_2/0.8) – pO_2
  - PiO_2 = 713 × FiO_2 at sea level. On room air PiO_2 = 150
  - Normal = 0.2–15 at 25 years of age, 1.5–30 at 75 years of age
- Causes
  - Respiratory acidosis
    - Acute: Hypoventilation, respiratory failure/depression—drugs, airway obstruction, pneumonia, CVA, APO, pneumothorax
    - Chronic: COPD, restrictive lung disease
  - Metabolic acidosis
    - NAGMA mnemonic: ABCDE
      - **A**ddison's disease
      - **B**icarb (HCO_3) loss: Diarrhoea, RTA
      - **C**hloride

    - **D**rugs: Acetazolamide, acids, spironolactone
    - **E**nd anastomoses/enterostomies: Uretero-pelvic shunt, pancreaticoenterostomies, ureteroenterostomies
  - High anion gap (HAGMA) mnemonic: LUKE (I don't like the MUDPILES mnemonic so I made up my own)
    - **L**actate: Fe, cyanide, theophylline
    - **U**raemia: Rhabdomyolysis, renal failure
    - **K**etones: DM, EtOH, starvation
    - **E**xogenous: Methanol, ethylene, salicylate, isoniazid
- Respiratory alkalosis
  - Hyperventilation mnemonic: CHAMPS
    - **C**NS: SAH, stroke
    - **H**ypoxia
    - **A**nxiety
    - **M**echanical ventilation
    - **P**rogesterone
    - **S**alicylates, sepsis
- Metabolic alkalosis
  - Loss of acid, excessively alkali mnemonic: CLEVER PD
    - **C**ontractions
    - **L**icorice
    - **E**ndo: Cushing's syndrome, Conn's syndrome
    - **V**omiting
    - **E**xcess alkali
    - **Re**-feeding
    - **P**ost hypercapnia
    - **D**iuretics

- VENOUS versus ARTERIAL gases
  - Correlation between arterial and venous
    - pH: Good correlation. Mean difference minimal
    - pCO_2: Good correlation in normocapnia. $PaCO_2 > 45$ levels don't correlate well, however, if $PaCO_2 < 45$ hypercapnia is almost ruled out. Poor correlation in severe shock

    - HCO_3: Good correlation
    - Lactate: Dissociation above 2
    - Base excess: Good correlation
    - PO_2: No correlation obviously
- THEREFORE: You need an ABG to:
    - Accurately measure $PaCO_2$ if hypercapnic
    - Accurately measure $PaCO_2$ in severe shock
    - Accurately know lactate (rarely needed)

CHAPTER 21

Retrievals, disasters, epidemics and pandemics

Preparing interhospital transfers of critically unwell patients

- Prepare the patient
  - Secure the airway, secure the ETT, secure an orogastric tube. Check the ventilator. Stabilise spine
  - Secure any chest drains, insert chest drains if any question of pneumothorax and transferring with altitude. Ensure $ETCO_2$, sats probe, ABG. Check a CXR
  - 2 × IVC checked, secured and visible. IDC. Transduce arterial lines and central lines. Prepare all infusions and medications that may be required including fluids, sedation, inotropes, analgesic, antiemetic, antiseizure and other meds
  - Record GCS and neuro exam before sedation
  - Record temperature. Splint fractures, control bleeding, bivalve plasters
- Document. Take any imaging with you
- Notify arriving team when you leave

Definition of disaster

- Major incident
  - Incident that causes so many casualties that special arrangements are needed
- Disaster
  - An event that causes serious disruption to the community through, for example, threat to or loss of life and/or injury and/or damage to property
  - Beyond the capacity of usual emergency resources; e.g. hospital, fire brigade, police
  - Special resources are required

On-site at a disaster event

Communication

- METHANE
  - **M**ajor incident declared
  - **E**xact location
  - **T**ype of incident
  - **H**azards involved
  - **A**ccess to site
  - **N**umber and type of causalities
  - **E**mergency services required

Zones

- Police (or sometimes fire brigade) has control of the site
- HOT zone: Immediate area. Trained people only, personal protective equipment (PPE)
- WARM zone: For decontamination
- COLD zone: Usually no PPE needed. Medical staff in this zone

Triage

- Use pre-made triage tags/cards for speed
- Sieve: Initial triage system. Usually performed by senior ambulance officer. Used for adults but can be used in children. Performed as patients moved to casualty clearing post
  - Walking, uninjured: Taken to designated survivor area
  - Green: Walking and injured
  - Yellow: RR 10–29, CR < 2, HR < 120
  - Red: RR < 10 or > 29, CR > 2, HR >120
  - Black/deceased: Patients without an airway after simple manoeuvres
- Sort: Used to order patients transport to hospital
  - Scoring system based on RR, sBP, GCS
  - RR 10–29 = 4 points, > 29 = 3, 6–9 = 2, 1–5 = 1 and RR 0 = 0 points
  - sBP > 90 = 4 points, 76–89 = 3, 50–75 = 2, 1–49 = 1 and sBP 0 = 0 points
  - GCS 13–15 = 4 points, 9–12 = 3, 5–8 = 2, 4–5 = 1 and GCS 3 = 0 points

- Calculate score for RR + score for sBP + score for GCS
- Green = score of 12
- Yellow = score of 11
- Red = score < 11
- Some systems include Blue = score 1–3, breathing
- Black = score 0 or 1, not breathing

- Performed in a casualty clearing station
- Treatments based on stabilising and lifesaving manoeuvres only
  - Examples: Airway manoeuvre, oxygen, decompress tension pneumothorax, control bleeding
  - No ETT, No CPR
- Triage is dynamic and patients should be reassessed

Managing a single disaster event (example: train crash)

- Notification: Usually via ambulance
- Prepare: Refer to individual hospital disaster plans
  - Confirm number of casualties and likely injuries
  - Cascade of communication: Notification of important teams (e.g. ICU, pathology, blood bank, radiology, patient flow coordinators, NUMs [nursing unit managers])
  - Prepare the hospital
    - All staff should remain on duty
    - Surgeons remain in OT, don't start new cases
    - Inpatient teams and NUMs to arrange patients. Those which can be discharged must be discharged
  - Prepare the ED
    - Inform the waiting room of incoming disaster. Any non-urgent patient should leave
    - All family and visitors should leave
    - Any patient that needs admission should be moved to the ward
    - New ED arrivals should be informed and asked to leave if possible
    - Some ED's plans will incorporate any new ED patients not associated with the disaster into the disaster cohort. Other ED plans allow for a virtually and sometimes geographically separate ED for non-disaster patients requiring urgent ED care

    - Allocate the ED spaces, define areas for triage and areas for red, yellow and green patients. Often green patients sent to a separate area
    - Plan patient flow. Once a patient leaves ED they should not come back; e.g. not go to CT then return to await report, instead go to CT on route to OT
    - Allocate staff, define teams, usually location based (i.e. one team per 1–3 bed spaces of yellow patients), define roles
    - Depending on the likely duration of the event, prepare a second round of staff
    - Ensure enough equipment. ID what you will be needing and ensure there will be enough
    - Establish a control centre. Need a senior staff member to control and not get involved in individual treatment
- Treatment
  - Patients begin to arrive
  - Keep flow through triage. Triage must be rapid
  - Triage with identification labels for speed
  - Control information management
- Stand down
  - Can be partial or total
  - Return ED to normal function
  - Re-establish normal patient flow
  - Debriefing, counselling

Managing a contagious epidemic or pandemic

- Usually there will be some time from first alert to clinical contact
- Very important to prepare
- Plan for a tiered response: Levels of action required based on case numbers; from small cases with minimal impact on systems to large case numbers overwhelming systems. Need to set triggers to progress to the next level

Strategies that can be implemented depending on what tier of pandemic plan is currently engaged

- The ED
  - Redesign ED to accommodate zones: Hot (potentially infective patients) and cold (non-infective patients—usual ED workload).

Consider position of resus rooms and patient movements from resus to hot or cold zones

- Ensure minimal interaction between hot and cold zones including pathways that patients/staff will traverse
- Decrease ED demand
    - Set up clinics for worried well, away from hospital
    - Triage before entry into hospital to divert patients where possible
    - Inpatient teams to take admission to ward before usual workup
- Increase ED capacity
    - Consider ability to open more ED space
    - Reassign other facilities that may have decreased workloads at this time to ED space
- Prioritise care
    - In times of very high demand, care will need to be prioritised to those patients most likely to have a good outcome. The strategies for this should be pre-determined to decrease the stress to the treating team

- The ICU
    - Redesign ICU to accommodate infectious and non-infectious patients
    - Decrease demand
        - Cancel elective surgeries
        - Change ward emergency call outs to not involve ICU staff
    - Increase ICU capacity
        - Open more facilities if possible (e.g. new ICU not quite ready yet, old ICU recently decommissioned)
        - Reassign other facilities that may have decreased workloads at this time to ICU space
    - Prioritise care
        - ICU reserved for patients that need specific ICU interventions such as ventilation
        - In times of very high demand, care will need to be prioritised to those patients most likely to have a good outcome. The strategies for this should be pre-determined to decrease the stress to the treating team

- Engage the assistance of other departments
  - Discuss with other departments especially those that may have decreased workloads
- Staffing
  - Consider assigning all staff to work in designated small teams. This means if a staff member is infected or potentially infected, only a small group of other staff will have to be checked/ quarantined
  - Clear advice on when staff need to be isolated and checked for infectivity if they become unwell
  - Consider sick leave and extra time staff will be off if staff need to be checked for infectivity
  - Remove at-risk staff from working in hot zones; e.g. pregnant women
  - May need to increase workforce: Consider retired staff, staff redeployed from other areas, medical students etc.
  - May need to cancel leave although consider staff will need breaks during potentially high-stress times
  - Staff may need accommodation on or close to site
  - Ensure psychological support for staff during potentially high-stress times
- Equipment
  - Identify what equipment will be needed
  - Identify equipment that may be too risky to use; e.g. BiPAP, nebulisers
  - Arrange to have equipment ready
  - May need to ration equipment and use
  - Consider what will be needed to transfer patients between departments and within departments including PPE (see below)
- PPE
  - Staff safety is paramount
  - Always use approved equipment. Do not use non-standard or improvised equipment
  - Use pandemic data to identify type of PPE needed; e.g. respiratory precautions, droplet precautions, airborne precautions
  - Ensure training for staff on how to put on and take off (don and doff) PPE
  - Avoid environmental cross contamination

- Communication
  - Communication is vital
  - Consistent information
  - Regular updates
- Visitors and family
  - Keep to a minimum
  - Screening questions +/– tests to ensure not infectious

Index

Page numbers followed by '*f*' indicate figures, '*t*' indicate tables.

D

Q

R